ROUTLEDGE LIBRARY EDITIONS:
ETHICS

Volume 2

APPLIED PHILOSOPHY

APPLIED PHILOSOPHY

Morals and Metaphysics in Contemporary Debate

Edited by
BRENDA ALMOND AND DONALD HILL

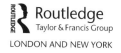

Routledge
Taylor & Francis Group

LONDON AND NEW YORK

First published in 1991 by Routledge

This edition first published in 2021
by Routledge
2 Park Square, Milton Park, Abingdon, Oxon OX14 4RN

and by Routledge
52 Vanderbilt Avenue, New York, NY 10017

Routledge is an imprint of the Taylor & Francis Group, an informa business

British Library Cataloguing in Publication Data
A catalogue record for this book is available from the British Library

ISBN: 978-0-367-85624-3 (Set)
ISBN: 978-1-00-305260-9 (Set) (ebk)
ISBN: 978-0-367-45720-4 (Volume 2) (hbk)
ISBN: 978-1-00-302495-8 (Volume 2) (ebk)

Publisher's Note
The publisher has gone to great lengths to ensure the quality of this reprint but
points out that some imperfections in the original copies may be apparent.

Disclaimer
The publisher has made every effort to trace copyright holders and would welcome
correspondence from those they have been unable to trace.

Applied Philosophy

Morals and metaphysics in contemporary debate

Edited by
Brenda Almond and Donald Hill

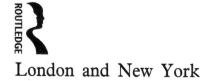

London and New York

First published 1991
by Routledge
11 New Fetter Lane, London EC4P 4EE

Simultaneously published in the USA and Canada
by Routledge
a division of Routledge, Chapman and Hall, Inc.
29 West 35th Street, New York, NY 10001

Printed in Great Britain by T.J. Press (Padstow) Ltd, Padstow, Cornwall

British Library Cataloguing-in-Publication Data
Applied philosophy: morals and metaphysics in contemporary
   debate.
   1. Philosophy
   I. Almond, Brenda   II. Hill, Donald
   100

Library of Congress Cataloging-in-Publication Data
Applied philosophy: morals and metaphysics in contemporary debate/
   edited by Brenda Almond and Donald Hill.
       p.   cm.
   Contributions previously published in the Journal of applied
philosophy, 1984–1990.
   Includes index.
   1. Ethics.   2. Social ethics.   3. Human ecology—Moral and ethical
aspects.   4. Medical ethics.   I. Almond, Brenda.   II. Hill, Donald
BJ1012.A68   1991
170—dc20   90–48664

ISBN 0–415–06015–X

Contents

Acknowledgements

The Editors would like to record their thanks to Anthony O'Hear who, as Joint Editor of the *Journal of Applied Philosophy* from 1984–90, helped to make possible the original selection and publication of the essays included here. They also wish to thank Roger Osborn-King, the publisher of the Journal, not only for his help and co-operation in the production of this volume, but also for his vision in recognising the need for such a journal and for fostering it from its inception.

Introduction

It may seem that there is a paradox at the heart of the notion of 'applied philosophy'. For philosophy is the most abstract of disciplines, while 'application' suggests the most practical, least abstract, of activities. And yet there is nothing unique about this kind of symbiotic relationship between theory and practice, for most disciplines, from physics to psychology, are termed 'applied' when they attempt to use their distinctive body of theory to solve practical problems. It is in this way that 'applied philosophy' is already widely understood as the name for philosophical engagement with the many issues of practical life that hinge upon ethical considerations, and are capable of being illuminated by deeper conceptual understanding and by critical analysis of the arguments they involve.

It is in this way, too, that philosophy is recognised as having a role in medicine and health-care, in business and management, in education, law and many other fields of public policy. Philosophy approaches issues in these areas not merely from a technical point of view, taking ends for granted and looking only for practically effective solutions, but from a holistic and humanistic perspective, sometimes challenging presuppositions, but always keeping in view the question of ends or ideals.

A willingness to do this marks something of a new departure for philosophy in the conceptual and analytic tradition. For this type of philosophy has frequently been accused of fence-sitting, of maintaining detachment in the face of compelling reasons for commitment. It has been caricatured for its fondness for such turns of phrase as 'On the one hand ... on the other hand' and 'It all depends what you mean by ... '. It has been perceived as promoting a damaging form of value-nihilism based on the trivialising of value-judgements.

And yet in many ways such criticisms are based on a widespread popular misunderstanding of the potential of a critical and analytic philosophical approach. This misunderstanding has been fostered by the tendency in the past of analytic philosophers themselves to insist that philosophy could have nothing to say about important moral issues. When they have made this disclaimer, it has been for what seemed excellent theoretical reasons: perhaps the most important of these was the fact-value distinction—the *logically* based claim that mere statements of fact—statements about what *is* the case—can have no implications *in themselves* about what people ought to do or to choose. But many events—perhaps the best known and most striking of these being the attempts of scientists working on the atomic bomb to prevent its use against civilian populations—have demonstrated in a compelling way the devastating consequences for human beings of allowing facts and values to remain marooned on separate islands, with philosophy—representing here people's reflective capacities and their striving for ideals—making no attempt to build a bridge between them.

If a theoretical objection appears to prevent this, then it may be preferable, while continuing to look for flaws in the theoretical arguments, to carry on demonstrating practically that the enterprise is viable and can provide a programme for a morally and practically 'engaged' philosophy. Nevertheless, it is worth making the theoretical point that one can insist that *values* must be informed by the *facts* of human psychology, sociology, biology and history without claiming that they must be, in a logical sense, a derivation from these facts.

This volume, however, represents the more pragmatic solution to the problem. In other words, it provides examples of the possibility of applied philosophy, by contributors from a variety of philosophical backgrounds and different cultural and geographical settings. And yet it would be a mistake to claim too much novelty for this enterprise. On the contrary, it represents in a sense a return to the earliest conception of philosophy, involving, not a claim to ethical expertise, but a commitment to the canons of clear argument and open debate, together with the moral qualities associated with these: honesty, courage and a willingness to *hear* what others are saying. In its origins—even before the time of Socrates—this philosophical tradition was concerned with questions of law, citizenship, social role and politics. In approaching these issues today, certain broad areas of enquiry dictate the pattern of reflection:

(i) First, philosophy in this vein must concern itself with what is perhaps the broadest and most pressing of contemporary problems: the quality of the natural world on which we depend for our existence, but threaten by our activities. Hence the first section in this volume is based on the theme of Environment.

In the opening chapter, R. M. Hare discusses the question of moral duties relating to environmental decisions and argues that these duties are owed only to sentient beings. It is necessary, he suggests, in reaching environmentally sensitive decisions, to set out the various interests which are at stake, strength for strength, and adjudicate between them. In reply, Donald Hill argues that it may be more difficult than it looks to set out these different interests fairly and impartially, and he suggests that one of Hare's own examples—that which concerns the building of new roads—overlooks some important interests.

Timo Airaksinen, writing from Finland, discusses conflicts of interest that may arise between the original populations of countries, striving to maintain traditional forms of life, and immigrants or newcomers with more developed technologies. These, having first introduced practices that threaten the natural environment may then, with growing ecological consciousness, attempt to impose a radically preservationist attitude, which is equally threatening to the way of life of the original population.

Unlike R. M. Hare, Timothy Sprigge believes that it is possible to offer a philosophic defence of the view that non-sentient nature has a value, independently of human or animal consciousness—a value which may be based on a pan-psychic or pantheistic metaphysic. Such a view would supply a metaphysical basis for the position known as 'deep ecology', which is the theme of the next two chapters. According to this view, the solution to the environmental crisis is to be found in a retreat from a purely human-centred perspective and a return to a non-technological paradigm, such as can be found in some non-Western cultures. William Grey, however, argues against this type of solution, claiming that a science-based world view need not foster manipulative and exploitative attitudes to the natural world. In the final chapter of this section, Alan R. Drengson rejects Grey's criticisms, arguing that deep ecology represents a change of perspective involving harmony with nature, a deepening of understanding, and an element of vision.

(ii) While securing the physical context for human life to exist at all must be a dominating concern, a second range of issues may seem equally pressing to individuals—matters which concern them more directly and more intimately on a day-to-day basis. Hence questions about directions for personal life, including questions of family and other relationships, provide the theme for Part II.

Brenda Almond discusses the various bonds that exist between human beings: biological, legal and social. She considers the philosophical arguments that may be advanced for or against deep personal bonds and argues that these have a fundamental moral priority in the lives of human beings. Edgar Page considers the particular bond that exists between parents and children, and argues for a justification of parental rights based on the special value of parenthood in human life.

Sexual relationships provide the theme of the next two chapters. Paul Gregory criticises the ideal of exclusivity—of a single, central relationship for sexual life. In contrast, J. Martin Stafford, taking as his theme homosexual relationships, defends the notion of 'sexual integrity'—sexuality as integrated within a life of personal affection and responsibility. He argues that homosexuals will find it difficult to achieve this goal unless education and social institutions make positive provision for them.

(iii) However, relations of conflict rather than harmony are a harsh reality of the world in which we live, and so Part III focuses on some of the disorders of political and social life, looking back, too, to the prime example in modern times of the almost complete breakdown of human ties, sympathies and responsibilities: the Holocaust.

Haig Khatchadourian addresses the fundamental issue of the morality of terrorism. He distinguishes four types of terrorism: predatory, retaliatory, political and moralistic, and argues that there are no circumstances in which terrorism can be justified. He finds support for his position in 'just war' theory and in the notion of human rights, rejecting utilitarian arguments to the contrary.

Gerry Wallace considers the issue of terrorism in relation to the bombing of civilians in conventional wars, since both cases involve the killing of innocent people. He argues against taking an absolutist stand, and suggests that the issue can be resolved only by weighing competing moral intuitions in particular cases.

Absolute condemnation is, however, appropriate when considering the evil of the Jewish Holocaust. But is this because of its sheer enormity or because it was an evil of a unique and distinct sort? Douglas P. Lackey considers this question and argues that the evil involved was neither qualitatively nor quantitatively distinct. M. Križan disagrees, arguing that the Holocaust cannot be evaluated from the standpoint of ordinary moral values, which deal in such categories as murder and torture. The Holocaust, Križan argues, involved an attack on culture itself. Here lies the necessary 'additional moral argument': to the destruction of life must be added the destruction of culture and the greatest ever man-made challenge to the Enlightenment.

Even this dark period of human history produced examples of moral courage, however, and M. W. Jackson considers the case of Oskar Schindler, a German industrialist who sheltered more than 1,000 Jews during the Holocaust. Jackson explores the difficulties involved in evaluating Schindler's case in terms of universal moral principles and suggests that this difficulty shows up limitations in standard moral theory.

The final chapter in this section, by Richard Norman, presents the case for pacifism based on respect for human life. Norman argues for a very strong, though not necessarily absolute, moral presumption against killing, whether in war or any other circumstances.

(iv) If war, terrorism and genocide represent the breakdown of human relationships, this should prompt a deeper and more reflective consideration of social relationships and social institutions. Hence Part IV offers a selection of essays on political, social, economic and legal questions, with the question of social justice forming a central theme.

Julian Le Grand points out that there is widespread disagreement about what would constitute just and equitable social arrangements. He maintains that it is because they ignore choice that most recent theories are flawed, and he argues in his chapter for a conception of social justice based on choice.

Antony Flew, however, suggests that Le Grand's difficulties, as well as the difficulties of those whose views he criticises, arise from taking equality of outcome as the standard by which to judge whether or not a just distribution has been achieved. This assumption is attacked by Flew as Procrustean—eliminating extremes in order to achieve a painful social homogeneity.

Anthony Skillen shows more sympathy for egalitarian ideals in his defence of the welfare state as an expression of community. He discusses the charge that welfare subverts personal and social responsibility, giving it an inbuilt tendency to self-destruct, but suggests that the same problem is also inherent in a capitalist state. He argues for some reconstruction of the welfare state as an articulation of 'community' and discusses the implications of this for class, gender and the age structures of society.

Martin Hollis argues that the liberal wish 'to pursue our own good in our own way', on which criticism of the welfare society may be based, involves a negative idea of equality or 'equity'. He argues that 'equity' viewed in this negative way cannot deal with the problem of public goods because the working of the market requires a moral commitment to a positive basic equality among citizens.

In the final chapter in this section, Richard Tur argues that law is, in some sense, a moral system. He challenges the view that law is not in the business of enforcing morals and also challenges the prevailing paradigms of legal theory: naturalism and positivism. He argues for 'normative positivism'—a theory that sees law as a community morality, and the legal system itself as applied moral philosophy in action.

(v) Part V constitutes applied philosophy in action in a different sphere, that of medicine. The first chapter, which is a collaborative undertaking by a group of physicians and philosophers working together at one American hospital, is a comprehensive overview of the relation between medicine and ethics. Making extensive use of examples drawn from routine case material, the authors identify various levels of critical reasoning within the medical setting and argue that there is a remarkable similarity between medical and ethical decision-making.

Sandra Marshall discusses the issue of medical confidentiality, starting from a particular case in which notes about a patient were used without her permission in an enquiry concerning the conduct of her physician. She argues that the patient's complaint can only be understood by recognizing that facts about one's body are intimately bound up with one's self, with one's identity and thus with one's autonomy. These considerations, Sandra Marshall argues, justify the patient's demand for privacy.

Questions concerning the transfer and donation of embryos and gametes also involve issues of ownership and identity, and Edgar Page argues that the Warnock Report on these issues overlooked an important underlying principle which sets the question of embryo-transfer apart from that of adoption or the transfer of children. As a result, he argues for well-regulated surrogacy with enforceable contracts as an acceptable route to parenthood.

His view is criticised by Jennifer Trusted, although she believes Page is right to object to the suppression of all forms of surrogacy, in view of the hope this offers to infertile couples. She insists, however, that donating gametes or embryos cannot be compared to donating blood or selling a house, and argues that a surrogate mother contributes so fundamentally to the development of the embryo she accepts that she should not be compelled to give up the child she has nourished.

Ruth Chadwick's concern is also with the transfer of bodily parts, particularly organs such as kidneys for transplant surgery. She argues that we do have duties to our own bodies, grounded in the duty to promote the flourishing of human beings, including ourselves. This provides a reason, she concludes, for opposing a market ethic in health-care provision and, in particular, the sale of bodily parts.

Alan Holland's theme is the 'pre-embryo', which is, he suggests, a term coined to remove the first 14 days after conception from the story of a human life. Important moral consequences may be drawn from this, in particular with regard to the permissibility of experimenting on such early-stage embryos. Without expressing a view on this substantial issue, Holland considers the arguments for recognition of the separate status of the 'pre-embryo' and concludes that they do not provide any good reason for denying that a human being exists from the moment of conception.

The question of when a human being ceases to exist is as important for medical practice as when it begins, but Alister Browne suggests that it is a mistake to try to redefine death. Changing the definition of death, he argues, will not help to solve the practical difficulties of terminal care, and may in fact generate new problems.

★

The essays included here do not, then, offer a single perspective, even when treating related themes. Nevertheless, whether by professional philosophers or practitioners in other fields, they do display a commitment to the philosophical ideal of pursuing truth through open and unbiased enquiry. In separating ends from means and subjecting both to critical scrutiny, in offering clear argument in support of clear conclusions, these essays demonstrate the way in which some of the better habits of mind connected with philosophy can be put to good effect in practical discussions.

The possibility and the opportunity to explore controversial social issues from an independent point of view, rather than *parti pris*, are rarer than the casual follower of newspaper or television reports may appreciate, for most media opportunities are opportunities only to defend some partisan position. So it is worth pointing out that the *Journal of Applied Philosophy*, which provided the original place of publication for all the essays in this volume, is independent of any source of pressure or partisan support—it exists by courtesy of its readership, in particular the members of the Society for Applied Philosophy—and was set up with the simple aim of 'making a significant and constructive contribution to public discussion of issues of general concern'. The reader will, we hope, find that the essays included here do indeed fulfil that aim. While each contribution represents, of course, the views of its author, the book as a whole can be read as a Socratic dialogue, a process of dialectic which leads to a clearer view of the issues involved.

But merely to clarify, as has often been said, is not enough. And we hope that because our contributors have in most cases defended a positive viewpoint, some lines of thinking will have emerged as more rationally defensible than others. On some issues, of course, we may be doomed to philosophical indecision, but even in these cases, the fact is that the requirements of life mean we are bound to take action—or non-action—*before* perfecting the arguments. So we believe that on the whole it is helpful that the authors in this volume take a stand, even if it is controversial, and even if, in some cases, a counter-view is also included.

There are many ways in which philosophy can have an impact in the world, so the ultimate meaning of the term 'applied philosophy' must be philosophy as a force and influence in the public arena. Not everyone who wears the label will accept this goal, but for some at least commitment and persuasion may form a legitimate, indeed necessary, part of the enterprise. If this seems too large a claim, it should be said that it is not intended to imply either that consideration of practical problems is the only business of philosophy, or that philosophers through argument alone can change the world. Far from it. On the contrary, this book is intended to show only that it is necessary and important that at least *some* people who take philosophy seriously should also take the enterprise of applied philosophy seriously. It is also intended to show, however, that, while the assembly of facts and collection of statistical data may be an essential part of practical problem-solving, they cannot in themselves provide the answers we need. Solutions to the problems of political and social life must in the end be sought in the kind of reflective consideration characteristic of an outward-facing philosophy.

Brenda Almond and Donald Hill
July 1990

Part I

The Environment

1

Moral Reasoning about the Environment

R. M. HARE

ABSTRACT   *This paper deals in the main with the problem of delimiting the classes of beings to which we have moral duties when making environmental decisions, and of how to balance their interests fairly. The relation between having interests, having desires and having value (intrinsic or other) is discussed, and a distinction made between entities which can themselves value and those which can have value. Its conclusion is that duties are owed directly to, and only to, sentient beings, and that these duties can be ascertained by weighing their interests impartially strength for strength. It ends with some suggestions about procedures for doing this. Examples are taken from proposals to develop a beach commercially, and to construct a new road in an environmentally sensitive area [1].*

I

Though philosophers can make a modest but useful contribution to environmental problems, it is important to be clear what this contribution is. Philosophers are above all students of arguments (how to tell the good from the bad ones); and they have their own techniques for achieving this, all part of logic in a wide sense. They ought to be able to sort arguments out with more expertise than many of them manage. And non-philosophers who address this essentially philosophical task often, in their innocence, simply fail to notice on what thin logical ice they are skating; and no amount of enthusiasm or commitment will make up for the blunders they then commit. What we need is some account of the way in which one should reason about environmental issues, and the principles that such reasoning leads to. It might go on to suggest political and administrative procedures to make the public argument run clear. Both conservationists and their opponents ought to be trying to make their arguments hold water. Unless they can do this, how can they expect reasonable people, who do not want just to listen to a lot of rhetoric, to be convinced by them?

I shall not be able in this paper to complete such an account, but I will discuss just two or three very crucial questions with which it would have to deal. First, since environmental planning is a way of adjudicating conflicts between various interests, we need a careful delimitation of the interests that have to be considered: and then we need to ask by what method of moral thinking the adjudication should be done. Since it is moral reasoning that we are discussing, we need consider only those interests which can generate moral duties and rights. I shall call these 'morally relevant interests', and sometimes in what follows abbreviate this to 'interests'. As we shall see later, there may be some kinds of entities (trees and bicycles for example) which have interests of a sort, or in a sense, that is not morally relevant. This complication I will ignore for the present.

In the literature a lot of things are credited with interests, and the first task should be to decide which of these things actually have morally relevant interests. Some people speak of the interests of 'Nature'. Others speak of the interests of the biosphere, of the ecosystem, and of non-living things in it, such as lakes, valleys and mountains. It is a controversial question whether such non-living things can have interests. Others, while denying that such things have interests, assign interests to plants and non-sentient animals, which are living indeed, but have no conscious experiences.

We could rule all these latter classes of things out of court if it is impossible to have interests without having desires for their furtherance or regrets if they are not preserved; for desires and regrets are conscious experiences which non-sentient things cannot have. One might be inclined to answer that it is not impossible, because obviously a small child might be harmed if its trustees made away with some of its money, and it never found out about the defalcation, and, because there was plenty of money left, never noticed the diminution in spending power even when it grew up. So the child would have interests without having any desires or regrets. This answer, however, misses the point I am trying to make. Presumably the child, when grown up, will have *some* desires which would have been realised if there had been more money, but as it was could not be realised. If this were not so, there really would be no harm to the child's interests. So even in this case the frustration of desire, now or in the future or possible future, is a necessary condition of harm to interests. Even if the child, in the event, dies before it has the desire that would have been frustrated, it might not have, and therefore its *expectation* of desire-satisfaction has been diminished, and that is harm.

I shall assume provisionally (leaving for later consideration an argument against this view) that there can be no harm to morally relevant interests without at least potential prevention of desire-satisfaction. So, on this showing, we ought not to attribute such interests to creatures such as plants and the lower animals, which could not have desires. Next, we have to ask about the interests of the higher animals, who do have conscious experiences including desires (or at least I presume they do), and lastly of people. The general question is, where in this list do we draw the line and say that, since the things below the line have no interests (at least of the kind that generate moral duties) questions about duties to them, and of their rights, do not arise?

II

A second dimension of controversy emerges when we ask, of things of any of these sorts, whether to have interests they have already to exist, or at least be definitely going to exist. It is easiest to take people as an example, though the question arises in principle for any of the things I have been listing. It seems reasonable to say that if it is the case that a certain person is definitely going to exist (say the person that the foetus in this normal pregnancy will turn into when born), then he or she will have interests in what happens to him or her after becoming a normal adult. But it is not possible to generalise from this clear case to the interests of posterity in general. The reason is that almost any adoption of an environmental or planning policy is going to affect people's actions in the future, and in particular the *times* at which they copulate to produce children. This in turn will affect the precise sperms and ova that unite to produce the children, and so the individual identities of those children [2].

The consequence is that there is no such thing as an identifiable set of people that we can label as 'posterity'—as if those and only those people were the ones that were going to be born. 'Posterity' is a set of people whose identities are not yet fixed, because they depend on actions not yet taken and policies not yet decided. If therefore (as some philosophers have done) we claim that no interests are harmed or rights infringed unless there already exists, or is definitely going to exist, an identifiable individual person whose interests and rights these are going to be, posterity in general will have no interests or rights and we can do what we please about the future of the world.

A particular case of this problem is that of whether we have a duty to bring people into existence. Most people think that we do not have a duty to bring into existence all the people we could—and there are arguments for this view which I shall not have room to go into. But have we a duty to bring *any* people into existence? Could we rightly, if it suited us, just stop having children altogether? I do not myself accept the view that, just because posterity does not consist of now identifiable individuals who could have interests and rights, posterity in general has no interests or rights. I do think that we have duties to posterity, and these may even include the duty to ensure that there is a posterity; but I shall not here give my arguments for this view, which I have set out in full in a paper that I hope to publish before long [3].

III

There is a relation between having an interest and valuing, which is a special case of that between having an interest and desiring. If *A* values *B* (or in other words if *B* is of value to *A*), then *A* has an interest (*pro tanto* and *ceteris paribus*) in the existence of *B*. And this implies that (again *ceteris paribus*) *A* desires, or will under certain conditions desire, that *B* exist. Valuing is one kind (I am not committed to saying that it is the only kind) of desiring. This relation between interests and values may help us in delimiting the class of entities which have interests, and to which, therefore, there is a point in attributing rights.

It does not follow, from the fact that an entity can value other entities, that it itself has positive value, even to itself. It is not self-contradictory to speak of a valueless valuer. A very unhappy man might value his childrens' continued existence, even though he did not value his own, and neither did anyone else. So, in classifying entities that have value, we do not need to include any entity just because it is capable of valu*ing*. The class of entities which have interests may therefore contain members which do not have value; for these members may value other entities though they themselves are of no value to any entity, even to themselves.

We must distinguish three classes of entities which can be said to have value. I shall call these classes *alpha*, *beta* and *gamma*.

Alpha. Pre-eminently, something has value if it has value *to* itself, as when *A* values the existence of *A*. Most humans fall into this class, because they value, and therefore have an interest in, their own continued existence. The same may be true of other higher animals. For example, it seems likely that cows, as sentient creatures, value their own existence. At the other end of the scale God, if he exists, values and has an interest in his own existence. To borrow a phrase from Aristotle, to all these things 'their own existence is good and pleasant; for they take pleasure in being conscious of [their own] intrinsic good' [4]. We may say that such entities are valuable *to* themselves.

Beta. There are other entities of which this cannot be said, but which, though not valuable *to* themselves, are valuable *in* themselves *to* other entities (e.g. to those in class *alpha*, or to other entities which can value). As examples of *beta* entities, we may give inanimate objects which are valued in themselves. For example, someone may value Wastwater in itself, and want it to exist for its own sake, even when he is no longer alive to enjoy the beauty of the lake. I am not discussing whether there could be any good reason for thinking like this about Wastwater, but only claiming that if somebody said it, we would understand him. The same might be said of some kind of tree of which we make no use: somebody might want giant sequoias to go on growing in California even after he is no longer there to see them, and perhaps even when there is *nobody* there to see them. But Wastwater is of no value *to Wastwater*, and the sequoias are of no value *to the sequoias*, because they are not entities that can value.

Gamma. Lastly, there are entities which do not value their own existence like those in class *alpha*, and which are not of value in themselves to other entities as are those in class *beta*, but which are valued by, or of value to, other entities *instrumentally*, for the use made of them. Into this class fall crops, natural commodities like gravel, and some artefacts.

IV

It might be objected that we are prejudging an important issue if we say that these are the only classes of things that have value. May there not be a class (let us call it *omega*) of entities which have value (are valuable) though they do not have value (are not valuable) *to* anything, even to themselves? I wish to argue that class *omega* must be empty, because to think that an entity has value although nothing is valuing it is incoherent. For to think that something has value is either to value it oneself, or to think that it has value to something else. To think that something has value although nobody and nothing, not even oneself, values it is like thinking that some statement is true although nobody, not even oneself, believes it. In thinking it true one *is* believing it. It is important, however, not to confuse this argument with the view, to which I can attach no sense that makes it acceptable, that we somehow *make* things valuable by valuing them. This is like saying that we make statements true by believing them.

Even if it be granted that it is incoherent to say that something is valuable though valued by nobody, does it follow (an objector might ask) that it is incoherent to *suppose* that there might be something that was valuable although valued by nobody? There could after all be a statement that was true although believed by nobody (not even the person who made it). I would answer that it is incoherent, because it is incoherent to suppose that the supposition could be true. For if it were true, we should be able to say of the thing in question that it was valuable, and in so doing we should either be valuing it ourselves, or claiming that something else valued it, and therefore could not, without the same pragmatic inconsistency as before, say that nobody was valuing it. In any case, such *supposed* valuable entities are not going to have a bearing on practical decisions unless and until it is established that they might *become* actual if certain decisions were taken.

It is true that we can coherently suppose the existence of an entity having certain specific properties, and say that it *would* be valuable *if* it existed. Then we should be valuing its existence hypothetically, and could not consistently say in the same breath that this was not valued by anybody. Hypothetical valuing as inescapably accompanies the hypothetical existence of valuable things as actual valuing does their actual existence. In each case we are valuing the existence of a thing having *those* properties *because* it has them. If, however, we merely suppose the existence of something valuable without specifying the properties that make it valuable, we do not know what we are supposing to exist, and our valuation is empty, because we do not kow what we are valuing, nor on what grounds. Even if such a supposition makes sense (which I doubt) it is at any rate clear that it is not going to affect any practical decision, because that would have to be grounded in our valuation of the properties that do, or would, make the thing valuable.

I conclude that the class *omega* is empty. I may add that if we are talking not about values but about interests, then the argument has even more obvious force. For even if it made sense to speak of something that had value although nothing valued it, it would make no sense to speak of there being interests which were the interests of nothing.

V

Reverting now to the problem of delimiting the class of beings that can have morally relevant interests and rights, I will suggest a possible way of solving it which looks promising. It is a generalisation of the method of moral argument known as the Golden Rule. We have to ask what we wish should be done to us, were we in the position of the victim of a certain action. The method, as a way of deciding moral questions, has a very strong affinity, not only with the Christian law of *agape* of which it is one expression, but also with the Kantian and utilitarian traditions in moral philosophy, which are supposed by some to be oppnents, but actually come to the same thing, at least in this area [5].

It certainly seems possible to ask what I want to be done to me if I am one of the people who occupy my house and garden when I have vacated it on my death. These are not yet identifiable people; but that does not stop me having regard to their interests: not, for example, polluting the garden by burying hazardous waste in it. I know what it would be like for this to be done to me, so I know what it would be like for my successors, whoever they may be, to have it done to them.

Though some will make objections. I myself do not find any difficulty in extending this argument to sentient animals who may suffer if I do not keep the garden free of pollution. I am not claiming that all sentient animals suffer from the same causes or to the same extent. For example, if the land is to be taken over by a farmer and occupied by cows, they will not mind, as a human occupant might, if the land is infested with some weed that is anathema to gardeners but delicious to cattle. But what about non-sentient animals and plants? If I ask myself whether I mind what happens to me if I become a tree in the garden, I answer (holding the view that I do about the physiology of trees and their lack of a nervous system, which I think to be a necessary condition of sentience) that I could not care less what happens to me if I am a tree, any more than I care if someone cuts off my limbs after I am dead. In consequence, a 'Golden-Rule' method of moral reasoning will not ascribe any morally relevant interests to trees, nor any rights that we have a duty to respect.

No doubt some will deny that the supposition that I could become a tree has any sense. If this were accepted, it would do equally well for my present argument; but since I do not actually think this, and wish in any case to give the opposition a run for its money, I shall not take advantage of this move. In my own view, the reason why I do not care what happens to me if I become a tree is not that it makes no sense to suppose this, but that when I do suppose it, as I certainly can, I know that in the tree's position I shall have no sentience, and therefore no suffering, any more than I shall when I am dead, and so what happens to me in the role of tree will not affect my experience for better or worse.

The crucial point here is that in making the moral judgement that we ought (or ought not) to treat something in a certain way, we are prescribing that anything of an exactly similar sort ought (or ought not) to be so treated in exactly similar circumstances. Where the thing in question is sentient, we shall be unwilling (*ceteris paribus*) to prescribe that we ourselves should, if in that situation with that sentience (including those desires), be so treated, if the treatment runs counter to the desires. So this will stop us saying that we ought to treat *sentient* creatures in a way that runs counter to their desires (unless there are countervailing considerations arising out of the desires of other beings in whose places we imagine ourselves). But in the case of non-sentient creatures that have no desires, this argument will not work, and we shall not be stopped from treating them in any way consistent with the furtherance of the desires and interests of sentient creatures. If I am right about this (and I have had to leave out a lot of the argument) it gives us a fairly clear cut-off point at which we can stop speaking of the morally relevant interests of the classes of beings I listed at the beginning: non-sentient animals, plants, ecosystems, the biosphere and the universe or Nature.

There is an argument against this cut-off point sometimes used by conservationists, which is Aristotelian in inspiration. It is an argument for including in the class which has morally relevant interests not only sentient, but also non-sentient living beings, while still excluding non-living beings. It is said, for example, that we morally ought to consider the interests of trees. We do, perhaps, speak of the good of trees. Trees have a nature, and grow in accordance with it, even if they are not conscious. The interest of the acorn is to become a full-grown oak, for example. That is what it would be for the tree to realise its own good. Robin Attfield, who maintains a view of this sort [6], has told me in conversation that he does not wish to go as far as Aristotle, and attribute *desires* to trees, or say that they are *trying* to become full-grown. There would indeed be no harm in saying this, in Aristotle's senses of 'desire' and 'trying' which do not imply consciousness.

But the question is whether such interests, desires and tryings have moral relevance, in that they constitute moral reasons for treating trees in one way rather than another. For it is possible to agree that we do speak of the good of trees without admitting that this has any moral relevance for environmental policy. If the basis of morality is the Golden Rule to do to others as we wish that they should to to us, then if, as I have said, I could not care less what happens to me if I am a tree, I shall not care in particular whether, if I am the tree, it realises its peculiar good or not. I no more care what happens to me if I am the tree than I do what happens to me if I am the bicycle that I knock over. The bicycle too has a good; one can harm it by knocking it over. But that does not entail that the bicycle has interests of the sort that could generate moral rights or duties.

From the premiss that we have no duties *to* trees or lakes or the biosphere, it does not follow that we have no duties *with regard to* these things. Harm to them may harm sentient beings including people, to whom we have duties. It is up to the conservationists, and not so difficult as some people think, to show that these inanimate things, though they themselves have no morally relevant interests, ought to be conserved in the interests of beings that do have such interests. Wise conservationists try to show this, instead of taking the short cut of assuming illegitimately that all kinds of things have morally relevant interests, and thus rights, which could not have them.

I suspect that what is happening when people attribute morally relevant interests and rights to non-sentient creatures is this. They are projecting their own values (their ideals) on to the things in question. They, the environmentalists, think certain natural objects like mountains valuable 'in themselves', as they would say; that is, they value them highly, which they are perfectly at liberty to do. Through a confusion between classes *alpha* and *beta* above, they slip from expressing their own valuation of the mountain in itself, which puts it only into class *beta*, to attributing an act of valuation to the mountain itself, thus mistakenly including it in class *alpha*. Entities in class *alpha*, it will be remembered, must be capable of having interests, because they can value; but this is not true of entities in class *beta*.

Although I would be the last person to rely on moral intuitions as proof of moral theses, it is perhaps worth saying that the classification I have suggested does seem to be in accord with the intuitive opinions of most people about where to draw the line between the entities to which we have moral duties and those to which we have not. If we ask, for example, why most people think it worse to devastate Wastwater than some lake in the remote Yukon which hardly anybody will ever see, the answer seems to be that we are giving weight to the interests of the people that will enjoy the lakes. No doubt we should add the interests of the sentient wild life that can enjoy them; and of course the preservation of the Yukon may be important environmentally because of its wider environmental effects, and because of the value it may have for posterity. But when all these interests, including the immediate interests of sentient creatures that can enjoy the lakes, are added up, it looks as if Wastwater wins. The same kind of reasoning explains why we value the preservation of some rare and beautiful species of butterfly over the preservation of the smallpox virus. Part of the reason may be that we think that the butterfly is sentient and the virus not; but more importatly, we think that the preservation of the virus, except for a few specimens safely locked up, would harm sentient creatures, whereas the preservation of the butterfly adds to their pleasure.

VI

I should like at this point to refer to a lecture I gave some years ago [7], and take up some problems that I did not then have time to deal with. I did deal at length with the problems of choosing between environmental options when only one party's interests are affected; and I suggested two contrasting models of how this should be done. In the first, the *means-end* model, what are called 'goals' are specified right at the start, and then it is determined on a factual basis, without further evaluative judgements, which option would most fully realise these goals. In the second, the *trial-design* model, the factual predictions come first; it is determined in sufficient detail what would actually happen, or what it would be like, if each of the various options were realised, and after that an informed evaluative choice can be made between the options, because we then know clearly in factual terms what we are choosing between.

The assumption that a single entity called 'the public' could make these choices would be too simple. Where there really is just one individual making the choices, he can proceed by the trial-design method, and need do no cost-benefit analysis; he can just choose, knowing what he is choosing between. But where the conflicting interests of individuals are affected, the question of what morally ought to be done cannot be answered without comparing the strength of the interests, and this involves some kind of cost-benefit analysis. Anti-utilitarians may not like this; but it is hard to see how else we can be fair to the different parties. Not only utilitarians, but anyone who needs to assess the amount of harm or good done to those affected (Rawls for example, with his difference principle, or Ross with his duties of beneficence and non-maleficence [8]), has to have a method for assessing it; and this will be cost-benefit analysis under another name.

The reason why even the trial-design method does not obviate the need for cost-benefit analysis altogether is that after we have put it into operation—i.e. after it has become clear to everybody just what the various options will be like in practice, which is of course a very difficult thing to achieve—the person or body that makes an environmental decision will have to find out from all the people affected, as best he can, *how much* they would like or dislike the various options, and then translate those likes and dislikes into a decision which is fair. I suggested jocularly, in the lecture I have referred to, that if everybody affected howled, and one could measure howls in decibels, one might thus arrive at a fair solution by choosing the option with the minimum of decibels against it. This too would be a kind of cost-benefit analysis. It would however be defective, because it would ignore posterity, which cannot howl yet, and also would give a false picture if, as is likely, the howlers were not accurately envisaging what the various options would be like in practice even for them.

Even less satisfactory, in theory, is any pure democratic method, not only because posterity cannot vote any more than howl, but because votes do not measure strengths of preferences. I shall later be using the example of the proposed construction of a new road. It might be that a huge majority was in favour of the road, because each member of the majority would benefit to a relatively small degree, but that enormous harm would be done to a few people who would be affected severely by the road, but who would be voted down because they had only one vote each. In some cases this could result in injustice; for it might be that the enormous harms to the few outweighed the relatively minor benefits, in time and money saved, to the many. This indeed is what the opponents of new roads sometimes argue. As a utilitarian, I am able to invoke justice here, because it is of dominant utility in a society that justice should be seen to be done, and also because it will actually *be* done in a particular case if interests are weighed in proportion to their strength, as utilitarianism requires.

In theory this problem could be overcome if people were able to buy votes and thus proportion the number of votes they had to the strength of their preferences. In the interests of social justice one would have to make the price paid for a vote proportionate to the voter's net income. I cannot see such a system working in practice; and perhaps it is a misuse of the democratic principle. What democracies ought rather to do is to vote for laws setting up principles for deciding such environmental questions —principles which would be accepted by all as just. The principles would include procedures for choosing the wise men who make or prepare the decisions (whether officials, or ministers, or inspectors at public inquiries), and, after choosing them, seeing to it that they decide fairly. This involves the power of the voters to turn them out if they do not satisfy the requirements of justice, as perceived by the voters.

VII

We have then to ask what the procedures ought to be in our own society—procedures for ascertaining the various interests affected and adjudicating between them when they conflict. The first thing, obviously, that the procedure has to establish is the relative strengths of the interests. There is an excellent device used in the United

States for this purpose, which we do not have in Britain, called the Environmental Impact Statement (EIS), which has to be prepared and published at an early stage before approval is given for major projects. This is then made the subject of a public hearing about the project. If either the statement or the procedure at the hearing has been defective, the project can later be challenged in the courts.

Our British system is not so good; government agencies have a habit of preparing schemes in the secrecy of their offices and only revealing them at a later stage when it is hard to change them; the 'public inquiries' that then take place often cannot have so much effect as the public process does in America. The necessity for publishing an EIS secures the *early* consideration of environmental dangers, and may result in greater care being taken at this early stage to avoid them, when it is not too late.

I know of a case in Britain where day-to-day intervention by a keen and influential environmentalist during the construction of a motorway, right up to the time of its opening, resulted in great improvements being made in the design and execution of a short length of it, but at very great expense, which could have been saved if the matter had been considered more carefully by the engineers who prepared the original design. But this is not likely to happen often, because such people are rare. The American system also does a lot more than the British to educate the public, so that these matters may be intelligently discussed.

The purpose of an EIS should be to make clear what environmental interests would be affected by a project, and to what extent. This at least sets the stage for an adjudication. Without going into a lot of ethical theory I shall not be able to substantiate this; but it seems natural to say that the strengths of the various interests, environmental and other, and the degree to which they are affected, should be the determining factor. We have to balance the interests against one another. A good procedure for adjudication would see to it that the interests were safeguarded, all in all, to the maximum degree possible, treating impartially all those affected.

It is sure to be claimed by some people that this way of looking at the matter leaves out the quality of the interests, and considers only their quantity, i.e. the strengths of the preferences. Imagine, for example, that it is proposed to develop a certain part of the sea-shore, adding various attractions, and that hordes of people will go there and enjoy it, but at the cost of entirely destroying its former natural beauty. It will be said (in many cases rightly as I think) that it ought not to be done. But it is very important to get the reasons for this right; for bad arguments in the long run defeat themselves politically. One reason is that the beauty of the shore is destroyed for ever and cannot be restored. So there is in principle an unlimited number of people whom you are depriving of that beauty in the future.

It might be said that there is also an unlimited, and larger, number of people in the future who could enjoy the popular attractions. Part of the answer is that the enjoyment of *these* people is often achievable without going near any shore. There are plenty of places which can be developed with these attractions without harming much natural beauty. So good planning would preserve the shore for those (we hope an increasing number within its capacity) who will enjoy it in times to come; and the others, even if more numerous, can be accommodated elsewhere. The only reason in the first place for proposing the development of the shore may have been a wholly mistaken belief that, to the people it would cater for, spoilt or even still beautiful shores have anything to offer that cannot be provided elsewhere. In that case, the interests of all parties could be preserved by keeping the shore as it is.

In Florida where I spend the winters there is a case which illustrates this argument.

If the developers of Disney World had chosen a site on the coast, as they easily might have, then that huge attraction, which gives innocent pleasure to vast numbers of people, would have had a far more adverse environmental impact than it has had. I might have said 'even than it has had'; this is a matter for dispute.

However, when all of that has been said, the environmental planning of the coastline remains a difficult task. Any theory that makes it sound easy must be wrong. It may be that there are large numbers of people who have a legitimate interest in spending their holidays by the sea, and enjoy them more when the attractions are provided. Fortunately coastlines are quite long, and it should not be impossible to preserve the wilder and more beautiful parts of them, while still providing agreeable recreation for the hordes (who luckily do not mind a lot of company). We can have Blackpool *and* Skokholm. This kind of decision is the stuff of environmental planning; and if the planner has been fair to all the interests affected, he has done his job.

VIII

I am going to end with another typical example of an environmentally damaging land use which illustrates the problems of planners even better: the building of new roads. This is a question which still excites enormous bitterness in Britain, but, I believe, less so now in America. In Britain there must be at the moment a half dozen or so major road schemes, and no doubt dozens of smaller ones, which are being bitterly contested. It may be that Americans are more tolerant of roads and automobiles; or that they have in general more room for roads, and so can avoid environmentally sensitive areas more easily than we can in Britain. Or is it just that they have been coping with the problem for longer and have arrived at a *modus vivendi* which satisfies most people?

I am not saying that new roads never excite controversy in America, where many more appalling things have been done by way of road-building than would ever be countenanced in Britain; but only that they now (perhaps as a result of past errors) seem to be better at resolving the controversies. The wiser part of the environmental lobby in America now rightly spends more effort getting the roads that have to be built put in the right places and made environmentally acceptable, than in trying to stop them altogether. What is most needed there is the kind of control of access to *all* highways that in Britain, since the Ribbon Development Act in the Thirties, has prevented the dangerous and disfiguring development that mars most American roads on the outskirts of cities.

What has to be done in this case, as in all cases of environmentally damaging land uses, is to do justice between the various interests affected; and I have already suggested, though only in principle, a method of doing this. We have to find out what the interests are, and then protect them to the maximal extent, treating the interests of all those affected impartially, strength for strength.

To see the problem of road construction in perspective, it is helpful to think, perhaps while one is driving along one of these new roads, what the great volume of traffic on them would be doing if the road had not been built. Would it be trying to force its way through the cities and towns which the road now avoids? That, I am sure, would harm more interests more severely than any road through open country, however beautiful the landscape through which it passes. Or would the freight and passengers that are now conveyed along the road be using alternative modes of transport? I am not going to have room to argue this, but I do not believe that there *are* any alternative modes of transport which could convey the same amount of freight and passengers to the same places without prohibitive cost. Or are the opponents of new roads just wanting there not to be this amount of transport of freight and passengers? So far as the freight goes, this entails accepting a sharply reduced level of economic activity, with all that that implies. I do not believe that even these people would like it if that had happened: they would have found their interests as adversely affected as everybody else's. They are only pretending to favour a life-style such as we would have if this freight were not transported.

As for the passengers, I am again convinced that interests would be more adversely affected by forcing nearly everybody to travel by public transport than by constructing roads. I am talking about motorways and major trunk roads through open country. It may be different when we speak of roads *through* and *into* towns and cities, though the extreme views on that question are, as I think, both wrong. No doubt a good case can be made for more provision of public transport in large cities, and indeed for the preservation of a viable and efficient railway system. But even if both these things were achieved, they could not possibly enable us to dispense with more than a small fraction of the traffic that now goes by road.

Those who oppose new roads simply because they impinge on the landscape are in effect asking that people should not make the journeys which now, for good purposes of their own, they wish to make. And that is to affect their interests adversely. I believe that if these people could not go in their own cars, they would not in most cases go at all. We have only to compare the state of affairs that obtained when no more than a few rich people owned cars (and I can remember that time). Though the majority who had no cars did travel sometimes by train, this did not happen often, and so they did not see each other, or see things they wanted to see, so much, or in general do things they wanted to do. So I think that to prevent them now travelling by car would be a deprivation more severe than any suffered by people who do not like looking at roads or having them built across their land. And many activities would just cease. For example, would the Royal Horticultural Society's gardens at Wisley be financially viable if people could not get there by road?

It is generally agreed even among conservationists that, at the time when the railways were built, it was on the whole beneficial to build them. The great increase in general living standards that occurred in the course of the nineteenth century would have been impossible without them. Yet in Britain at least there was just as much opposition to the building of the railways in the nineteenth century as there is in the twentieth to the building of roads. We should remember Ruskin who thought it monstrous to build a railway so that every fool in Buxton could be at Bakewell in half an hour and every fool in Bakewell at Buxton. That line was built, and conservationists fought its recent closure, just as they do that of the line from Leeds to Carlisle across the Ribblehead viaduct.

I am very ready to admit that a lot of roads in Britain, and no doubt elsewhere too, have been built in the wrong places. And I am prepared to admit that, even when they were put in the right places, they were built sometimes with great insensitivity to the landscape. In the early days when these roads were planned, the economics of road location and the aesthetics of road design were little studied. But we are learning more about how to get these things right. If those who oppose all roads on principle would instead spend more time studying how the job could best be done, and less saying that it should not be done at all, it might be that it would be done better. I think that this is beginning to happen even in Britain.

R. M. Hare, Department of Philosophy, University of Florida, Gainesville, FL 32611, USA.

NOTES

[1] This paper was given in Spring (1986) to conferences on the environment of the Society for Applied Philosophy, and of the Center for Applied Philosophy, University of Florida. Although revised and expanded, it is far from being the last word, or even, I hope, *my* last word on the subject. I am also grateful to the working party on these questions of the Ian Ramsey Centre at St Cross College, Oxford for allowing me to use material I wrote for its meetings; and to its members, especially James Griffin and Robin Attfield, for helpful comments and improvements.

[2] See D. PARFIT (1982) Future generations: further problems, *Philosophy and Public Affairs*, 11, especially p. 115, and ch. 16 of his *Reasons and Persons* (Oxford, OUP, 1984).

[3] Possible people, discussing D. PARFIT's 'Repugnant Conclusion' in *Reasons and Persons*, ch. 17.

[4] Aristotle, *Nicomachean Ethics*, 1170b 4.

[5] My own ethical theory, as set out in my *Moral Thinking* (Oxford, OUP, 1981) is at once Kantian and utilitarian. See especially pp. 4 f. In this paper I rely heavily on the arguments of that book.

[6] See R. ATTFIELD (1981) The good of trees, *Journal of Val. Inq.*, 15 (1981), reprinted (abridged) in D. VAN DE VEER & C. PIERCE (Eds) *People, Penguins and Plastic Trees* (Belmont, Wadsworth, 1986), p. 96.

[7] Contrasting methods of environmental planning, in R. S. PETERS (Ed) *Nature and Conduct* (Royal Institute of Philosophy Lectures, 1974; Basingstoke, Macmillan, 1975), reprinted in K. GOODPASTER & K. SAYRE (Eds) *Ethics and Problems of the 21st Century* (Notre Dame, University of Notre Dame Press, 1979).

[8] J. RAWLS (1971) *A Theory of Justice* (Cambridge, Mass., Harvard University Press, 1971), pp. 76 ff.; W. D. ROSS (1930) *The Right and the Good*, p. 21 (Oxford, OUP).

2

On Reasoning Morally about the Environment
—Response to R. M. Hare

DONALD HILL

ABSTRACT   *R. M. Hare argues that moral reasoning about the environment requires the setting out of the various interests at stake and adjudication between them, strength for strength. Though there are possible objections to some aspects of his programme, it is clearly intended to be fair. However, it is not clear that in his concluding discussion, of the building of new roads, the interests at stake are set out with total impartiality. Some further relevant interests are listed, in an attempt to redress the balance.*

I

R. M. Hare seeks to establish the classes of beings to which we can have moral duties when making environmental decisions, and the basis of those duties [1].

The beings to which we can have moral duties, he explains, are those with morally relevant interests, interests which can be harmed only if the satisfaction of those beings' desires is at least potentially prevented [2]. Such beings, then, have desires: they are sentient beings. They do not include non-sentient animals, plants, ecosystems, the biosphere, nor the universe or Nature [3]. They do, of course, include human beings alive now, as well as human posterity [4] and other sentient beings [5]. The morally relevant interests of such beings include interests which may be furthered or damaged by planned changes to their environment.

The proper job of environmental planners, from a moral point of view, is, according to Hare, to identify those interests "and then protect them to the maximal extent, treating the interests of all those affected impartially, strength for strength" [6]. Where the interests conflict, the strengths of those interests must be compared. The comparison, whatever the terms used to describe it, will, in effect, involve some form of cost-benefit analysis [7]. Hare recognises [8] that it will be objected that there are problems in comparing the strengths of *qualitatively* different interests; but he does not see this as a sufficient objection to the utilitarian programme he has in mind. Such a programme would be facilitated in Britain, he thinks, if Britain were to adopt a device something like the Environmental Impact Statement in use in the USA. This attempts to set out relevant interests and their strengths at an early stage in the planning of any project which may significantly affect the environment [9].

II

Hare's formal analysis is cogent and likely to command assent. It is open, however, to the following objections. The problem of comparing qualitatively different interests [10] strength for strength [11] is rather greater than he is here prepared to allow. One might object further on the pragmatic ground that the outcome of a quantitative cost-benefit analysis of an environmentally sensitive project is likely, other things being equal, to favour the party which can pay the costs of a favourable presentation of its case; and that this party will normally be the sponsor of the project in question. Again, one might object, more fundamentally, that no cost-benefit analysis can be realistically expected to take adequately into account all the relevant interests affected; in particular, those represented by the 'externalities'—predictable, if unplanned, adverse side-effects—of new projects [12].

Nevertheless, it is clear that Hare intends his programme to be fair. It is therefore surprising, on reading his Section VIII [13], in which he explores an example of a planning issue, to find oneself asking whether he himself is setting out the interests at stake with total impartiality. The problem is the building of new roads; in particular, new motorways (freeways) and trunk roads through open country in Britain. Hare is evidently in favour of such roads, as long as they are built in the 'right places' [14], and he puts forward some considerations in support of new roads. He is, of course, entitled to do so. Philosophers are not debarred from holding views about the world. However, in the context of his formal analysis, which the example of road-building is intended to illustrate, one might have expected as much attention to have been given to the interests which are *adversely* affected, as to those which are furthered, by the building of the roads.

The interests picked out by Hare for *sympathetic* treatment are the interests of those who would *benefit* from the building of new roads, whether as consumers dependent on road freight, or as people making journeys they would not otherwise make so conveniently, or at all [15]. To prevent people travelling by car "would be a deprivation more severe than any suffered by people who do not like looking at roads or having them built across their land" [16].

There are interests, not mentioned by Hare, which may be *adversely* affected by the building of new roads, interests which go beyond a superficial dislike of the look of the roads, or an objecting landowner's taste. Examples of such interests are indicated below; might they not be taken into account among all the interests at stake in the building of new roads?

First, there is an interest, shared by all the sentient beings on Hare's list, of not being killed or injured on the roads. This is one of the interests taken into account in Mayer Hillman's evaluation of British transport policy in the 1970's. There were more than 85,000 deaths and serious injuries on roads in Great Britain in 1980, of which 19,000 were pedestrians' [17]. The road lobby frequently maintains that motorways have a relatively low rate of deaths and injuries per 100 m. vehicle kilometres, but the fact that journeys do not begin nor end on motorways, but typically in towns and cities, tends to be overlooked, as does the fact that motorways generate longer-distance patterns of travel.

Secondly, there is a general interest in breathing clean air. If one assumes that new inter-urban roads increase traffic overall and in the towns they join, then, other things being equal, they will increase air pollution by road vehicles. The pollutants include carbon monoxide, hydrocarbons, oxides of nitrogen, sulphur dioxide, particulates and lead. In Great Britain there was a marked increase in road vehicle emissions of all these pollutants, except for sulphur dioxide, between 1970 and 1980 [18].

Thirdly, there is an interest in not being subjected to noise nuisance from road vehicles, and, more positively, in being able to hear things one may wish to hear, such as conversation, music, or birdsong. Noise from traffic may be taken to be proportional to total traffic mileage, which is used by Hillman as an index of traffic noise. Road traffic mileage in Great Britain increased by 36% between 1970 and 1980 [19].

Fourthly, there is an interest in freedom of movement. Children and the elderly (characteristically pedestrians), for example, find this interest adversely affected by road traffic, since it is not safe, let alone pleasant, for them to cross the road. Their movements tend to be curtailed for this reason, or made by car or other vehicle instead of on foot [20].

Fifthly, there is an interest in the conservation of ecosystems which are diminished by the building and use of new roads.

Sixthly, there is an interest, damaged by the building of new roads, in the conservation of landscapes perceived as landscapes of the past. The motives are complex [21], but it is hardly to be doubted that for some people the interest is a *strong* interest, and so, on Hare's own account of moral reasoning about the environment, should be taken into account.

Seventhly, there is an interest in good health, and it is far from clear that, other things being equal, an increase in road traffic will do more to promote it than to damage it. Cycling, for example, a good way to stay fit if one can stay alive, is problematical in cities inundated by ill-driven motor traffic.

Eighthly, there is an interest in not paying the high economic cost of road transport. This cost should, of course, be offset against the claimed economic benefits road transport gives. Part of the economic cost, of freight or of company cars for example, is passed on to the consumer and so paid indirectly; part is paid directly. The true economic cost includes the cost of public provision of the roads, as well as the costs of vehicles, fuel, and the quantifiable costs attributable to deaths and injuries.

Finally, there is, in addition to the economic cost, a less easily quantifiable cost of the using up of non-renewable natural resources: in particular of fuel. There is an interest in conserving such resources.

In listing some examples of interests which may be adversely affected by the building of new roads I am not assuming that no adequate cost-benefit analysis could ever show the building of a new road to be justified under any circumstances. Nor am I recommending a footpath society forthwith [22]. I am maintaining only that, if the analytical programme favoured by Hare is to be followed, then interests such as those I have listed should go into the mix. Otherwise, the outcome will be unfair.

It may be worth adding that on three matters of empirical fact, Hare appears to be making assumptions which may not be well-grounded.

First, he appears to think that the volume of traffic using a new road would exist—on the old roads—even if the new road had not been built. "Would it", he asks, "be trying to force its way through the cities and towns which the road now avoids?" [23]. There is, however, evidence that, not surprisingly, new roads generate new traffic [24], so that if the new road had *not* been built, the new increment of traffic would not have come about. Nor does all the traffic on new roads outside the city stay outside the city [25].

Secondly, Hare appears to find it odd [26] that while conservationists (such as Ruskin) once opposed the building of new railway lines, conservationists now oppose closure of some of the lines that were built, while opposing the building of new roads. That would indeed be odd, if the environmental impact of railways and roads were the same: but it is not. Railways have less land-take, for instance, are safer, and more fuel-efficient. They are also more equitably available: to all, rather than to car-owners.

Thirdly, in referring to new roads "built through open country" [27], Hare might be taken to be assuming for the purpose of his exercise that the open country will remain—apart from the roads—open country. In fact, new motorways in a road-dominated economy tend to generate pressures for 'development' along their routes. (In Britain, the Department of Transport itself is reported not to be objecting to a massive out-of-town shopping and leisure centre on land half of which it now owns, in the 'Golden Triangle' at the interchange of the M1 motorway and the newly completed M25 London orbital [28]. It will be interesting to see what planning enquiry procedures are followed in this case. The interchange is in the 'Green Belt' of protected countryside around London.) The development generated by new roads outside cities, and the impact of such development on the economic life of cities like London, which have by and large resisted the building of urban motorways, should be taken into account in any assessment of the environmental impact of new roads, such as the M25 motorway [29].

III

It may seem peevish to have homed in on Hare's handling of the example of new road building, rather than to have paid more attention to the substance of his formal analysis of moral reasoning about the environment. The analysis may well survive the example; but in *applied* philosophy, is not the application crucial?

Donald Hill, 6 Mansfield Place, London NW3 1HS, United Kingdom.

NOTES

[1] R. M. HARE (1987) Moral reasoning about the environment, originally published in *Journal of Applied Philosophy*, 4, pp. 3–14.

[2] Ibid., p. 4.

[3] Ibid., p. 8.

[4] Ibid., p. 5.

[5] Ibid., p. 8.

[6] Ibid., p. 12; cf. p. 11.

[7] Ibid., pp. 9–10.

[8] Ibid., pp. 11.

[9] Ibid., pp. 10–11.

[10] cf. J. S. MILL (1910) *Utilitarianism*, pp. 8–12 (London, Dent) (originally published 1861).

[11] COLIN BUCHANAN found difficulty in quantifying the negative value to be placed on the proposed demolition of a medieval church on a proposed airport site: see his minority report in (1971) *Great Britain. Commission on the Third London Airport (Chairman the Hon. Mr. Justice Roskill), Report* (London, HMSO). See also Note [12] below.

[12] On one aspect of this question, see J. G. U. ADAMS (1974) . . . and how much for your grandmother? *Environment and Planning*, 6, pp. 619–626. Adams, a geographer interested in transport planning, is writing about the problem faced by enlightened environmental planners who, for purposes of cost-benefit analysis, seek to put a cash value on human disablement and loss of life. Adams praises the economic rationality of a precursor, Swift: see JONATHAN SWIFT (1729) *A Modest Proposal*, reprinted in (1968) *Jonathan Swift* (New York, Random House). "The value of human life was, (Swift) demonstrated, simply a function of supply and demand. Further, the optimal time to end it was that at which the selling price minus the cost of production was a maximum. This time he computed to be one year and the net profit on a plump yearling child he calculated very precisely at 40p (1729 prices)" (Adams, op. cit., p. 619). Adams, deploring Swift's having been read ever since, except by some recent economists, as a satirist, drily concludes his own piece: "We must not be deterred by the soft-hearted among us who prefer not to think of death and disablement in terms of money. Rationality and efficiency demand that we reduce everything to cash. If we refuse, we throw away all the inestimable benefits of the cost-benefit calculus" (ibid., p. 625).

[13] HARE, op. cit., pp. 12–13.

[14] Ibid., p. 13.

[15] Ibid., loc. cit.

[16] Ibid., loc. cit.

[17] MAYER HILLMAN (1982) An evaluation of transport policy in the 1970s, *Policy Studies*, 3, Table 4, p. 78. For data on road accidents see Department of Transport (annually), *Road Accidents Great Britain* (London, HMSO). For an extended discussion of accidents see STEPHEN PLOWDEN & MAYER HILLMAN (1984) *Danger on the Road: the needless scourge* (London, Policy Studies Institute).

[18] Ibid., Table 1, p. 73.

[19] Ibid., loc. cit. Hillman's figures are taken from Department of Transport (1981) *Transport Statistics Great Britain, 1970–1980* (London, HMSO).

[20] See, for example, MAYER HILLMAN, IRWIN HENDERSON & ANNE WHALLEY (1976) *Transport Realities and Planning Policy* (London, Political and Economic Planning).

[21] —and very human. To recapture the past entirely is impossible, but to retain symbols of it is necessary to some sense of personal identity. David Lowenthal comments, "The past has no doubt taken place; we ourselves stem from it". The past not only predates us, but includes our lives up to the present. Lowenthal quotes Margaret Drabble: "We feel such profound and apparently disproportionate anguish when a loved landscape is altered out of recognition; we lose not only a place, but a part of ourselves, a continuity between the shifting phases of our life". See DAVID LOWENTHAL, Revisiting past landscapes, in: JOHN R. GOLD & JACQUELIN BURGESS (Eds) (1982) *Valued Environments*, pp. 91 and 94 (London, Allen & Unwin), and M. DRABBLE (1979) *A Writer's Britain: landscape in literature*, pp. 270–1 (London, Thames & Hudson).

[22] —though footpaths have their uses. There are also, for many journeys, effective or potentially effective public transport options which, if attractive enough, would be taken up without the 'forcing' referred to by Hare (op. cit., p. 13). In Great Britain, this may well require an increase in public transport subsidies. In recent years, when London's public transport subsidies have increased, enabling fares to be lowered, private car traffic has diminished. When the subsidies have been reduced, and fares raised, private car traffic has increased. London has much lower subsidies than some other metropolitan cities such as New York or Paris. See, for example, STUART COLE An integrated transport policy—a public transport solution, in: STUART COLE & DONALD HILL (Eds) (1986) *Astride the A1 Corridor: report of a conference on traffic problems in the Holloway Road and the A1 corridor*, pp. 66–80, especially Table 6, p. 77 (London, Polytechnic of North London).

[23] HARE, op. cit., p. 12.

[24] See, for example, United Nations Environment Programme (1987) *Environmental Data Report*, p. 261 (Oxford, Blackwell). On this issue in general the report states that " ... it may be expected that the increasing numbers of vehicles *and the increasing lengths of roads* would result in increased distances driven" (my italics).

Increased use of roads is given in turn as a reason for building yet more roads. For example, Steven Elliott of the British Roads Federation (a pressure group of the commercial vehicle operators) urges (*Sunday Times*, 15 November 1987) that "the Government has to start designing roads for future traffic volumes. By 1991 the M1 will be carrying 160,000 vehicles a day—double its design capacity. No sooner is a road completed than it is out of date". Does the road lobby, or (if that is a different question) the Department of Transport, have a model which spells out the long-term environmental impact of this self-feeding process? Would demand for the use of roads grow so fast if their use were not free at the point of consumption?

[25] See, for instance, HUGH COLLIS (1986) Through traffic/local traffic, in: COLE & HILL (Eds), op. cit., pp. 28–30. One survey showed that nearly two-fifths of the traffic on the Holloway Road, part of the A1 in inner London, had origins or destinations well outside the city, beyond the new M25 orbital motorway.

[26] HARE, op. cit., p. 13.

[27] Ibid., loc. cit

[28] *The Independent*, 7 November 1987.

[29] See JOHN ADAMS (1986) A view of the strategic context, in: COLE & HILL (Eds), op. cit., pp. 11–22.

3

Original Populations and Environmental Rights

TIMO AIRAKSINEN

ABSTRACT   *This paper deals with a conflict between our sense of social justice and the need to protect the environment. It is argued that original populations do not own the land and other relevant aspects of their environment. However, immigrant newcomers will work on them and claim them for their own. The original populations are an integral part of the environment. When the newcomers realize that they must protect the vanishing natural environment, they must also control the lives of the original populations. The problem is that the newcomers have brought about the problems which will harm the others, too. In order to analyse this situation I distinguish between different types of rights, the value of nature and our alienation from it. The basic dilemma is described in normative terms and it is suggested that the rights claims of the original populations are quite strong. At the same time it is clear that it is impossible to return to any 'original position'. Some piecemeal solutions are suggested.*

1 Introduction and Examples

In many countries an original population lives alongside some immigrant 'newcomers'. I shall focus on situations where the original population is a minority and also less developed both technologically and politically. I shall give several examples of relevant cases in order to show how the original population is dependent on its natural environment (hunting, fishing, primitive agriculture), which is also valued, preserved and protected by the members of the *non*-original population.

Tragic conflicts emerge when the original population tries to maintain its traditional forms of life which in the new circumstances, due to the technology and the politics introduced by the immigrants, have already become harmful and even potentially destructive to the natural environment. The presently fashionable ecological consciousness—paradoxically—reinforces this trend, sometimes without even hinting at solutions. Such a vicious causal cycle was started by the same people who now try to reverse its direction because of their own changing values and priorities—moving from exploitation and economic imperialism towards a radical preservationist attitude.

The problem is that the original populations are left alone in no-man's-land, between nature and modern society where their environmental rights tend to become crushed. Such a tendency is familiar all over the world as the sad heritage of European 'imperialism'.

I am not, however, referring to the 'dirty hands' of imperialist politics. Sheer exploitation and large scale violence against original populations is an historical fact. But its negative moral message is much clearer than that of the environmentalist cases. An example is salmon fishing rights in the rivers of Northern Finland. The local peasant population had developed a distinctive, rich and flourishing fishing culture. This was instantly destroyed by the dams and power plants constructed in the rivermouths after the Second World War when rapid industrialisation of the southern part of the country started. The new economy in the far-away South made an age-old life-style impossible in the North.

Now, my purpose in this paper is twofold. First, I shall analyse in terms of rights and welfare claims a given historical situation. The newcomers want to protect the environment, and this cancels some of the traditional rights of the original population. But their life-style has already changed because of the new technology they have started to use. The new technology does not allow one to exercise one's full environmental rights—especially when the environment is already depleted.

Secondly, I shall try to say something about the question of how such problems may be alleviated. They cannot be solved, however; it is a moral dead-end. My suggestion is, roughly, that one should provide compensation for the losses and also possibilities for new and alternative life-styles through education. The mainstream society should be *open* to the members of the original population. We shall discuss also political contracts.

My first example of the old-style practices which appear so strange and difficult to justify is this:

> In the northern United States, snakehunting and sacking are by far most popular in Pennsylvania, where prizes are awarded to hunters bringing in the largest snake, the snake with the most rattles (. . .). The biggest prizes go to the hunters catching the most snakes and the smallest snake, usually the hardest to handle.... For the competition, the sacker is presented with a canvas sack filled with five poisonous snakes, usually two copperheads and three rattlers. After dumping the snakes into the pit, he is allotted three minutes to calm them down,... Meanwhile a partner holds the sack. At the sound of the bell, the sacker plunges his hands into that hissing, squirming mass, picks up the snakes, and tosses them tail-first into the sack. The quickest time... wins [1].

These games have been condemned by environmentalists as 'brutal and uncivilised', as well as detrimental to the snake population. Such negative reasons are very revealing. Snake-sacking has survived in a newly regulated and controlled context.

Let us forget the problems of cruelty and focus on the survival of populations. Prevention of cruelty to animals is a valid motive: it is nowadays illegal in Finland to castrate reindeer in Lappland by biting their testicles. Indeed, many traditional methods look cruel to the modern man. Sometimes this constitutes a peculiar problem as one's moral 'intuition' demands that cruelty be stopped and yet one knows that ascriptions of cruelty are culture-dependent. However, cruelty is wrong and it is one's prima facie duty to prevent what one knows is cruel. The relativist ramifications of such norms do not interest us now.

My second example is the seal, whale and bear hunting rights of the Eskimos in their old hunting areas where some species tend to become more and more depleted and closer to outright extinction. The hunters may nowadays use powerboats, rifles, and snowmobiles. The poaching of rhinos and elephants in Africa because of meat and their valuable horns and ivory should also be mentioned.

Then, finally, think of some nomadic tribes whose herds tend to impoverish their own environment by overgrazing, about which the tribes themselves cannot do anything. They may have received heavier, more demanding but more productive cows. The range of their traditional migrations is limited by new borders and regional warfare. They are lured into selling and not using their own products in order to buy goods from incoming merchants. The people will ultimately destroy their own environment for good.

Similar examples are easy to give. But what is their significance and how can we analyse them correctly? The practical implication is clear: given the need to protect the environment, in a tragic fashion the original populations are supposed to change over from their old ways to a modern life-style, even without their own free and informed consent and often with negative consequences to themselves. They seldom reach full political and economic equality with the dominant newcomers anyway. Yet, their life-styles become ecologically disastrous so that the extra pressures of legal control and social paternalism are easy to legitimate.

2 Rights and Property

The members of the original population may refer to their natural right to utilize their own environment. I call such rights *weak environmental rights*: the subject of these rights is free to take advantage of the environment, its opportunities and its products. It is a simple liberty. Typically one does not become conscious of such a moral fact before this customary enjoyment is challenged. Let me clarify this idea.

My basic point is simple: one has been born to the natural environment and one is free to use what is available for one's own good. Actually this is a kind of *collective* right which applies at the level of groups and, moreover, there seems to be no need to conceptualise it in terms of ownership and property. Originally no one owns the birds, the plants and the rocks, valuable as these may be to the members of the original population. One may perfectly well utilise and enjoy them without owning them either collectively or privately. We may find no genuine property rights in this context. We are dealing with basic welfare which is grounded on the fact that one is *entitled* to it.

The following hard facts are of interest.

> In simple horticultural societies, as in hunting and gathering societies, there are no gross inequalities in material possessions. The reasons for this are twofold. First, most material necessities are readily available to all. In most of these societies plenty of land is available and anyone willing to work can supply his own needs. (The abundance of land may well be a by-product of the chronic state of warfare which is so common among these societies ...) The second factor ... is the relative absence of capital goods.
> [But] in nearly all ... [advanced horticultural] societies there is no clear distinction between the personal wealth of the king or chief and the people's surplus with which he is entrusted [2].

Such empirical considerations point to the *common* nature of the original 'simple' means of survival and their relation to war and the exercise of power. Affluence, shortages and disasters influence everyone in the same way.

In the next stage, when the given political organisation allows, the structural position of the king may entail a valid demand to the effect that most property rights belong to its current placeholder. This is the first drastic move away from the weak environmental rights towards communal property rights and even individual ownership. I do not intend to derive any definite conclusions on the basis of such empirical generalizations. They only make us aware of the complex descriptions of the forms of organised moral life.

All people, except slaves, possess some private property. I am, however, now focusing on things which lack the status of property. The members of the original population simply cannot go and sell the birds. There is no market. What they may be able to do is share, exchange or give away bird hunting opportunities. They agree that other people may hunt if they themselves can, say, travel through their territory. In such situations we observe again a move away from the weak environmental rights towards genuine collective property rights, or successful claims to respect for ownership.

Somehow it seems natural to think, however, that in many cases when such weak environmental rights are surrendered to (say) another original population, this transaction is simply a gift or an exchange of assets not owned but only *effectively controlled* by some organised group. If, say, hunting opportunities are wanted by all but available only to the stronger of two groups, it does not follow that this stronger group would hold a property right over the opportunity.

It is highly suspect to maintain that any newcomers—whose culture is directly comparable to that of the original population—should bargain with that population: we now presuppose that there is no mechanism suited to the conduct of negotiations and their subsequent enforcement and control, as well as no systematic way of fixing the value of the privileges exchanged. Also the *duties* of the newcomers towards the other population cannot be easily conceptualized. It simply does not make sense to say—without strong qualifications—that the newcomers' acts of apprehension and the resulting possessions entail a failure to observe some duties towards the original population. No valid environmental (deontic) claims exist; all we see are some weak rights as liberties. The level of conflicts is basic and concrete and it embodies power and control.

The original population defends its freedom against the newcomers; this is a relation of *power* and not of morality. Both groups defend their own claims which are perceived to be important both on the basis of their temporal span and the urgency of need satisfaction. One group was there earlier but the other's motives for acquisition may be even stronger. The result is *war*.

These facts do not become clearly visible until a modern state moves in and asks for valid proofs of ownership and legitimate transfer. Such proofs are not forthcoming and the signs of transfer remain invisible. Therefore, what the original population uses and enjoys is based on weak environmental rights; and even if they bargain with other original groups with regard to some amenity, it does not prove that property rights and collective ownership are in question. All parties share the opportunities to gain satisfaction and equal welfare.

Suppose two groups both qualify as original populations and present claims over territorial matters; it is impossible for them to exchange rights so that the new distribution of assets could be assumed to be binding, just, and permanent by a third similar group. If the third group joins forces with one of the former groups, the new coalition is in a good position to claim the assets for itself. The demand is effective because it is enforced by a power advantage. Every distribution of territorial privileges appears valid only in those given circumstances in which the deal was actually made. The distribution is situationally specific; or in other words, it is devoid of moral meaning.

My basic premise that all property logically presupposes its own type of politics can be denied. One may try to say that even the original population owns its environment as collective property, in the full-blown moral sense of having a claim right over it. There is much to say in favour of this view, as one might argue. The members of the original population have mixed their labour with their natural environment and they tend to defend their 'rights' as if they were property rights in a collective but otherwise Lockean sense. There may be at least a strong analogy with claim rights. I have already argued that this is not so: property indeed presupposes politics.

3 Equilibria, Alienation and Justice

It is a natural liberty to act out one's intentions and goals in one's environment in the manner specified and justified by one's own culture. In the same way, it is plausible to maintain that if the original population has reached an *equilibrium* with the environment its members are free to keep the situation stable without possessing any claim right against newcomers. One's range of actions, its planning and success, depends on one's relation to natural forces. The existence of this equilibrium guarantees some basic action possibilities whose range depends on the type and nature of the equilibrium. If a disequilibrium is created, this fact entails one's inability to take care of one's welfare in the long run.

I shall clarify the notion of equilibrium by means of an example: in Finland, if the hunter uses only a bow and arrow or a very primitive gun, he can kill moose mainly in special weather conditions when firm snow carries the hunter on skis but prevents the mooses' running away. There is an equilibrium between man and moose and it is determined by the regularity of the weather and the low level of technology. The hunter is not able to kill moose too frequently. Nowadays one is able to exterminate moose by helicopters and machine guns. The natural equilibrium is replaced by hunting laws.

The basic point is that one's *original position* is an *environmental equilibrium* which entails a (weak) right to utilize the resources. One is part of the environment, and it is difficult to distinguish between the natural, human and social environments and their ecology. What a person does is part of the dynamics of the global environment. This includes all kinds of degrees and variations, but human action together with its causal consequences is an integral part of some equilibrium.

An equilibrium tends to obtain whenever the original population is directly dependent on environmental changes. If they destroy an aspect of the environment these developments influence their own living conditions within a relatively short timespan. By cutting all trees they create a lack of firewood and dustier surroundings, without any compensatory methods to cope with these problems. Here *technology* would be exactly the factor that creates a more mediated and complex equilibrium, which I shall call *alienation* from nature.

Lack of technology makes one's causal responsibility for the environment rather direct. In other words, the feedback loop between one's actions and their effects on the agent's own welfare is relatively short and isolated. Overhunting causes hunger very soon. One must pay the price for destruction and misuse immediately. Modern societies pay through some delayed costs—like those pollution problems and increase in cancer rates which result from corrective efforts, substitute measures and their side-effects. This is characterized by an almost complete environmental alienation. We can control natural processes but ultimately we always pay.

The equilibria may suffer from *social* impacts which are superimposed on natural factors: given a non-alienated original population, imagine some politically and technologically more advanced groups entering their territory. The first group's equilibrium state should be able to incorporate yet another disturbing causal factor which is now of a new, social kind. Thus the original simple equilibrium is either destroyed by the newcomers or, what is equally likely, it is incorporated into the technological complex of control and environmental alienation.

In this way, the original population will form one additional factor within the more advanced, complex system and create an additional problem of control and management. Modern socio-technological systems will contain cells which the original populations occupy, presupposing that they can survive the initial shock of the impact. How do these systemic controls work?

We earlier assumed that the newcomers possess sophisticated political and technological systems. They are then independent of any natural equilibria and also capable of enforcing the relevant moral relations, including contracts and property rights. Such newcomers are able to extend their concept of private property everywhere: individuals consider the environment vacant, appropriate it and mix their labour with land, air and sea. Everything is turned into property and private property rights are ascertained as both morally and legally binding.

Such an argument refers to the balance of power as the necessary but never sufficient condition of the mutual acceptability of a distributive pattern. Justice is needed, too. (Between two original populations the balance of power was both necessary and sufficient.) Private property rights extend over those possible changes which affect resource advantage and power. Property is a stable moral relationship, based on a set of norms of justice.

The original population contrasts its environmental rights against the demands of the technologically and socially more sophisticated newcomers. Magic, tradition, and force are opposed to the moral claims of the newcomers. The latter may therefore feel justified in using violence against the original population whose social and economic system does not embody the moral application of the relevant conceptual categories. The original population appears ultimately defenceless against the newcomers. Its weak rights will disappear. The newcomers are not committed to respect its weak rights. Moral arguments are one-sided.

4 Duties towards Nature

Original populations have been seen as lacking in regard to their social relations, such as participation in democratic and competitive political and economic processes which form the basis of property rights. It can be argued, however, that the same reason which explains their failure to establish property rights is sufficient to establish their *strong* environmental rights, or moral claims against newcomers. Perhaps there is a way to defend the original population against the kind of rather traditional view I have sketched above.

Suppose one cannot participate fully in the complex social life of the non-original population. Now the same argument that grounds this claim may also justify the further claim to strong environmental rights without going all the way to the concepts of property and ownership. To make sense of this suggestion, I shall try to show that the more advanced newcomers have *duties* towards nature and hence towards the original populations, who can therefore refer to these duties in order to validate their corresponding claim rights.

The basic presupposition must now be, obviously, that the equilibria of the natural environment are intrinsically valuable so that they should be allowed to subsist and flourish, in the sense that it is one's duty to refrain from exploitation and interference. Such a duty would entail the corresponding rights of the original population.

In other words, I call a *strong* environmental right of a weaker party such a normative position (claim right) as follows from the corresponding duty towards the environment and which binds the stronger and more advanced party. One can present a *valid claim against* the more advanced party because that party is committed to the care and preservation of the environment.

This is exactly what many radical environmentalists are saying: Nature is a teleological process, a principle of intrinsic value and Technological Man has duties towards Nature. This is indeed radical, but the fact that it is a surprising way of thinking does not make it automatically false. Modern science has necessitated only one way of approaching nature; perhaps it is time to consider another side of the matter: Nature is not only a collection of hard facts but is in itself an intrinsic value. And it seems that the normative property of the environment allows for degrees. One may reject the exploitative attitude towards Nature, adopt either a moderately protective position or a full-blown environmentalist one and maintain that Nature is valuable as such, non-instrumentally and independently of man and man's needs and welfare.

Something like this has been recently argued by Hans Jonas in his book *The Imperative of Responsibility*:

> Now, this we can say with certainty of a 'subjectivity' of nature, that it is neither particular nor arbitrary, and that over against our private desirings and opinings it has all the advantages of the whole over the parts, of the abiding over the fleeting, of the majestic over the puny . . .
> I can *legitimately* dissent from nature only if I can appeal to a tribunal outside it—that is, to a transcendence which I believe to possess the authority I deny to the former [3].

Perhaps this ethical project makes sense. However that may be, such arguments are becoming more and more popular alternatives and some philosophers place weight on them.

My suggestion is as follows: the bipartite division of right-elements into liberties and property rights above is too simple. We should admit that the original position is, as such, value-laden. The original population has its strong environmental rights simply because it is part of the environmental equilibrium and its constitutive force, Nature, is seen to be intrinsically valuable. If one is committed to protect natural equilibria and their intrinsic value, one cannot exclude the original population from the sphere of duties (on restrictions to this thesis, see below). The stronger the intrinsic value of Nature and the duties thus generated, the stronger are the rights of the original population.

Such rights need not be political. Neither need they rest on any extreme eco-philosophical theses. All my argument needs is the proposition that the natural equilibrium has some intrinsic value. Such a *minimal* point is hard to deny. Moreover, environmental duties follow from one's commitment to the protection of Nature. This fact characterizes the modern ecological attitude.

Now, here is a basic thesis: the original population has no political rights, and just this fact gives its members—paradoxically—strong environmental rights. The idea is that the only possible reason why one may not have political rights and, consequently, cannot present a claim to one's environment as property, is that one's social status is based on one's original position; and this entails strong environmental rights.

As a cynical counter-measure, one might suggest that when general environmental considerations become more sensitive issues in modern society, one should provide political opportunities for the original population. This would eliminate an aspect of one's duties towards the original population and, hence, their disturbing strong environmental rights. Is this feasible? The case looks like a trap: as I shall argue, one cannot have both strong environmental rights and political rights at the same time.

5 Political vs. Strong Rights

We may well be tempted to say—graciously and benevolently—that the rights of the original populations are strong environmental rights. But when the natural environment becomes too profitable to leave unexploited, the rights of those people may be reduced into mere *prima facie* political ones. The people are shifted into a new social position.

The dominant view deteriorates all too easily towards some kind of social *paternalism* where the original population is seen as divorced both from its own environmental equilibrium and our political processes. However, as a compensation they are offered physical safety, economic security, medical care, free education, entertainment and a limited access to the natural environment. All these are outside their own control but considered desirable by those who have full political rights. Such openly paternalistic suggestions are certainly dubious.

The following is an illustration of the political processes: American Indians did not get their US-citizenship before 1924, after a fair number of them had participated in the Great War. Before this conflicts between the Indians and the newcomer immigrants were handled by treaties and, after 1871, by 'agreements'. Territorial ownership problems antedate the reception of political rights by a wide margin indeed.

My basic question is: what happens when an original population gradually loses its environmental position and becomes more and more dependent on politics and technology? Modern weapons, agricultural tools, fertilizers, new breeds of animals and new production techniques change their situation, bringing them closer to the life of the non-original population. Can these developments take place in such a way that some environmental rights will stay intact? Shall such rights survive regardless of the (partial) alienation from the 'natural' environmental equilibrium?

One can claim that the strong environmental rights of an original population will stay intact only on condition that its members both (i) *need the exploited natural resources for their survival or basic welfare* and (ii) *they had no chance to acquire modern technology to help them to reduce and eliminate damage*. The point is both simple and familiar: if the original population destroys an aspect of the environment which should be preserved even against their will, their demands can be refuted, for example by referring to the possibility of replacing the protected item by means of a harmless method—should they accept its use. There are many examples. This is a fictional one: a ritual use of rare local eagle feathers can be replaced by imported substitutes.

A crucially important methodological fact can be seen here: I have not given any argument to support the view that politics and technology are closely connected social facts. This can be corrected now. If the proposition (ii) above is false so that the original population *had a chance to acquire technology*, such a fact automatically follows from their participation in political processes. Political power makes techno-logy (in principle) available to its wielder. The political man can acquire technology. And technology entails politics because one cannot understand and apply technology without money, training, legal responsibility, and power. When one buys a gun one needs a license, and one must learn how to handle and maintain the weapon. Modern technology cannot be mastered without the proper 'attitude'.

The original population need not accept the consequences of such an argument from the 'equivalence of politics and technology'. Its members may well claim that even if they had more sophisticated alternatives but chose freely to live their traditional life their rights would still stay valid. They may maintain that their cultural values or even their social identities are at stake. Such is the fundamental conflict.

It seems that there is no answer to be given in any absolutist terms. We need a *comparative approach*, in the way I shall sketch now. Full political rights imply a zero degree of the strong environmental rights, because then the alienation is complete. The traditional way of life is only an expensive hobby. Right-grounding duties do not apply to such alienated life-styles, even if they still apply to Nature and natural equilibria. Technical education is presupposed by one's political existence, and under these conditions one cannot claim any special environmental status along with its privileges. One's environmental equilibrium is mediated through the use of technology so that one always has alternative approaches to the solution of one's practical problems. One can always find a different route to one's goals and, therefore, need not harm the surroundings.

A complete *lack* of political rights entails full, strong environmental rights. One's simple equilibrium state dominates one's life and choices so that disturbances tend to be harmful. One has only one road to follow and this should be respected. Non-interference is a duty. However, after contact with modern legal and social systems, such a 'pure' social status is definitely fictional.

Between the two extremes we can locate an inverse proportion of the strength of these two types of rights: when (say) political influence increases, strong environmen-tal rights decrease correspondingly; and vice versa. The main question involves the correct moral attitude towards such an inverse rule. Empirically it seems to have some plausibility. Moreover, if it is in normal historical circumstances the only open possibility, we can hardly condemn its advocates.

6 The Scope of Contracts

Environmental alienation creates the further problem of the re-establishment of rights: is it possible to make a *contract* between the different parties to the effect that the environmental rights of the original population would again become valid? With this question we return to the themes of paternalism. An explicit contract may look desirable because full cultural integration into the newcomers' society seems unlikely or painful.

I have argued that environmental rights are either *liberties* or *strong* rights but the contract would allow for political rights only. The contract could not re-establish the lost original position which is exactly what is desired. Alienation is beyond contract because contracts seem to presuppose a political viewpoint towards the environment; therefore, the system that follows from contracts demands *political* participation.

However, if we apply the comparative approach here, we can say that the more alienated a group is, the more it can utilize contracts with the dominant groups. All contracts have some bite and can help the original populations support their claims over their lives and environment. Still in case of a conflict of interests where one party has less political weight on its side, no contract avoids the danger of bias. The comparative approach explains the fact that contracts can be made and they are useful, but it cannot avert the accusation that these contracts are always made between unequal parties and from unfair bargaining positions. If the parties are politically equal, the original population can no longer be called 'original' and no contract is needed.

Certainly it is disturbing that the new ecological consciousness which emphasizes the detrimental effects of technology should be unable to understand and handle conceptually the problem of the contracts. Original populations are virtually trapped if they cannot get full political rights without losing their cultural identity. It seems to me that the original populations do not have a choice: even at the risk of environmental alienation they must insist on their political status and power. Such a second best alternative is the only way, especially after technology has made their traditional lifestyle almost impossible. The basic rule is, however: the better the contract, the stronger the alienation.

The new technology has already changed the world and destroyed the original natural equilibria. Yet the original population is not fully equal with the newcomers in terms of political rights, actual scientific knowledge and technological know-how. This is the tragic dilemma to which the original population tries to find a solution by returning to their alleged strong environmental rights which are denied by the new environmentalists and politicians alike.

It is difficult to see what the moral judgment should be: the newcomers did not violate the weak rights of the original population when they entered their territories; they were simply able to do so. Imperialism cannot be condemned in this way. No property rights obtain and the strong rights become basically void because of alienation. Of course we may say that Europeans should have left the original populations alone a long time ago for reasons which do not include a direct reference to rights, but to the environmental duties of the newcomers.

If this move is valid, it entails *guilt*. The only thing left to do is, perhaps, to provide some utilitarian compensation, educate the people so that they can understand the new lifestyle and, finally, make a serious attempt to respect the remains of the culture, as well as the demands and desires of the members of the original populations. The original populations should find the correct balance between their political rights and the environmental equilibrium. The more advanced social system should also be economically and politically *open* to everybody.

But there is still another complication: for instance, in the case of nomadic Lapps' demand to get rid of the local bears and wolverines, the dominant Finns have lived in the same territory as long as the Lapps and they are willing to tolerate the beasts. In the same way, to speak about the original population is often quite metaphorical and hides a relationship based not on the party being a newcomer but being simply more dominant within the limits of their shared territory.

According to such a view, the real problem is cultural dominance and political power in dealing with partisan issues. This makes it extremely difficult to see how one could reach a consensus concerning compensations to those whose life-style has become impossible because of the changed environment and the new technology.

If social dominance is the *problem*, the return to full equality cannot be the key method of reaching towards the better world; equality means and actually *is* the same as the better world itself. Equality is not a means. It is the goal.

7 An Illustration: limits of property

In Finland all citizens have their so-called 'everyman's rights' in relation to the use of certain environmental privileges. The point is that if someone owns a forest, everyone may use this forest under the condition that no harm is done to the property. One may not cut timber, kill moose or fowl, or go fishing; but one can freely hike and camp there, pick berries and mushrooms—even sell them. These everyman's rights can be interpreted as limiting cases of the environmental contract in the sense used above.

One cannot assume that all aspects of the natural environment belong to the sphere of private property. There are, therefore, certain assets which are necessarily excluded from the contract, which cannot be owned, and which embody the original environmental liberties. From the Finnish point of view, strict trespassing regulations are a consequence of too extensive applications of power outside the sphere of property rights, simply because certain aspects of the environment cannot be owned, or at least their ownership is such a fleeting affair that it need not be respected. Why can't I walk through your wood and pick mushrooms which will be rotten tomorrow? The answer to the effect that all is yours is not at all convincing within the environmental context.

I cannot deal with the real meaning of this legal phenomenon here. Let me add one feature: everyone is supposed to know the limits of such basic environmental rights; for example, one does not approach anyone's house or yard so closely that one can be identified. Then one would be violating the occupant's right to privacy, and that must always be respected. Everyman's right is limited by the right to privacy, which is an important consideration in traditional Finnish social life.

Timo Airaksinen, Department of Philosophy, University of Helsinki, Unionink. 40B, 17, Helsinki, Finland.

NOTES

My thanks are due to Dr Gerald Doherty (University of Turku) and Ms Maija-Riitta Ollila (Academy of Finland). This paper is my contribution to the Annual Conference of the Society for Applied Philosophy: *The Environment*, May 1986, Sussex, United Kingdom.
[1] LEE GUTKIND (1984) *The People of Penn's Woods West*, p. 116 (Pittsburgh, University of Pittsburgh Press).
[2] GERHARD LENSKI (1966) *Power and Privilege: a theory of social stratification*, pp. 134 and 166 (New York, McGraw-Hill).
[3] HANS JONAS (1984) *The Imperative of Responsibility: in search of an ethics for the technological age*, pp. 85–86 (Chicago, University of Chicago Press).

4

Are there Intrinsic Values in Nature?

T. L. S. SPRIGGE

ABSTRACT   *Some think we should look at aspects of what is commonly thought of as non-sentient nature as having a value in themselves apart from the use or recreation they provide for humans or even animals. But to what extent does nature, in the character it presents to us, exist apart from presence to consciousness such as ours? Surely at least many of its aspects cannot. However, that does not stop them having a genuinely intrinsic value, just as works of art do, whose existence also is impossible apart from their display to a consciousness such as ours. But can nature, as it exists quite apart from human or animal consciousness, have any intrinsic value? It is suggested that only a panpsychic, and perhaps pantheist, view of nature (a view for which there are excellent metaphysical grounds) can give a positive answer, and even that must be a very vague one [1].*

There are three main sorts of position on questions as to man's obligations towards the non-human. There is the view that ultimately all that should matter to man is human welfare, and that right and wrong in the treatment of the non-human turn ultimately on how this affects human welfare. Let us call this human welfarism. Then there is the view that ultimately all that matters is the welfare of beings commonly recognised as being sentient, namely animals, so that man has direct duties towards animals but no non-derivative duties to anything else. Let us call this human and animal welfarism. Thirdly, there is the view that not only what happens to humans and animals but also what happens to various realities, not commonly thought sentient, matters of itself, and that man's duties include those of direct concern with the flourishing or survival of such things because they matter in themselves and not merely for their effects on men and animals. For the lack of a better word I shall call this universalism.

Human welfarism has its proponents still. To me it seems utterly irrational. The joys and sufferings of animals are quite sufficiently the same sort of thing as ours for it to be irrational not to see them as bearing on the rightness and wrongness of actions in the same way as those of fellow human beings do. There are, indeed, specious arguments which would deny that animals really have a conscious mental life in the sense in which we do. However, both common sense and an intelligent metaphysics unite in ridiculing the idea that a dog cannot feel bored or feel pain or enjoy a run in a way quite comparable to the human. There seems no doubt therefore that human welfarism should give way to one of the other two views. That still leaves the question whether human and animal welfarism is an adequate ethic, or whether it should give way to some form of universalism.

What is known as a deep ecological ethic, as opposed to a shallow one, seems to be some form of universalism. But what form? One form of universalism is the doctrine that absolutely everything is of intrinsic value and even of equal intrinsic value [2]. The only difference lies in the ease with which creatures like ourselves can see the value of a thing. Such a universalism would be of little use to those in search of an environmental ethic since there would be equal value whatever one did, unless it was possible to reduce the amount of sheer being in the world, which presumably it is not. The idea of a deep ecological ethic seems to be rather that there can be intrinsic value, and presumably disvalue, to states of, or objects in, the natural world which cannot be cashed in terms of any valuable states of human or animal consciousness which they either include, produce or in any way help to constitute. Thus the existence of an eco-system of a suitably rich kind can have a value which we should seek to sustain, or at least refrain from upsetting, quite apart from any practical or recreational use it has for any human or animal.

This kind of universalism seems perverse to many sensible people. There is something highly compulsive in the view that patterns and processes which are not themselves conscious can only matter in so far as they affect some form of conscious life. Yet, on the other hand, part of the appeal of many apparently non-sentient parts of nature seems to lie in the way in which they take us out of ourselves and show us how we belong to a vast scheme transcending the interests of man, and in this mood we are inclined to feel that there is some kind of value in the world beyond the human and the animal.

One way of bringing out the problematic nature of universalism is to think about the universe before there was any consciousness in it, which many will think means, in practice, before there was any life. Let us assume for argument's sake that once there was no life on any planet but that stars and solar systems were being formed and that atoms danced their dances. To the cosmologist who reconstructs those events in thought they are vastly exciting, but the question is whether any of it mattered while it was going on, so that the different processes would have been of various different degrees of value even if no one had ever been going to know about them. Most people think it faintly absurd to think in these terms.

Now if there could be no value, no way in which one state of affairs could be better than another, before consciousness came on the scene, how can one state of affairs be better than another now except in so far as it affects consciousness? Yet the universalist, and in particular the deep ecologist, does think that the variety of different plant species (especially when considered as parts of a rich eco-system) is something which matters for its own sake independently of its relation to any human or animal consciousness.

Deep ecologists might say that the valuelessness of the universe before consciousness came on the scene was due, not to the lack of consciousness, but to the lack of life, and hence of anything which can flourish or otherwise. Value, it may be claimed, pertains only to life, both to individual living things and to biotic communities of inter-dependent living things. Or if value pertains to things which are (at least as usually conceived) neither alive nor exactly communities of living things, it is only when these are things of which, when they are in a condition which can be suitably described as flourishing, various forms of life are an essential constituent, such as a lake or the whole earth or the so-called biosphere. But if we think of living things which are supposed not to be conscious it is not too easy to see why they can have value and different degrees of value and yet there be no value or degree of value where there is not life. I am not convinced that, in the absence of life, there can be no ground for talking of things as flourishing. My very vague idea of what modern physicists say about atoms and sub-atomic particles suggests that what is going on at that level of nature might possibly be described in such terms. It is at least doubtful how far one who could take in every detail of what was going on in nature and on every scale, would find a break of any absolute significance between life and not life [3].

There are two sorts of reply a deep ecologist might give to these challenges. He might allow that there can be differentiations of value in the absence of life. What matters, he might say, is the existence of a certain kind of variety in unity and this can vary in degree even in the absence of life. Nevertheless, by far, the greatest such values and those about which humans know most, and which they can most affect, are those which involve life and it is sufficient for the present if man can extend his concern to the safeguarding and perhaps promoting of these values. The second possible reply would be to the effect that there is something quite special about life which means that it can be the locus of value. But what can this be? If the deep ecologist could embrace some kind of vitalist biology he would have an easy answer available, say that living systems have a self-developing and self-maintaining entelechy or power not found in the merely physical, and that this has a unique claim to respect. Unless some such vitalism can be revived I am not at all clear how this second reply could be supported. However, the point I wish to emphasise above all is that this reply needs support on the basis of some metaphysico-biological thesis about the special nature of life.

Upon the whole, it seems that the deep ecologist who wishes to claim that there is value, and degrees of value, in life which cannot be cashed in terms of the value pertaining to the states of consciousness of sentient individuals must think that there are better and worse states of affairs of the physical world at large, whether life is present or not. This, then, is the view with which I want to engage.

Adequately to decide on the wisdom of such a view one needs to do two things. First, one needs to have a defensible view as to what value is, and what marks its presence, and secondly one needs to have a defensible view as to the nature of the realities whose value is at issue. If, for example, somewhat after the fashion of Kant, you believe that nothing can be good or bad except an individual *will* then you must both have a view as to what a will is and a view as to what goodness and badness are and what marks their presence.

Let us consider first how the deep ecologist might deal with the question as to the nature of the things to which he ascribes value. He has two tasks. First, he has got to persuade doubters that there can be value there at all. Secondly, he has got to say something as to what determines the degree of value. In answering the second question there may be talk of the value of certain sorts of whole in which there is the maximal variety of individuals with a power of self development and self preservation existing in mutual interdependence and symbiosis. But it may also be said that finally there just is a certain value to certain things such as may reveal itself to the sensitive observer but which cannot be detected on the basis of a formula. Thus Tom Regan has spoken of the intrinsic value of certain stretches of the Colorado river in which it is wild and free [4].

Such answers may be of some use, so far as they go, but in the end I suggest that the whole matter is left in the deepest obscurity unless a point of view is taken on two deep metaphysical questions. The first concerns the extent to which natural objects exist independently of us in the character they wear for us. The second concerns the extent to which various wholes have a genuine individual existence not derivative from a synthesising observing mind [5].

When Tom Regan thinks of a wild rushing river as of something intrinsically valuable, does he think that anything very like what he sees, hears and perhaps feels, exists independently of his seeing it? Personally, I find few things more soothing than to walk along the sides of a river with overhanging trees, bubbling over stones and rocks, down which a variety of branches and driftwood float. Concerning that whole scene which is revealed to my sight and hearing, and which carries suggestions, which may or may not be realised, of the wetness of the water which I would feel if I put myself into it, I ask whether it exists except as a vista, or felt environment, for a human being. Doubtless something which God might recognise as essentially another version of the same exists for the birds who skim around it, and more remotely even for the fish who swim within it. But physics and chemistry describe the water as H_2O in a manner which quite moleculises or atomises the water into discrete or at least wavy ingredients in a manner which seems quite incompatible with the special wateriness of water as element in our experience. How much, when it is envisaged in terms of a basic scientific account, is left of that which seems to make such a river something of intrinsic value? If little or nothing, then the ascription of a value of any type with which we are familiar to it must turn on the belief that there is more to it, as it is in itself, than physics and chemistry can say, and that is a strong metaphysical claim. If it is replied that science does not tell us how to envisage things I answer briefly that that is a mere 'cop out' from a problem which has to be faced [6].

But perhaps the value of a beautiful peaceful riverside will seem rather obviously a human value, and not an example of the aspects of nature which the deep ecologist proclaims as possessing an intrinsic value independent of its effects on the consciousness of creatures like ourselves. Yet is the situation really so different when we think of the value of some complex eco-system? In some sense that whole system exists undoubtedly, but if the ecologist really tries to give himself some kind of intuitive sense of the whole system he must either imagine it in some kind of sensory way, or he must form the conception of some abstract structure which it exemplifies as a whole. What he strictly imagines seems as much a merely human vision as the river, while if he only thinks in terms of an abstract structure, he must acknowledge that this is but the bare bones of what is really there. He then has, or should have, the problem of what concretely fills out the structure. If he thinks of it as including a particular kind of tree with a particular kind of leaf, does the colour of one of those leaves, or even its shape, as that presents itself to sight or tactile feeling, really exist except as registered in some sensory mode and synthesised by a unifying mind? Well, I could go on for ever putting these questions, but let me try to move on a bit.

There are a number of different views as to the way in which our perceptual and conceptual experience of the physical world relates to that world. For *phenomenalism* the physical world just is actual and possible sensations on the part of minds like ours; for *naive realism* the physical world has the variously perceived and felt dynamic energy, the crashing and bashing, and the qualities and forms (colour, over all shape, noisiness of various sorts, bristliness and fragrance) which occur in our experience, and these somehow exist alongside the fine-grain properties and abstract mathematically conceived structure, movement and force of which science speaks; for *scientific realism* not the manifest image but the scientific image is the truth of the matter; for *theistic idealism* the physical world is the content of a divine experience in aspects of which we can participate, and so forth. Doubtless these are not the only alternatives, but what I wish to insist on is that there can be no sensible opinion about the existence of values in nature which does not take up either one of these positions or an alternative which does not duck the problems to which they are alternative solutions.

Since I can hardly argue the case here, I shall give a brief sketch of my own views about these matters, and indicate how they might bear upon the question of values in nature. First, however, a word about what it is for something to possess value.

Some think that there is a human activity which we can call valuing, but that values are not actual properties which things can possess. Such thinkers often point out, quite correctly, that there is nothing against a deep ecological approach in this opinion. We human valuers may well value non-human things for their own non-human being and not for their effects on us or other sentient beings. However, I do personally think that value and disvalue are real properties which certain things possess. The most obvious species of intrinsic goodness are the various forms of joyfulness. The joyfulness of an experience is a real property of it, but it is a property with an inherently magnetic force, so that one cannot imagine it without finding that it motivates action which promotes it. Joyfulness or pleasure bridges the usual fact/value gap because it is a fact with necessary effects upon the will. Now I do not say that pleasure is the only form of intrinsic goodness, but I do say that whenever one values something one thinks of it as having a property which bridges the fact/value gap in the same kind of way in which pleasure does. Now it seems to me that no property could do this except one which could only exist within a consciousness. Thus in my opinion there cannot be intrinsic value where there is nothing at all akin to pleasure and pain, joy and suffering. This may seem to make me necessarily an opponent of a deep ecological approach.

However, it does not make me an opponent. This is because in the end I believe that none of us can really conceive of a world divested of consciousness. Whenever we seriously try to bring into clear consciousness the nature of any situation in the existence of which we believe, we imagine it either as a form or a content of some consciousness, actual or possible. I can imagine your grief as a form of consciousness, and I can imagine your garden as an object of consciousness. If I try to think about what some complex eco-system really is I must do so either by envisaging it as presented to some consciousness which can take it in as a whole or as somehow composed of all sorts of interacting streams of experience which form the inner being of the natural objects involved.

I cannot take seriously the notion that the vast panoply of nature only exists as an object for human consciousness, or is only a system of actual and possible sensations on our part. On the other hand I cannot make sense of the idea of its existing in some unexperienced manner. That leaves Berkeleyan idealism as one possibility, but—to put the matter briefly—that makes nature rather too much of a divine con trick to seem plausible. That leaves me with a panpsychic view of nature. According to this the inner 'noumenal' essence of all physical processes consists in streams of interacting feeling. Our own experiences are streams of high level feeling which emerge out of the low level streams of experience which are the inner essence of the enduring existence of the neurons in our brain and these emerge from the lower level streams of experience which form the inner essence of atoms and so forth. Thus the nature, which existed before life, consisted of streams of experience of comparatively low level. In so far as this experience waxed and waned in its own felt satisfactoriness there was a variation of the value there.

This panpsychic view, which represents more or less the position of Whitehead and Hartshorne, makes feeling the inner essence of the ultimate constituents of nature. But is there a higher level feeling pertaining to wholes made up of certain systems of these ultimate constituents? There are two cases where it certainly does. First, in the brains of animals the feelings of the neurons—in virtue of the teleological system they are so wired together as to constitute—somehow give rise to the over all consciousness of the animal. Secondly, in my opinion, there is an over-all experience which the universe itself enjoys as a single individual. Unless there was, there would be no way in which there was any real wholeness to the universe at all. It (so far as one could then talk of an 'it' at all) would have consisted of disconnected monads such as Leibniz would have postulated if he had not given God a unifying role incompatible with his basic conception of relations. Things can only relate to each other through making up a *whole* together and the only *whole* which feelings can form together is that of an overarching feeling. So the things in the universe can only relate as aspects of one overarching experience.

But are there any wholes (short of the one universal whole) which have feelings and can thus be the loci of intrinsic value other than animals? Another way of putting it, from my point of view, is this. Does the one universal consciousness which nature possesses as a whole articulate itself into any other subsidiary wholes, not simply wholes for an external observer, besides those which constitute either the inner being of the ultimate constituents of matter or the individual consciousness of men and animals? I shall not give my tentative answer to that question now, but only indicate that it is important for the question of the existence of the kinds of value in nature which deep ecologists seem to cherish. However, there is another way in which a whole might have value. Consider the wholes we call nations. One does not have to believe in a kind of over soul to a nation in order to make sense of there being such a thing as a kind of national consciousness. In so far as the conscious lives of the citizens are permeated by particular modes of thinking and feeling which turn on their being so related as to form a nation, the value of that aspect of their conscious lives is, in a sense, a value of the whole rather than of the individuals. So the flourishing of an eco-system might be regarded as a good of the whole in so far as it was realised in the distinctive forms of conscious flourishings within it of individuals who could only exist in such a system.

Now I realise that my metaphysical point of view will seem fanciful to many, especially if they have no real idea of the considerations which lead such thinkers as Josiah Royce, Gustav Fechner, Whitehead and myself to adopt it, or of our answers to the more childish objections to it. To me this kind of view gives the only possible answer to a whole gamut of metaphysical questions, including that traditionally called the problem of mind and matter. But even if people have what they think some better alternative answer to these questions, I do not see what other metaphysical point of view can make much sense of the notion of values inherent in nature. If this view does not make sense of it, I think it is without sense. Thus, if one has some intuitive sense that there is some value there in nature, this may be another pointer to the truth of panpsychism.

But there is an immense qualification to be made to all this. The panpsychic view of things is a view about the inner noumenal essence of nature. But nature also exists as a phenomenon for the human mind and as such it has a value. Beethoven's string quartets, as aesthetic objects, only exist for a human mind, but their value is not that of your conscious states or mine or even Beethoven's. Rather, one thing that gives value to a conscious state is that such an aesthetic object can exist within it. Now in the same way natural phenomena can exist as objects for a human mind, and the value they have as such is neither the value which pertains to their inner essence, nor simply a matter of the value of personal conscious states. They have a value as objects of consciousness and one can want to preserve them not as a means to certain conscious states but as something of value in itself which, all the same, cannot exist except as a conscious state.

The value of a beautiful city is a good example here, because it is easier (I should expect) to agree on the essential matters than in the case of nature. I would think it a tragedy if the New Town in Edinburgh was destroyed. That which I regard as valuable here cannot be thought of as existing without its value if no one with an appropriate cultural background was there to perceive it. On the other hand, it is not mere psychological states of those who wander round Edinburgh which have value. The value pertains to a common object which can exist for their consciousness. The mere physical stones, as science might describe them, have surely no special degree of value. What would be there without human consciousness would have no particular value; yet it is not exactly the value of states of consciousness which is in question.

I think it somewhat like that in the case of nature considered as a panorama. That panorama cannot exist as a panorama unless there are appropriate humans to take the panorama in. Still, granted that the panorama needs us if it is to be wholly actual, it still has its own value.

However, aspects of nature which have special value as a panorama may also be parts of nature which have some more or less special hidden value in terms of the inner psychic life of nature which is going on there. This may be partly the relatively transparent life of animals, or it may be something more mysterious belonging to certain stretches of land, sea and air. Moreover, even if there is nothing very special to the noumenal psychic essence of what is going on in certain places, they may be of especial value in promoting a human sense of the larger inner psychic life of the universe. The vista and the feel of stretches of solitary countryside, or the sea dashing itself wildly on rocks, give us a sense of oneness with nature, which, on my view, is not an illusion. Philosophers talk of man's responsibility for nature, but a deeper truth is that of nature's responsibility for man. We are elements in a larger whole, which has its own inner psychic life, and some aspects of that whole bring us back to that sense of belonging to the whole, and stemming from it, which too artificial an environment cuts us off from, thus stultifying the deeper levels of our being.

In spite of what I have been saying, I should like to emphasise the obvious fact that we do not have all to agree on one metaphysical, religious or ethical scheme in order to find intermediate goals around which many rational persons can rally. A neglected masterpiece on the dangers of thinking that one must agree on ultimate goals and values in order to resolve ethical issues rationally is the chapter on 'Intrinsic and extrinsic value' in C. L. Stevenson's *Ethics and Language*. All the same, one must sometimes try to think out things on the basis of fundamentals, and I do not think a deep ecological ethic can avoid encountering the metaphysical issues I have briefly aired, and asking itself questions of a kind which still embarrass academic philosophers. As such, even answers to the most abstruse questions of metaphysics are relevant to a philosophy which would be applied.

T. L. S. Sprigge, Department of Philosophy, University of Edinburgh, David Hume Tower, George Square, Edinburgh EH8 9JY, Scotland.

NOTES

[1] This was read as a paper at the conference of the Society for Applied Philosophy on environmental ethics held in May 1986.
[2] Thus it has been contended that to have a 'valid ethic of nature' we must affirm 'the equal value of

every item in creation' (see *Ethics and the Environment*, Eds DONALD SCHERER & THOMAS ATTIG, New Jersey, Prentice Hall Inc., 1983, at p. 15. where W. H. Murdy is quoting C. Birch. This collection is a very useful one for a general conspectus of current views).

[3] This is not to doubt the especial significance which life, at large, must always have for us as urged, for example, by EDWARD O. WILSON in his *Biophilia*, (Cambridge, Mass., Harvard, 1984).

[4] See *All that Dwell Therein* by Tom Regan, California, University of California Press, 1982 p. 200. Compare also this description of the perhaps more persuasive views of ALDO LEOPOLD by J. BAIRD CALDICOTT, in his important article comparing animal liberationism and environmental ethical views, 'Animal liberation: a triangular affair' in the Attig & Scherer volume cited above at p. 56. "Yet there is no doubt that Leopold sincerely proposes that land (in his inclusive sense) be ethically regarded. The beech and chestnut, for example, have in his view as much 'biotic right' to life as the wolf and the deer, and the effects of human action on mountains and streams for Leopold is an ethical concern as genuine and serious as the comfort and longevity of brood hens."

[5] For a very interesting and still relevant discussion of this see *A Pluralistic Universe* by WILLIAM JAMES (N.Y., Longmans Green) p. 186 et ff.

[6] For a more technical development of these points see my *The Vindication of Absolute Idealism* (Edinburgh, Edinburgh University Press, 1983). See also 'Non-human rights; an idealist perspective' in *Inquiry*, 1984, Vol. 27, pp. 439–461.

5

A Critique of Deep Ecology

WILLIAM GREY

ABSTRACT   *Our environmental crisis is commonly explained as a product of a set of attitudes and beliefs about the world which have been developed by post-Cartesian technological society. Deep ecologists claim that the crisis can only be overcome by adopting an alternative non-technological paradigm, such as can be discovered in non-Western cultures. In this paper I (a) express misgivings about the use of the expression 'paradigm' by deep ecologists, (b) question the claim that a science-based world-view inevitably fosters manipulative and exploitative attitudes to the natural world, (c) suggest that non-technological cultures do not necessarily provide exemplary and superior models for relating to the natural world, and (d) defend a scientific naturalism as a satisfying way of realising our unity with the natural world.*

A popular story which recurs in the annals of environmental philosophy runs something as follows. The development of science and technology over the past few hundred years, and especially in the past few decades, has been responsible for producing the modern industrial state. This comparatively recent mode of social organisation has generated seriously skewed life-styles which are too violent, too stultifying, too alienating, and which are, except in the very short term, unsustainable. In order to correct the potentially catastrophic, pathological, social habits of humanity, it is not enough to modify our technological and industrial practices: these are merely symptoms of a seriously deficient set of attitudes and beliefs which stand in need of drastic modification.

In particular, the evils of the modern industrial state are produced by a particular set of *anthropocentric* attitudes and beliefs, which can be uncovered by examining the deep psychology of technological society. An examination of the deep psychology of present Western society reveals a constellation of attitudes and values which we can call the 'technocratic' paradigm [1]; it is essential that this paradigm be replaced by an alternative which will enable human societies to develop sustainable modes of living in co-operative harmony with our human and non-human companions within the complex and integrated biosphere which we share. A satisfactory alternative constellation of beliefs and values which would permit a harmonious, non-alienating form of life involves the acceptance of an alternative paradigm—the 'person-planetary' paradigm [2]. The recognition of the need for a radically different paradigm is the distinguishing mark which separates shallow 'reformist' environmentalism from 'deep ecology'. Shallow environmentalism remains imprisoned by the dominant anthropocentric attitudes which are (or tend to be) mechanistic and reductionist, in comparison to the holistic, biocentric, non-reductionist conceptions which are advocated by deep ecology.

Two pre-eminent anti-heroes who have done much to foster the ascendency of the technocratic paradigm are Descartes and the Christian Church. Descartes' infamous contribution is the mechanistic conception of the non-human world, and its sharp separation from the world of mind (or spirit) which humans occupy, and which (on the Cartesian view) is the sole repository of intrinsic values. Christianity has reinforced a conception of humankind as the locus of moral concern, and as the rightful authority over the rest of nature. The attitudes which have emerged from the unholy alliance of Descartes and the Church are, to a large extent, responsible for the present-day ascendancy of the technocratic paradigm with all its destructive consequences.

Deep ecology emerges from the realisation of the inadequacies of this essentially anthropocentric conceit and suggests, by way of corrective, that natural systems and the non-human world are utterly different to the technocratic conception. Biological systems, and biological organisms are nothing like bits of clockwork, which can be completely understood by analytic dissection into physical component parts. They demand essentially holistic modes of conception: natural systems consist of intersecting fields of processes rather than separate individuals-with-properties.

In this paper I draw attention to some internal tensions in this picture, and question several of its features. I begin with a difficulty which arises from the expansive use of the expression 'paradigm'.

Kuhn's appropriation of this term to explain some features of the way scientific (in particular physical) theories develop produced sharp critical response [3]. This led Kuhn to refine his account so that the notion 'paradigm' could be put to useful analytic work [4]. Unfortunately many writers who have made free use of Kuhn's expression have not been so careful and scrupulous. Rodman for example uses the expression, not untypically, to indicate what he calls a "cultural paradigm", explicated as "the basic beliefs, values, political ideals, and institutional practices of a cultural epoch" [5].

Rodman's use of the expression 'paradigm' is too general to function as a useful analytic tool. We can speak of, say, the Newtonian or Darwinian paradigm because the theories associated with these eponymous names consist of a relatively unified and structured set of beliefs. However this is not the case with so-called 'cultural paradigms'. They are not thus unified and their elements are readily detachable [6].

The Kuhnian story is (or should be) well-known, and it is unfortunate that it needs to be raised once again in connection with the deep ecology literature. It is important in particular to resist the polarising manoeuvre which makes it appear that we must accept *either* the technocratic *or* the person-planetary constellation of beliefs and values. We should, I suggest, keep open the possibility of discriminating *within* each of these roughly delineated sets of beliefs and values, and consider alternative combinations of the standard components. The central claim of deep ecology [7], namely the rejection of anthropocentric systems of value, is in fact consistent with a range of positions. Instead of talking of *the* 'deep ecology' position we should speak rather of alternative deep ecologies. A major defect of paradigm-talk is that it makes deep ecology appear to be a single, well-defined, normative standpoint, rather than a class of related positions. In fact deep ecology involves a number of independent claims, not all of which can be uncritically accepted.

The first item in the standard deep ecology package which I will consider is the conception of dominant scientific attitudes as mechanistic, reductionist, and fostering manipulative attitudes and practices with respect to the natural world. Secondly, I will express some reservations about the popular call to return to the old wisdom of non-technological cultures, which are often supposed to provide a superior basis for our relating to the natural environment. Finally I will suggest, combining both these points, that a purely secular, scientific naturalism can provide a thoroughly satisfying way of realising our unity with the non-human world. Certainly religious, animist and pantheistic beliefs have been historically important in providing a basis for the wholly laudable business of recognising a commonality or community with the natural world; but it seems to me that there are to hand other belief-systems which can do much the same job, and—I will suggest—a good deal better.

I said above that there is an internal tension within some common articulations of the deep ecology paradigm. What I have in mind is a tendency to denigrate the systematic, piecemeal, empirical approach to a study of the natural world. Far from being shallow, such a science-based, analytical approach is not (or need not be) an objectionable and manipulative way of interacting with the natural world; it is on the contrary quite indispensable for the development of a satisfactory conception of its nature. An adequate understanding of the destructive predations of technological society, and the development of satisfactory, softer alternatives based on the use of renewable resources, can only be based upon systematic, scientific conceptions. It is all very well to say that we must tread lightly upon the earth, but this cannot be based upon a turning away from the methods of science and controlled experiments, for it is precisely to these we must turn to determine what is and what is not treading lightly. This analytical approach, 'counting commas' in the book of nature, as Needleman [8] has expressed it, is indispensable for the systematic understanding of complex systems. It does *not* preclude the equally indispensable treatment of complex systems as unitary wholes, which is necessary for experiencing and valuing nature, as well as for its proper understanding [9].

The second point which I want to make is that not all primitive resource-use is wise, and not all technology is destructive: what is and what is not environmentally acceptable can be determined only by developing insights into the effects of our actions (for act we must); it is hardly credible that these insights could be gained by the use of, say, intuitive empathy alone. The maintenance of equilibrium of dynamic living systems requires, *inter alia*, continuous inputs of energy and the recycling of essential nutrients. To understand how human interference with natural systems perverts both energy flow and the recycling of nutrients, we should not abandon our science-based conceptions but embrace them. Nature may indeed know best, but how, except through systematic empirical inquiry, can we determine what it is that nature tells us?

In practice much of the deep ecology critique of human predations is based precisely on the sorts of empirical studies which, in other passages and other moods, those same critics are prone to denigrate. This seems to me to be an unresolved tension which occurs in a number of articulations of deep ecology. Scientific understanding is not of course a sufficient condition for wisdom, but the insights of science are certainly necessary for acting wisely.

A major alleged vice of the technocratic world-view is its tendency to regard organisms and living systems as organised structures of material components. This is supposed to be a mechanistic picture of such systems, and reducing an organism to a mere aggregation of material parts is supposed to be tantamount to denying that such systems can be objects of value. Thus it has been suggested that materialist conceptions—the product of Descartes and his successors—have 'desacralised' the natural world, which thereby ceases to be a subject for respect and is transformed into an object for manipulation. We can counter this materialist thrust, it is suggested, by becoming 'future primitives', and by reinstating older and wiser systems of belief, found in non-Western cultures, for example, which can provide a basis for non-alienating and empathetic relationships with the natural world.

The ambition of fostering a harmonious relationship with the natural world is wholly admirable, and if a culture believes that the natural world is a repository of ancestral or totemic spirits, then the upshot of these beliefs is, thus far, to be applauded. But it seems to me that just as not all technology is pathologically destructive, so not all spiritual empathy with the non-human world is benign. We might characterise the Aztec belief that large-scale human sacrifice was essential for the maintenance of the diurnal cycle as a particularly vicious and pathological conviction: it is hard not to see faith in the diurnal cycle based upon physical theory as a distinct improvement. Life-wisdom is not the prerogative of primitive cultures any more than it is that of cultures of the modern variety. I am not suggesting that we have nothing of value to learn from other cultures and their beliefs; other cultures can certainly serve as an inspiration, and the development of a satisfactory critique of our own cultural vices can certainly be aided by comparison with alternatives. But we are certainly not obliged to accept such belief-systems *in toto*. Calvin Martin has persuasively argued that it is misguided sentimentality to suppose that we can simply transplant the values and beliefs from other cultures to our own [10]. His attitude contrasts with views expressed, for example, by Marshall Sahlins [11] and Paul Shepard [12], who suggest that these views provide an appealing alternative model to the industrial-technocratic life style which we are presently locked into. But these alternatives are not accessible to us—at least not in the short term [13]. And even accepting the desirability of emulating the ecologically sound practices of low-technology cultures does not entail taking on board every one of their beliefs about the natural world.

A final difficulty which I raise about the proposed 'resacralisation' of nature is that it seems to depend on the acceptance of one of the objectionable legacies of Descartes. The Cartesian conception of minds as the only items of intrinsic value, and material objects as of no moral consequence, has certainly led to an exceedingly objectionable set of anthropocentric values. However it seems to me that the urge to spiritualise nature is perhaps the result of an unconscious acceptance of the Cartesian view: if only spiritual substances have intrinsic value, then the spiritualising of nature is the route to reinstate non-anthropocentric values. A better approach, surely, is to reject the Cartesian presupposition and to (at least attempt to) develop a secular alternative to provide the basis for non-anthropocentric values. I will conclude with a few preliminary remarks about this project.

Modern physics, chemistry and biology, can, I think, provide us with a wholly satisfying basis for a sense of unity with the natural world. Living systems are temporary, stable, dynamic structures whose material components were forged inside stellar furnaces. Life is one of the many levels of organisation assumed by the world-stuff as it develops from its initial incomprehensible singularity through the primaeval fireball of the 'big bang', through the eras of hadrons, leptons, and plasma until it expanded and condensed into the stable nuclei which came to form the galaxies and stars. As the universe evolves—either to a slow heat death of empty, black, expanding space some 10^{100} years hence, when the whole cosmic machine will have run to a standstill and the second law of thermodynamics will have claimed its last victim, or to be remorselessly crushed into oblivion in a final, catastrophic, gravitational collapse —tiny and temporary islands of organised chemical complexity arise [14]. These poignant oases of complex chemistry are one of the most fascinating and beautiful modes of organisation of world-stuff as the universe winds down—or winds up. Our scientific eschatology tells us that in the long run (and we should not forget that it is a *very* long run) these, and indeed all, islands of complex organisation are doomed. What

Spinoza called the *conatus* of living systems—their striving to maintain their integrity—is bound, ultimately, to be frustrated. We are collectively, as we are individually, bound for extinction.

The nuclear, gravitational, and electromagnetic forces which we have now begun to comprehend, are responsible for the structural arrangements of the universe, including the rare and isolated pockets of chemical organisation which give rise to living systems. It may be, as Paul Davies has suggested, that "intelligence as a cosmic organisational activity may eventually be regarded as natural, and as fundamental as gravity, in the later stages of cosmic evolution" [15].

Within the living world we have further discovered, through advances in biochemistry over the last 50 years, a profound and strict unity on the microscopic level. All organisms, from microscopic bacteria to blue whales, rely on chemical machinery which is the same in its structure and its function. The unification of the biological world, which received its first solid theoretical foundation from Darwin, has been deepened and entrenched by the discovery that all living beings without exception are constructed from the same macromolecular components: proteins and nucleic acids. As well as this underlying structural unity, there is a functional unity of all living systems, in that all organisms rely on the same sequences of reactions for their mobilisation and storage of energy and for their biosynthesis of components [16]. A unified conception of the biological world has been given further theoretical support by the compelling arguments put forward (in particular) by James Lovelock, according to which the individual components of biosphere act in a collective and co-ordinated way to produce optimum conditions for the continuation of life [17]. This is the *Gaia* hypothesis, which provides a solid foundation for the often-intuited essential interconnectedness of the biological world. The work of ethologists has also revealed intriguing behavioural analogies and patterns across species, providing another dimension in which scientific inquiry, while expanding our knowledge of the world, serves to uncover deep unities and continuities.

In this way scientific investigations have provided us with a marvellous conception of our unity and interdependence with the natural world which is, I suggest, as rich and profound as any which has been provided by any animistic or pantheistic world view. It reveals also a unity and integrity which, *of itself*, in no way fosters disrespectful or manipulative attitudes. It is very puzzling to me how anyone can find a science-based view of the world to be shallow and disappointing [18]. Eric Ashby has suggested that whereas other cultures have identified with their environment through animism, our culture has enabled us to identify through scientific understanding [19]. One of my aims in this paper has been to argue in favour of this claim. The realisation that we are part of the natural world is an important preliminary to acting wisely within it (as has been repeatedly stressed), but there is no need to turn to exotic traditions to find a solid foundation for this first important step.

William Grey, Department of Philosophy, University of New England, Armidale, N.S.W., 2351 Australia.

NOTES AND REFERENCES

[1] ALAN R. DRENGSON (1980) Shifting paradigms: from the technocratic to the person-planetary, *Environmental Ethics*, 2, pp. 221–40; see also GEORGE SESSIONS & DEVALL BILL (1985) *Deep Ecology: living as if nature mattered* (Layton, Peregrine Smith).

[2] DRENGSON, op. cit.

[3] T.S. KUHN (1962) *The Structure of Scientific Revolutions* (Chicago, University of Chicago Press); see DUDLEY SHAPERE (1964) Review of *The Structure of Scientific Revolutions*, *Philosophical Review*, 73, pp. 383–94.

[4] See T.S. KUHN (1970) Postscript—1969, *The Structure of Scientific Revolutions*, pp. 174–210 (Chicago, University of Chicago Press, 2nd edn), and (1973) Second thoughts on paradigms, in: F. SUPPE (Ed.) *The Structure of Scientific Theories*, pp. 459–99 (Urbana, University of Illinois Press).

[5] JOHN RODMAN (1980) Paradigm change in political science, *American Behavioural Scientist*, 24, p. 75.

[6] The attempts to articulate cultural paradigms by W.R. CATTAN & R.E. DUNLAP (1980) New ecological paradigm for post-exuberant sociology, *American Behavioral Scientist*, 24, pp. 15–47, and S. COTGROVE & A. DUFF (1981) Environmentalism, values and social change, *British Journal of Sociology*, 32, pp. 92–110, provide further examples of constellations of beliefs and values which certainly do *not* invite acceptance or rejection *in toto*, whereas scientific paradigms *do*.

[7] As the notion was originally developed by ARNE NAESS (1973) The shallow and the deep, long-range ecology movement, *Inquiry*, 16, pp. 95–100, and developed by SESSIONS & DEVALL (see [1] above).

[8] JACOB NEEDLEMAN (1975) *A Sense of the Cosmos: the encounter of modern science and ancient truth*, p. 36 (New York, Doubleday).

[9] I suspect that one underlying worry about science is based on a conception of theories as constructs which inevitably stand between us and reality, and serve not to illuminate the world but to distort it. These misgivings about science are basically the same as Plato's misgivings about art, viz. that it is a vehicle for the perversion of truth and the distortion of reality (*cf.* IRIS MURDOCH (1979) *The Fire and the Sun* (Oxford, Oxford University Press)). It seems to me, moreover, that both the Platonic rejection of art and the present rejection of science are in the final analysis mistaken for the same reason: in each case they fail to appreciate the indispensable role these different modes of cognition can play in enriching our conceptions of the world.

[10] CALVIN MARTIN (1981) The American Indian as miscast ecologist, in R.C. SCHULTZ & J.D. HUGHES (Eds) *Ecological Consciousness*, Ch. 7 (Washington, DC, University Press of America).

[11] MARSHALL SAHLINS (1972) *Stone Age Economics* (Chicago, Aldine/Atherton).

[12] PAUL SHEPARD (1973) *The Tender Carnivore and the Sacred Game* (New York, Scribner's).

[13] The difficulties of the transition to a sustainable society are frequently underestimated: E. F. Schumacher is one thinker who was acutely aware of the formidable problems which arise here (see GEOFFREY KIRK (Ed.) (1982) *Schumacher on Energy* (London, Cape)). Schumacher is also very difficult to categorise on the standard shallow-deep parameters.

[14] FRANCIS CRICK (1982) *Life Itself* (New York, Macdonald).

[15] PAUL DAVIES (1978) *The Runaway Universe*, p. 178 (London, Dent).

[16] JACQUES MONOD (1971) *Chance and Necessity* (New York, Knopf).

[17] JAMES LOVELOCK (1979) *Gaia: a new look at life on earth* (Oxford, Oxford University Press).

[18] Though this perhaps has been true of *some* science-based world views. Certainly the nineteenth century attempt to reduce all theoretical knowledge to the science of mechanics was a conspicuous failure: as is well known mechanics failed to provide a satisfactory basis for physics, let alone other areas of science. Nor am I suggesting a 'scientistic' claim that the methods of empirical inquiry are adequate to provide answers for every human perplexity: my claim is the fairly modest one that it supplies a positive and enriching conception of our world, and can serve to enhance our relationship with it. Rejecting the hard-won conceptions which have been painstakingly forged over the last few millenia would be good neither for us nor for the non-human world. The way in which scientific naturalism has been perceived as inimical to important values is explored from another perspective in my 'Evolution and the meaning of life', *Zygon* (forthcoming).

[19] ERIC ASHBY (1978) *Reconciling Man with the Environment* (Oxford, Oxford University Press).

6

A Critique of Deep Ecology? Response to William Grey

ALAN R. DRENGSON

I

William Grey sets out to criticize deep ecology by first presenting his version of how deep ecology diagnoses the environmental illness of industrial society [1]. The picture he presents is a caricature drawn from the work of a number of contemporary authors, my own included, not all of whom claim to be followers of deep ecology. To show how this picture is inaccurate should require detailed textual analysis, but this is beyond the limitations of this space. It is possible, however, to bring out some of the inaccuracies in Grey's picture by evaluating the main criticisms of deep ecology that he bases on it.

Grey characterizes how followers of deep ecology diagnose the origins of our current environmental illness in the following manner. He claims that deep ecologists find the roots of our environmental problems in a shallow technocratic philosophy which has its deeper taproot in the subsoil of Cartesianism and Christianity. This orientation is essentially anthropocentric, and as a result it lends its science and energies to the exploitation of the natural world. It removes from the world anything of intrinsic value by its desacrilization of nature, and because it views nature as a source of only resources. He intimates that followers of deep ecology think that the division of the world into mind and body, where body represents the machine of nature, and mind represents spirit, is part of our current problem context. Deep ecologists think that accepting a different picture will enable us to solve our environmental problems. He calls all of these elements part of the "standard deep ecology package", as if deep ecology were a finished system.

The picture Grey paints has a number of familiar shapes, some of which I and others would recognize, but some of them are obscure. For example, not all claim, myself included, that Christian values helped to form the technocratic picture. Some might claim that Christian theology and philosophy helped to set the stage for the development of modern western science and technology. There is some merit in this claim. And yet, to be sure, the history of Christianity is very complex, and there are traditions in it that encourage respecting nature. Perhaps some followers of deep ecology would find some elements of the latter helpful.

When I sketched the picture of the contrasts between the technocratic (non-ecological) and the person-planetary (ecological) orientations, which Grey criticizes, I was trying to illustrate how certain conceptions of the world can interact with dominant political, economic, military, social and scientific institutions to produce a tacit philosophy of nature, which when pushed to certain extremes (as in the technocratic) will transform itself, since it undermines its own rationale for being [2]. In the paper to which he refers, I was not as clear as I might have been about what I was trying to do. I would now put the matter as follows.

Many followers of deep ecology would probably agree that certain philosophical and religious ideas and concepts, pictures and paradigms, models and metaphors, play a role in our overall relationships to one another and to nature. But how do we get at this? How do we develop a truly ecological form of knowing and understanding—an ecological consciousness? What is involved in knowing nature by means other than one narrowly defined method? Is not ecological knowing interdisciplinary, intradisciplinary, process, activity, inquiry-oriented? Can it be ecological and be static? To what sort of cosmology (if any) does it lead?

II

Let us suppose that we are captives of, or at least seem to need, pictures. Do our pictures promote healing of our relationships or not? Do they lead us to an understanding of nature that is ecocentric, not anthropocentric, transpersonal and not merely intersubjective? Are there dominant images and metaphors that inform (or misinform) public opinion, policy, goals, one's own life, etc.? What are they? What practical value can philosophy serve in environmental matters, if not at least to displace unwholesome pictures? Can wholesomeness be defined apart from pictures and stories? What sustains picturing? Can we live fully without picturing? (i.e. telling stories, creating theories, making models, etc.?) What would this be like? Would one then be aware of the world immediately?

Deep ecology is a philosophical activity, an inquiry, and also a social movement that aims to reopen the conversation with nature and between communities of beings that has been largely interrupted by certain developments in modern industrial society. As a way to an ecologically sound life it involves three elements: experience, practice and theory (stories and pictures, for example). Even though many of us recognize that there are environmental problems, there are different levels or degrees of movement thought necessary (possible) to deal with these problems. There is a spectrum from narrow reform to major change. Within this I do not think anyone has the illusion that pictures or theory alone will do the job. Theories and leading pictures can be of value, but only if they are part of a self-correcting practice. A useful model can outlive its usefulness. It can become a hindrance.

From an ecological standpoint there is no one right picture of the world. The world is rich and deep in the multitude of ways in which it can be known, felt, seen, appreciated, and responded to. The human self, nature and communities together create forms of life. It is our form of life that we hope to understand in its context. We do this by means of a variety of practices, some critical, some analytic, some therapeutic, some aesthetic, some moral and spiritual. The aim is to use (or use in a certain way) pictures that are not alienating.

One source of alienation of a person from nature involves alienation from one's natural self. Along these lines, Naess, for example, has suggested that the practice of extended self-identification can help lead one to realize a much larger Self [3]. As Spinoza observed, we are as large as our loves. The love of which he spoke was not romantic and self-directed, but realistic and self-giving. Naess has pointed out that this sense of extended self-realization is part of an ongoing inquiry, a deep ecological questioning and seeing.

In another paper Naess suggested this example of how one might approach deep ecology [4]. A child sits by a pond and grows more and more silent. After she has stopped stirring the waters, and has stilled her own noise, she begins to see and hear the other beings. As time goes on she sees more and more deeply into the pond. The meaning of the example is clear, but we could put it in another way. We could say: if folk in modern industrial society would get out of its rush and its structures, into the wilderness or in silent meditation, they could open to a larger world. Their focus of attention might be deepened and broadened. As a result the quality of their experience would change. They might discover a deep Self, not just ego. They might see nature as it is, not as they think it to be.

A whole range of practices can be undertaken that help make explicit our limiting pictures of things, our mental knots can be untied and the nature of our activities in industrial society can be seen from ecological perspectives. These practices will, it is hoped, lead us to ecosophy, i.e. to ecological wisdom as a way of living. If deep ecology is a way that leads to ecosophy, then its practices should have an affect on our ecological sensibilities. For example, our capacity for empathy might be increased by the receptivity it makes possible (but not inevitably, for different things work in different ways for different persons). As our understanding deepens (and our whole understanding involves at least all of the elements we mentioned above), we attempt to describe the features of this emerging vision, but these descriptions will never be complete or wholly systematic. The vision emerges; it has a moving horizon. The world as an ongoing process reveals itself most originally to us in its creativeness. Contrary to what Grey thinks, deep ecologists do not want to reinject the old Cartesian spirit into the world, but instead want to cut this matter/spirit dualism at its very root. Human intelligence is very much related to the human form of embodiment.

Deep ecology as a way aims to enlarge our appreciation for the intelligence, creativity, power, beauty, goodness, harmony and vitality of the whole of nature, of the human person and of other person kinds. Following deep ecology one would try to see with the eyes of many, not just with one's own. This is why it is by its very nature eclectic, open-ended, incomplete, creative, and developing. It is a form of inquiry and practice that is alive in its activity and receptive in its listening. Contrary to what Grey intimates deep ecology does not commit one to the claim that there have never been hunter-gatherer cultures that abused nature; nor that we have to take over all of their Old Ways (as Gary Snyder calls them) in total. (Ask, what is meant by neo or future primitive?) Nor does it advise us to reject all modern technology.

III

One way to use creative ecophilosophy as a design process to aid in developing ecological modes of reflection and imagination would be to create alternative ways of seeing things, alternative pictures. This is part of the idea behind 'shifting paradigms'. The play on words in the title was intended to refer to historical but also to intentional 'shifts'.

Kuhn first analysed changes in scientific outlook of a fundamental kind as shifts in paradigm [5]. His original definition of the term 'paradigm' was quite broad. However, before he introduced the term to the philosophical lexicon from the history of science, it already resided in philosophy in the slightly earlier idea of paradigm cases in linguistic philosophy, but also in medieval philosophy and ultimately in Plato and Socrates. Wittgenstein, N. R. Hanson and others have illustrated the ambiguity of graphic pictures and the type of perceptual shifts involved in 'seeing as'. Karl Jaspers also used 'paradigm' in his history of philosophy to refer to paradigmatic individuals, persons such as Socrates, Buddha, Jesus, and Confucius, who were founders of practices and traditions based on realization of a certain way of life [6]. These persons embodied the ideals of various schools of applied philosophy and religion. (The master artisan is for the apprentice a paradigm of the way to do the art, but eventually when the apprentice is a master in her own right, she becomes a paradigm to others. She shows the way, embodies the craft, etc.)

Rodman and I have used the term 'paradigm' to stand for constellations of certain ideals, images, models, measures, beliefs [7]. This is certainly legitimate and useful in the context of the above. My aim in describing technocratic and pernetarian (persons-in-networks-of-planetary-relationships, i.e. whole, person-planetary, etc.) paradigms and root metaphors was illustrative. I was trying to illustrate a design approach to applied ecophilosophy by sharp contrasts between ecological and non-ecological paradigms. I do not think that all persons in industrial society can be nicely sorted into technocrats and pernetarians. In most of us aspects of both of these probably lurk. The aim was to sharpen the contrast to bring out what direction different lines of thought take when pushed to extremes. It was not meant to polarize politically.

In my book *Shifting Paradigms* I tried to make more clear that I was trying to illustrate a certain approach [8]. In addition, in it I wrote about going beyond paradigmatic thinking, beyond shifting paradigms. Here is an explanation of what I meant in part. We try to quiet our selves so that we can hear nature's softest voices. But we are busy in our minds, restructuring the world according to habitual patterns of thought and perception. We can resist these pictures, especially the unhealthy ones, we can go with them, or we can see between and through them by means of experimental and experiential shifts in perspective, using creative comparative philosophy.

IV

Grey states at the end of his paper "(t)he realisation that we are part of the natural world is an important preliminary to acting wisely within it . . ." One could hardly take issue with this. But what is at issue is what constitutes this wisdom, and how deep this realization should be. Of the cosmology he sketches we must say, not yet deep enough, for we have not heard from other beings, from artists, musicians, poets, or from our whole selves. Let us practice so that our minds are as clear as crystal and as receptive as the soft sand . . . what is left in this silent clarity? Could it be a Self no longer lost in its subjectivity, nor paralyzed in its feelings by objectivity? No picture divides them, and there where subject and object meet in unique personal relationship is a unity in diversity, a harmony, an ecosophy.

I thank William Grey for his critical efforts, for they have helped to bring some of these issues into sharper focus.

Alan R. Drengson, Philosophy Department, University of Victoria, P.O. Box 1700, Victoria, British Columbia, Canada V8W 2Y2.

NOTES

[1] WILLIAM GREY (1986) A critique of deep ecology, originally published in *Journal of Applied Philosophy*, 3, pp. 211–216. What appears here is a condensed version of my response to Grey, based on a pre-publication draft of his paper. A full response is available from me on request.

[2] ALAN R. DRENGSON (1980) Shifting paradigms: from the technocratic to the person-planetary, *Environmental Ethics*, 2, pp. 221–40.

[3] ARNE NAESS (1985) Identification as a source of deep ecological attitudes, in: MICHAEL TOBIAS (Ed.) *Deep Ecology* (New York, Avant Books).

[4] ARNE NAESS (1986) Deep ecology in good conceptual health, *The Trumpeter*, 3, pp. 18–22.

[5] THOMAS KUHN (1970) *The Structure of Scientific Revolutions* (Chicago, University of Chicago Press).

[6] L. WITTGENSTEIN (1953) *Philosophical Investigations* (Basingstoke, Macmillan), esp. Part II; N. R. HANSON (1953) *The Patterns of Discovery* (London, Cambridge University Press); KARL JASPERS (1962) *Socrates, Buddha, Confucius, Jesus* (New York, Harcourt Brace).

[7] DRENGSON, op. cit.; and JOHN RODMAN (1980) Paradigm change in political science, *American Behavioral Scientists*, 24, p. 75.

[8] ALAN R. DRENGSON (1983) *Shifting Paradigms: from Technocrat to Planetary Person* (Victoria, BC, Lightstar).

Part II

Personal Relationships

7

Human Bonds

BRENDA ALMOND

ABSTRACT *There are three kinds of bonds between human beings: biological and natural; legal and artificial; social and voluntary. Marriage can be seen as an artificial and legal means of shifting the loose bonding of the third category of relationship into the deep and inescapable bonding of the first. The desire to create bonds of this type is widespread, but non-bonding, too, has been recommended either as good in itself—a way of achieving peace of mind or personal emancipation through wider relationships—or as necessary self-denial for some higher cause. In the latter case, the bonds of family are seen as a positive good, a view shared, though for different reasons, by religious and political conservatives and by revisionist feminists.*

In contrast to this, three philosophical conceptions which would favour unbonding, or detachment from emotional ties, are categorised here as (a) the Stoic, (b) the Existentialist and (c) the Feminist. Within the Feminist ideal, it is radical, rather than liberal or socialist feminism that has most in common with Stoic or Existentialist ideals. These ideals are considered, together with various alternatives to marriage, and are judged not to override the need for deep personal bonds between human beings. These personal bonds of love and commitment are compared with the alternative bonds of religion and politics and it is concluded that, whatever forms they take, personal bonds have fundamental moral priority in the lives of human beings.

Invisible bonds exist between people, knitting them into groups, communities or pairs, destroying their atomicity, making them interdependent rather than independent, parts rather than wholes, joined together rather than solitary. These ties are sometimes a matter of pride, sometimes of shame; they provide opportunities for heroism, but also for cowardice; for loyalty as well as for betrayal; they are sometimes a burden; sometimes a matter of satisfaction and support. They may be a source of grief and pain, but are potentially the locus of the greatest human happiness. People sometimes long to be free from their bonds, but then, if they achieve this, instead of flourishing in freedom, they may wilt and die in their self-sought isolation. Or, enmeshed within the stranglehold of unsought obligations, they may never achieve their own potential. Others again, accepting the inescapability of their situation, may use it to achieve a potential of a different order and in a direction not of their choosing.

There are many ways in which people seek happiness through unshackling: the husband seeks freedom from his unloved wife; the feminist independence from domestic ties; parents from the perpetual responsibility of dependent children; adolescents from the cloying pressures of family living; the wage-slave from the tyranny of the time-clock; the Jew from a racial identity that may be not chosen but externally imposed by others; the Northern Ireland Catholic or Protestant from a religious bonding he or she may have intellectually renounced; the left-wing intellectual of aristocratic origins from a despised social class. Sometimes, however, people seek happiness in the *acceptance* of bonds: perhaps through admission to an admired social class; or through identification with an employer or firm; or through commitment to a political party or religious movement. They may also seek it through *creating* new bonds, of marriage or of parenthood.

This webbing that knits our lives together is not, however, woven of one sort of thread. There are essentially three kinds of bonds between human beings:

[i] biological and natural
[ii] legal and artificial
[iii] social and voluntary

These categories may in some cases be disputable. For example, are the bonds of common membership of a race biological, or are they social? Are the bonds of common nationality legal and artificial, or are they social and voluntary?

Other cases may be taken as paradigms for settling such demarcation disputes. The first kind of bond is clearly represented by, for example, relationships like those of parent and child, or brother and sister; the second could be represented by a standard business contract creating a 'company' *persona*, or by a trade or professional apprenticeship; while the third type of bond may best be represented by friendships, or by short-term sexual relationships, or by membership of a voluntary group serving a common purpose.

Some would see it as a fact of human nature that the more widely shared a bond, the weaker its force. But this may be less an objective finding than a perception coloured by the perspective of individualism, and made more secure by certain curious linguistic habits of liberals. For where such bonds as religion, race, or country count for *more* with someone than family or friends, the liberal individualist will refer to that person as a fanatic. Fanaticism, to the liberal temperament, essentially consists in taking too seriously these wider bonds.

Nevertheless, it is true that the more intimate and closer bonds have the most natural and immediate force, and that they are to that extent prior. Thus, the wider bonds are frequently understood in terms of the narrower ones. It is, for example, a feature of religions and of political movements that they attempt to secure the intimate effectiveness of family bonds to weld together 'in one', as they sometimes say, their disparate membership. Hence, the use of terms like 'father', 'brother', 'sister', 'son', 'daughter', as ways of addressing fellow members of church or party. The religious or political aspiration to brotherhood or sisterhood is a way of attempting to transfer these deeper bondings to a wider circle without dilution. But as the terms show, it is an imitative venture. The quintessential network of bonding is the family; and at the heart of *that* system, the nuclear family, lies a central relationship between two people which, unlike all other family relationships, is *not* based on a biological or blood-tie—it is not natural but created, whether by the will of the two people themselves, or, in some cases, by external agencies or circumstantial constraints.

It is a curious feature of the marriage-bond, then, that it fits only with difficulty into the three-fold framework just outlined. It is a quasi-biological bond without a blood relationship. It is a legal bond, but the widespread reality of common law or *de facto* marriage shows that it does not have to be this. It is social and voluntary, but clearly much more than that.

Two main characteristics differentiate the lesser bond of friendship from the kind of biological bond that marriage aspires to become. To begin with, unlike ties of preference such as comradeship or friendship, biological ties are ready-made. Not only are they not chosen, but they often run counter to inclination. In this way they provide a setting in which people accept a shared existence with people whose characteristics they neither admire nor like—a situation which, of course, has both advantages and disadvantages. And secondly, they are inescapable: they cannot be dissolved: a person's 'sisters, cousins and aunts'—narrow-minded uncles, bad-tempered brothers or handicapped son or daughter—are part of the baggage of life.

Marriage can be seen, then, as an artificial means, perhaps all we have to hand legally and socially, to shift the loose bonding of the third non-binding and voluntary category of relationships into the deep and inescapable bonding of the first. Adoption is another legal device in which this is a visible and overt aim. But marriage is the paradigmatic case and one which aims at the creation of a relationship as close to the biological as law and effective practice can make it.

The nature of the bond may be spelled out in terms of duties, obligations and rights. And yet the bond is strong enough to override situations in which duties are disregarded, obligations ignored, rights violated; it can survive, too, those other cases in which the onset of illness, or the inevitable process of ageing, prevents the fulfilment of the marital transaction. Since in some cases there may be nothing left but the bond itself, irrationally persisting when all external indications are absent, those who want to recognise its continuing efficacy may describe it as mystic, and it is only to be expected that people with a narrowly empiricist or positivist orientation will refuse to recognise it at all. For them 'marriage' will begin and end with a legal transaction; for them there is a genuine possibility of divorce, while for others, the ending of a marriage, while technically and legally feasible, will never be so in intuited reality [1].

An institution like marriage, then, like that of adoption, gives expression to a desire to create bonds whose efficacy transcends the legal, and to use the medium of law itself to do this. It would be wrong, however, to assume that this desire can be understood only within the context of the existing social convention of marriage. Indeed it may be more illuminating to illustrate the sentiment I have in mind with an example taken from outside conventional or traditional relationships. Douglas Kramer's play, *The Normal Heart*, ends with a death-bed 'marriage' between the two partners of a long-term gay relationship. What sort of claim does this involve, and what sort of satisfaction could such a last-stage 'joining' be expected to offer? There hardly seems to be an answer in terms of practical commonsense. But if this is irrationality, it is deep-rooted: one of the oldest sagas of Western civilisation, Homer's *Odyssey*, displays the strength of what may seem as, by contemporary standards, equally irrational aspirations from the more familiar arena of heterosexuality. Why did faithful Penelope's suitors have to die? Why could she not have settled down with one of them? Why was her husband Odysseus compelled—and in what sense 'compelled'?—to struggle over twenty years of wandering to return to home, wife and unknown son? The difficulty of dealing with such questions is not a matter of mere changing mores and expectations—it is not simply that these are questions posed now, by us, about people remote in time and place. Whilst the story has made sense and carried conviction over two and a half millenia, there were, even within ancient Greek traditions, more 'rational' conceptions to be found. The Stoics, in particular, recommended non-bonding for peace of mind, as in this passage from Epictetus:

> Whenever you grow attached to something, do not act as though it were one of those things that cannot be taken away, but as though it were something like a jar or crystal goblet, so that when it breaks you will remember what it was like, and not be troubled. So too in life; if you kiss your child, your

brother, your friend, never allow your fancy free rein, nor your exuberant spirits to go as far as they like, but hold them back, stop them ... remind yourself that the object of your love is mortal; it is not one of your own possessions; it has been given to you for the present, not inseparably nor for ever, but like a fig, or a cluster of grapes, at a fixed season of the year, and that if you hanker for it in winter, you are a fool. If in this way you long for your son, or your friend, at a time when he is not given to you, rest assured that you are hankering for a fig in wintertime. [2]

The Stoic aim, then, was to find peace of mind in the detachment that arises from not clinging emotionally to that which must be taken away—not wanting what one cannot have, whether this is an object, a place or a person. The appeal of the Stoic attitude may be a consequence of external circumstances: just as the Stoic philosophy itself is often considered to have been a response to the extreme external constraint of slavery, a struggle to looser links is more likely to appeal to those who have been unfortunate in respect of a central exclusive link. And life inevitably in the end tears every human being away from whatever he or she holds dear. However, there can be reasons other than necessity for preferring wider bonds or rejecting closer and exclusive ones.

One such reason is portrayed in Kramer's play, which effectively, if unconsciously, reveals some of the ambivalence of feeling people have in sexual matters, whether heterosexual or homosexual. Earlier in the play, tribute is paid to the liberating effect of multiple, free and varied sexual relationships. And in general, gay liberation, like some conceptions of female liberation, is associated with an openness to other people and other lovers outside the constricting limits of, in the first case either abstinence or secrecy, in the second of a closed marriage. So some may advocate unbonding in the interests of personal emancipation and a richer, more varied fabric of relationships.

The second reason may be more austere: a perceived sacrifice accepted for what is seen as a more worthy and more compelling goal—as, for example, the acceptance of celibacy by Catholic priests. In this case, non-bonding may be seen as the deliberate renunciation of a good, rather than as a good in itself, and there would be endorsement of the attitude expressed by the British philosopher Roger Scruton that:

> The family bond is dispensable only in the way that pleasure, industry, love, grief, passion and allegiance are dispensable—that is, only in the case of the minority which can persuade itself (for whatever reason) to renounce these things. [3]

That the family should be seen as something of value from a religious or politically conservative point of view is perhaps not surprising. What may be more surprising is the way in which such a valuation seems to coincide with revisionist feminist perspectives on the institution. And yet one of the early advocates of female liberation now reassesses the family as:

> ... that last area where one has any hope of individual control over one's destiny, of meeting one's basic human needs, of nourishing that core or personhood threatened by vast impersonal institutions and uncontrollable corporate and government bureaucracies. [4]

This may be another version of that movement described by Isaiah Berlin as a retreat to the 'inner citadel' [5]—not this time a retreat to an atomistic inner individual, but rather to the family as a convivial multi-person entity, bonded by nature's most effective bonding agent, the sexual relationship, which also simultaneously invisibly binds to its two central agents the presexual beings who are its natural consequences.

The Liberation Circle

The way in which these personal and social questions flow into each other suggests that sexuality, gender questions and the institution of the family constitute a circle which may be entered at any point, one issue leading to the next and inevitably leading back to the starting-point. Let us call this the Liberation Circle. For in it questions about sex and sexuality are indeed, as they are often perceived to be, feminist questions, notwithstanding the indisputable fact that they do, of course, concern both men and women. This is because of the fact, stressed by feminists, that the sexual transaction exposes women to the possibility of exploitation by men, the reverse being true only exceptionally, with rape, violence and pornography as the ugly extreme manifestations of this general tendency.

Questions about sex and sexuality, however, naturally and inevitably lead to questions about marriage and the family—two institutions which radically affect the roles of men and women in society, generating a potential conflict between artificially-created separation of function and natural and necessary divisions. It is this that is called by feminists, Marxists and others, the gender issue. Settling it involves forming a conception of what are, for women and for men, the ideal terms and conditions of work, leisure, education and retirement. But changes in the social roles of women and men may themselves require or bring about changes in our conception of sexual relationships, and in particular of the key institution of marriage. For social and economic equality, if that is the goal, may not be compatible with traditional patterns of family-living, in which men work for economic gain outside the home and women bear the burden of domestic, and, in particular, child-care tasks. So sex, gender, family and society form a merry-go-round of considerations, on which people may ride such horses as female liberation; a wider conception of sexual relationships, including the homosexual; and conflicting demands for either the abolition of marriage and the family, or the reinforcement of the family as a legal and economic structure.

At their base, the questions that are generated are moral questions, at least in the sense that they insistently force us to consider what we *want*, what we *value*. But then, unless we find that the world already conforms to our values, they become social and political questions: What institutions should society protect? Are there any which it should outlaw? Two differing ethical conceptions of how to settle these questions compete for priority. According to one, it is only necessary to consider what will make most people happy—if indeed this can be discovered with any degree of certainty. According to the other, it is important to have respect for principles and institutions, like, for example, marriage and the family, even if there is a price to be paid in terms of individual happiness.

But there is a paradox at the heart of each of these two ethical positions where this particular issue is concerned. For the utilitarian, the obligation to promote the happiness of others extends indefinitely to remote persons, and it is difficult in purely utilitarian terms to justify preferring the indulgence of close family in non-essentials to charitable giving that secures necessities for remote strangers. At the same time, the universalistic rigorism of the alternative position seems in a different way to exclude special obligations to close family-members, since this would be to enshrine a principle of particularity within a universal morality. The dilemma is reflected in two competing political approaches: while capitalistic individualism may seem to neglect the needs of other people's children, socialist egalitarianism allows you to do for *your* child only what you can secure everyone's agreement to doing for *everyone's* children.

Although their defenders may offer ways of resolving this paradox, it seems clear that these broad moral and political positions do not deliver unambiguous answers to questions about family, marriage and close relationships. They may provide a setting and a framework for reflection, but they still leave open many questions of detail and practice. A possible ethical basis on which to proceed, however, would be to derive from utilitarianism the principle that the aim of social living and social organisation should be human flourishing; and to accept from the universalistic approach the importance of holding to certain long-term moral and spiritual values: for example, love, loyalty, honesty and respect for others as centres of need, will and desire.

On whatever basis decisions are made, however, it is clear that Western liberal societies like those of Western Europe or the U.S.A. *could* look very different: indeed there have already been very considerable changes affecting the area of personal relationships over the last twenty or thirty years. Current proposals could accelerate this process of change. For example, if the age of consent (to both heterosexual and homosexual relationships) were to be dropped, say, to fourteen; if incest were no longer to be illegal; if the category of homosexuality were to cease to feature in the law; if prostitution were to be municipalised; if surrogacy and transfer of gametes were to become commonplace. How are questions in these complex areas to be settled? This is a characteristic problem of applied philosophy, and as is typical with such problems, it is characterised by a convergence of facts and values. The facts themselves are the product of a number of disciplines, and value-judgements arrived at without taking account of this factual background are bound to be inadequate.

It is worth setting out what these factual areas are, comprising, as they do, most of the areas investigated by the social sciences. To begin with, sociological perspectives supply statistical patterns relating to sex, marriage and divorce, with information about the consequences of the latter for children; sociology compares groups and subcultures, tracing complex patterns of behaviour. Next, psychological perspectives may supply information about stress or breakdown, about family conflict and ways of resolving it. From law, there is the specification of rights, duties and obligations: while economic considerations radically affecting the family are linked with political decisions as to how provision is to be made for the non-earning members of society: the young, the old, the ill or disabled. Finally, beyond these 'internal' considerations, social anthropological perspectives draw attention to the different practices prevailing in other communities and cultures. Faced with this vast network of relevant facts, it may be that a case needs to be made for the claim that philosophy has a distinctive contribution to make. And yet it is the philosophical and more particularly the ethical that is the concern of most ordinary people who want to reflect on this fundamental aspect of their lives, as opposed to merely *living* or *experiencing* it.

The philosophical contribution may take the form of conceptual analysis: of sex and sexual desire, for example [6]; of the concept of marriage [7]—is 'open marriage', for example, a contradiction in terms? [8]—but while such discussions follow a path familiar from other areas of philosophy, it is arguable that considerations of a deeper and more profound kind are what are really demanded here. A comparison might be made with environmental philosophy, where again it may be hard to isolate a distinctively philosophical contribution from the thicket of facts. In the area of environment, there is no reason why philosophers should not join with others to draw attention to relevant facts about animals or ecology, for example. But when they go beyond these facts to appeal to the inner respect for nature latent in humans, and when they argue as to whether there may not be value in the physical universe independent of its human observers, then they behave most distinctively as philosophers. In a parallel way, the task of philosophy in relation to questions concerning human relationships must involve consideration of the rival ideals of bonding and un-bonding from an ethical and indeed, in some modest sense, metaphysical perspective.

Unbonding as a Philosophical Ideal

There are three powerful magnets in human affairs, any of which can strongly bond the individual. These are:

(i) sex and family;
(ii) religion;
(iii) politics.

Either of the latter two can replace the first as a focus for commitment, but I will consider the unbonding ideal here, mainly in relation to the first, returning briefly at a later stage to the question of these two other extremely powerful forces. The two reasons so far considered for the renunciation of bonds—promiscuous indulgence or ascetic self-denial,—were essentially practical or instrumental reasons. But unbonding —that is, emotional independence of other people, places and objects of attachment— may also be offered as a philosophical ideal. I want, then, to look at the philosophical case for unbonding, before making reference to some of the facts that are peculiarly relevant to the case for the most intimate of human bonds, those of marriage and parenthood.

The unbonding ideal can be reached through three diverse philosophical approaches, which might be loosely categorised as Stoic, Existentialist and Feminist.

(i) *The Stoic Ideal*

This may be derived from the ancient Stoic doctrine, already mentioned, which seeks to achieve liberation through freedom from emotional and mental commitment to person or place—the realm of the contingent. It is an ascetic ideal, also to be found in such diverse sources as the beliefs of some North American Indian tribes; in the acceptance of necessity that is at the root of so-called Mohammedan determinism, and in Buddhist doctrines. For the Greeks themselves and perhaps for others, it had its origins in ancient Orphic doctrines of reincarnation, with release from the wheel of birth and death as the ultimate goal.

(ii) *The Existentialist Ideal*

Second is the very much more recent Existentialist ideal, both the 'official' French variety and Californian derivatives. This is the view that makes a moral ideal of the notion of being yourself, or 'doing your own thing'. It is the ideal of the self-created free personality, independent of emotional ties beyond those of immediate inclination, and moving from relationship to relationship in strong and unregretful isolation.

(iii) *The Feminist Ideal*

Thirdly there is the feminist goal of liberation. Not all forms of this ideal are involved here, for its different forms have different consequences as far as the issue of bonding and unbonding is concerned. There is a liberal tradition, for example, represented by such writers as Mary Wollstonecraft [9], or Harriet Taylor and John Stuart Mill [10], in which female liberation need not imply emotional independence: in this tradition, the emphasis is on legal and political change only: on the achievement of political rights, equality of opportunity, freedom of choice and economic independence. In this respect, it is significant that while Mill endeavoured to renounce the legal inequities embedded in the Victorian marriage-contract on his marriage to Harriet Taylor, their relationship—most of it outside the framework of legal marriage—in fact represented an ideal of human bonding as an equal and permanent intellectual and spiritual partnership [11].

Socialist ideals of female liberation may also be compatible with the centrality of personal and family bonds; women's liberation for socialist feminists is linked to the achievement of a structured socialist society in which *private* domestic cares, obligations and ties are transferred to the *public* sphere. This is why such importance is attached to, for example, creche and child-care provision, and the sharing of domestic tasks.

So it is within the *radical* feminist tradition—a tradition which may include separatism and lesbianism, that liberation is most likely to be conceived as the shedding of bonds. Like socialist feminism, radical feminism also demands the restructuring of society, but where the socialist ideal tolerates the man-woman bond, only seeking equality by the removal of child-care commitments, the radical feminist is more truly committed as far as this bond, though not necessarily the maternal bond, is concerned, to something that can be compared to the Stoic or Sartrean ideals of detachment.

These traditions or ideals have both positive and negative aspects. The Stoic approach involves the recognition of necessity, and clearly such a goal is to be commended on rational grounds. But it is worth bearing in mind that the necessity involved in nature is decay, and the ultimate extinction of the individual. Therefore, the logical consequence of Stoic and other ideals of *apatheia* is the complete cessation of feeling and experience that can be attained only by ceasing to exist at all: in other words, in death. It is not surprising, then, that suicide as a practice was associated with Stoicism in ancient times. Bonds keep people alive, so that if we value life we value the 'ties that bind'. There are many examples of this truth in accounts of concentration camp survivors. Perhaps the strongest such account is given by Elie Wiesel of the way in which the bond between himself and his father kept him alive against all odds in the rigours of Auschwitz and Buchenwald [12]. It is worth reflecting, too, that a person's sense of self is built to a very considerable extent, possibly entirely, on that person's sense of others in relation. Divested of any intensity of care for close others, a person's sense of self-hood diminishes, perhaps vanishing entirely, until the will to continue in existence expires.

These considerations are also relevant to the Existentialist ideal. For this depends on the notion of a self-created self. It does this in the context of an assumption which reverses that of Stoicism. For it is based on the belief that people or individuals *can* control their fate, shape their character, be, unaided, whatever they want to be. This aim has sometimes found its application in the field of personal relationships with real attempts to put unbonding into practice as a way of life. The relationship between Sartre and de Beauvoir, recounted in detail by the latter, is a concrete illustration of this [13]. But it is often remarked that the arrangement appeared to suit Sartre better than it suited de Beauvoir, who found his relationships with other women set up strains in her own life. The relationship, too, depended on its non-consummation as a child-producing and therefore family arrangement.

This approach to unbonding is essentially particular. It is arguable as to whether it is satisfying as a psychological goal; as a moral ideal, however, it is clear that it is flawed by its very particularity. It fails, in other words, to link a concept of what is good or right to some broader conception of human flourishing—a conception capable of transcending transitory whim, preoccupation with personal gratification, and unjustifiable partiality for self.

The radical feminist approach provided the last example of belief in unbonding as a matter of principle. At its most extreme (for example, in Shulamith Firestone's *The Dialectic of Sex*) this may involve a Utopia in which artificial reproduction releases women, and men too, not only from their bonds to each other, but also from the deepest of natural bonds. This conception of freedom from familiar bonds is, however, if not less *revolutionary* than it appears, at least less *new*; for Plato proposed achieving the same result without benefit of modern technology by state-organised mating-festivals, followed by the communal rearing of babies, whose mothers would feed indiscriminately any baby presented to them by the nurses [14].

Here again, psychological considerations obtrude. There is the difficulty in modern Western societies of replacing what is lost in unbonding with 'comradely' bonds, expressed in such slogans as 'sisterhood is powerful'. It may be, but except for true lesbians, who are less common than lesbians *faute de mieux*, it is not as powerful as the natural bonds it seeks to replace.

The Ideal of Bonding

Are we to conclude, then, that (a) the family as an institution and (b) bonds of deep emotional attachment between people—let us accept the term 'love'—are cultural and moral universals? Anthropological evidence may be advanced that this is not so. Israeli experiments with kibbutz living are often put forward as evidence of alternative possibilities to traditional family-living [15]; there are also diverse examples from other cultures: Spartan boys and men lived together in common houses; amongst the Nayar, a warrior-caste of India, sisters and brothers formed a household, and biological fatherhood, husband-status and legal and economic fatherhood were conceived of as separate. It is often pointed out, too, that the family is a more recent conception than Western tradition takes it to be: that 'household' was the older concept, in which reference was made not to the nuclear family, but to all living beneath a roof, including servants, lodgers and so on. As one text-book on these matters puts it "the social facts of family life often violate the biological in various ways" [16].

Nevertheless, a certain network of connections is implied: common residence, economic co-operation, socially approved sexual relationships, reproduction and child-rearing. The family is, in other words, generally conceived of as an economic unit involving sex and child-raising, and essentially existing under a common roof. Sometimes, indeed, the roof itself may keep the family together—a thought given form in Amy's speech in T.S. Eliot's *The Family Reunion*:

If you want to know why I never leave Wishwood
That is the reason. I keep Wishwood alive
To keep the family alive, to keep them together,
To keep me alive, and I live to keep them. [17]

As for love, it is often pointed out that the elaborate concept of love familiar to Western traditions is barely recognised in other cultural traditions. On this view, romantic love is seen as essentially connected with individualist capitalist and Puritan societies. Other traditions may recognise the occurrence of irrational passion, but they would not regard it as a basis for marriage, but more like an attack of epilepsy—a madness struck by the dart of a playful or malicious god.

The rejection of love as a basis for marriage has, however, also found expression within the Western philosophical tradition. As Carole Pateman points out, Rousseau and Wollstonecraft, notwithstanding their polarity as far as the position of women is concerned, both make a distinction between sexual passion on the one hand and friendship and mutual respect on the other, and both assert that the latter is a better basis for marriage than the former. Pateman quotes Rousseau: "people do not marry in order to think exclusively of each other, but in order to fulfil the duties of civil society jointly, to govern the house prudently, to rear their children well" [18].

But it would be unnecessary to separate love and marriage for these sorts of reasons if it were not that the institution of marriage is seen as embedded in and integral to that of the family. Modern technology makes possible a separation of the two latter that could hardly have been anticipated by Wollstonecraft and Rousseau, although Hume clearly had the distinction in mind in his dry remarks on chastity as a moral ideal for the middle-aged, when he suggested that its continuing justification at the non-procreative stage of life could only be in terms of example to the young, and not for its intrinsic merits.

In the light of modern developments, however, it is possible to take seriously the possibility of separating marriage and the family, as do Joseph and Clorinda Margolis in their article on this subject. Rejecting the position of the Catholic Church as expressed in the views on contraception, abortion and sterilisation set out in *Humanae Vitae*, they propose the introduction of new types of marriage based on breaking the link between marriage and family. One such type is already common: their proposal simply amounts to recognising it *as* a type of marriage: this is *informal* marriage: the second type they propose is a 'term' marriage, which would involve a time-limit renewable by consent.

As a consequence of these new types of marriage, they propose also a new type of family—the contractual family—which could involve any number of persons of either sex or both, and be based on either adoption or begetting. As they put it: "Marriage ... need not entail families, and families need not entail marriage" [19]. In consequence, they continue, "marriage cannot on the hypothesis given, fail to become a relatively transient institution, at least for many. It would be a source of continuing personal freedom and renewal for competent parties, weaving in and out of contact with more permanent and more fundamental family relations" [20].

But a number of considerations count against accepting this essentially devalued concept of marriage, and, notwithstanding the much-publicised failings of the nuclear family, this attenuated and weakened notion of family. To begin with, the psychological assumptions on which it is based are at least questionable. 'Competent parties', where deep emotions are involved, are almost certainly less common than the authors suppose, and *less* competent parties may fail to find personal freedom and renewal in the new conventions. In addition, it may be unrealistic to seek to introduce what are naturally-occurring patterns of life in some primitive societies into complex and fluctuating Western societies. Finally, there is, it must be said, a certain illogicality about the suggestion: divorce may not be a contradiction in terms, but marriage with the *intention* of a limited commitment comes close to being one. Of course, there is nothing illogical about recognising, on marriage, the *possibility* of later breakdown, but this is not the same thing as forming a union with that *intention*.

One advantage put forward for these proposals is that they open the way to non-standard or deviant marriages such as, for example, marriages between homosexuals. But the demand for the possibility of marriage between homosexuals is precisely *not* met by a legal agreement for temporary cohabitation, since the essence of this demand is that homosexuals should be able to experience the deep and not easily relinquishable bonding characteristic of heterosexual marriage. This has as minimal defining features at least the *intention* of permanence, as well as a willingness to engage in a partnership which may, perhaps, while it lasts, exclude others. So if the homosexual demand is to be met, it would be best to meet it on the terms and conditions on which it is sought, rather than in some devalued currency.

Of these two defining characteristics, however, exclusivity may not be as essential a feature of the kind of relationship in question as is the intention of permanence. For sometimes, as another writer on this theme has pointed out: "Our sexual lives fail to go hand in hand with our friendships, our love and the alchemy of erotic attraction" [21]. So while promiscuity of the type reputedly common amongst California's gay community before the morally irrelevant but practically compelling advent of AIDS, involves an extreme depersonalisation, more varied relationships, if they are relationships in the fullest sense, may in some circumstances be necessary and also enriching.

Nevertheless, the search for enrichment may for many people have lower priority than the need for stability—stability not merely for the sake of the children involved in a relationship, but also for the central parties too. When, either as a result of human decision, or of natural intrusions such as illness, death or protracted separation, the bonded individual is suddenly cut free from that bonding, the effect is indeed freedom, but it is the freedom of a ship in a storm-tossed sea, cut free from its anchor [22]. In a 'couple culture' like those of America and most European countries, the bond-free individual is at risk of loneliness, mental breakdown, illness triggered by the collapse of the network of dependency, and of death either from such illness or directly by suicide. It is well-known that women in their later years are overwhelmingly over-represented in psychiatric institutions [23]: perhaps less well-known but equally pertinent is the fact that it takes nine years for the death-rate of widowed *men* to return to that of their married opposites, a fact linked illuminatingly, if coincidentally, by Jonathan Gaythorn-Hardy, with Bertrand Russell's comment on his own marital breakdown: "It takes me nine years to recover the freshness of feeling that is wanted for love" [24]. Little wonder, then, that the same author speaks of "Those terrible cries of pain which rip through our late twentieth century prose and distort the faces on our screens . . . " [25].

Unbonding, then, may be less harmoniously accommodated to human nature than the ideal of bonding, though necessity may drive some people, or perhaps most people at some stage in their lives, to seek for a form of cold comfort in Stoic or other conceptions. And there will always be some who will place other intellectual or spiritual goals higher than personal ones. While some of these alternative goals will merit the sacrifice, it will be useful, in conclusion, to consider to what extent this is true of those alternative magnets in human affairs which have most popular mass appeal: religion and politics.

Alternative Bonds

Religious and political movements of every variety press their frequently competitive claims, appealing to people to place allegiance to church, party or state above personal loyalties. It is worth remembering in this connection that, notwithstanding the widespread perception to-day of Christianity as a family-centred religion, its leader and founder was himself explicit on the conflict between family ties and religious commitment, saying: "Whoever will not leave father, mother, brother, sister and follow me will not enter the kingdom of Heaven", while his follower, Paul, recommended marriage only in preference to damnation. Other sects and religions contest the individual's family loyalties equally, if not more, strongly with, in the case of some fringe sects, kidnappings and counter-kidnappings, programming and deprogramming.

As far as the bonds of religion are concerned, then, these can undoubtedly be harnessed against, as well as *for*, personal relationships. However, that the former represents the true underlying order of priorities is strikingly revealed in the story of Abraham's testing: that he had to be willing to place his son on the altar in obedience to God's command—a story which may be compared with one from another tradition, the story of Agamemnon, who was called upon to sacrifice a daughter on the altar of another god.

Divesting themselves of cloying personal bonds, then, the truly religious of every faith are ultimately confronted with the necessity of turning their faces away from the claims of intimacy—the bonds of nature and of love—towards their chosen other loyalty.

Although women, like men, may choose a religious framework for their lives, it may nevertheless be the case that women are more reluctant than men to espouse this ordering of priorities—that they are more likely to take the personal as pre-eminent, preferring, for example, the life of a son to the demands of abstract religion, morality or justice. Possible even the apocryphal Spartan mother who told her son to come back *with* his shield or *on* it, hoped for his life even whilst appealing to his courage. Such speculation is supported by findings of recent research in which a feminist critique of neo-Kantian ethical assumptions is beginning to emerge—research which has its roots in examination of responses to the peculiarly female moral dilemma represented by individual abortion decisions [26].

As far as the realm of the political is concerned, it is, by now, a literary and historical commonplace that political movements seek their recruits young and encourage them to place loyalty to group or state above loyalty to family members. Political Pied Pipers are aware of the competitive pull of natural and biological bonds; they are aware, too, of the strength of sexual love, which they often subvert for their own ends. And any group which aspires to totalitarian political control knows it must first tame and curb this otherwise ungovernable network of loyalties. It is this that makes the family, in political terms, an ultimately subversive institution.

Political systems may be in conflict with the family structure in two ways: socialist systems by removing too many of its functions; conservative or traditionalist systems by leaving too many of its functions to be fulfilled by one (usually female) member, whether or not this is her choice. This produces a dilemma for those who wish to combine humanity and compassion with the preservation of the family structure. On the one hand, no philosophical or ethical ideal is compatible with watching people starve or suffer. And not only the needy, but also those who take on the care of helpless others—the young, the old, the chronically sick or suddenly disabled—need support from the wider community. However, if a solution is sought in universal publicly-provided care—a cradle-to-grave underwriting of all the contingencies of life—different problems arise: responsibility, if it is *shared* by the state, is actually *transferred*, for responsibility essentially means 'This will *not be done* if I don't do it'. Consequently, support for deserted wives or abandoned children may be counter-productive. Indeed, it may provide the very conditions that make desertion or neglect realistic alternatives for people who would otherwise have been restrained by their consciousness of others' dependency.

It there is to be a solution to this dilemma, it is most likely to be found in compromise and calculation, avoiding, however, strategies that reduce people to social atoms. The task of settling responsibility for categories of care is a matter for reappraisal in the light of women's needs, as well as the needs of those who traditionally benefit from their care. But the family is the ultimate private sphere, and the state should intervene in its affairs and take on its functions only with hesitation, respecting this privacy. There is, indeed, a valid political and ethical reason—liberal in the classical sense—for guarding family ties as an essential protection for individual liberty.

Both political systems and political loyalties that attempt to take precedence in the life of the individual, even if they use the *language* of liberation, are offering a stone in exchange for bread. The instinct which sites a person's true loyalties on the intimate human scale, and that unerringly places the political under the governance of the personal, is a sounder guide in human affairs than the brave new worlds of political ideologies. In terms of its political effects, such a reordering of values would reduce much of that very considerable part of the tragedy of human existence that is the result of the actions of people rather than of nature.

Consideration of the Liberation Circle, then, has ended with what may seem a paradoxical conclusion. It is one familiar, however, from other areas of political philosophy. This is that freedom, where human relationships are concerned, must include freedom to live within the bonds that make human existence bearable and worthwhile. These bonds are not always to be found in stereotyped or conventional settings: the forms and objects of love take different shapes. But set within the wider social and political context, these deep personal bonds have an ineluctable moral priority. State, law and economics are merely the canvas on which the picture of an individual's life is painted; and for the great majority of human beings, that life acquires meaning and purpose from the bonds of love and commitment.

Brenda Almond, Social Values Research Centre, University of Hull, Hull HU6 7RX, United Kingdom.

NOTES

This paper was delivered as the Conference Address to the Annual Conference of the Society for Applied Philosophy at Gregynog, Wales, on 22 May 1987, and subsequently to the Societas Ethica at Debrecen, Hungary on 2 September 1987.

[1] Alys, Bertrand Russell's first wife, reputedly refused to acknowledge their divorce in the sense that I have in mind, although she accepted it as a legal reality. At the age of 82, she wrote to Russell: "I am utterly devoted to thee, and have been for over 50 years ... But my devotion makes no claim, and involves no burden on thy part, nor any obligation, not even to answer this letter". Letter dated 14 April 1950. *The Autobiography of Bertrand Russell*, Vol. III (London, Allen & Unwin, 1968, 1971), pp. 48–49.
Explaining her inability to meet him face-to-face after their break-up, she wrote of their marriage: "I was neither wise enough nor courageous enough to prevent this one disaster from shattering my capacity for happiness and my zest for life" (ibid., p. 47).

[2] Epictetus: *Arrian's Discourses of Epictetus*, trans. W. A. OLDFATHER (1985, 1928), (London, Heinemann), Book III xxiv, pp. 84–87.

[3] R. SCRUTON (1986) *Sexual Desire*, p. 31 (London, Weidenfeld & Nicholson).

[4] B. FRIEDAN (1981) *The Second Stage*, p. 229 (New York, Summit Books).

[5] I. BERLIN (1970) Two concepts of liberty, in: *Four Essays on Liberty* (Oxford, Oxford University Press).

[6] See, for example, R. SCRUTON op. cit.

[7] For example, J. MARGOLIS & C. MARGOLIS (1977) The separation of marriage and family, in: M. VETTERLING-BRAGGIN, F. A. ELLISTON & J. ENGLISH (Eds) *Feminism and Philosophy* (Totowa, N.J., Littlefield, Adams).

[8] See Is adultery immoral?, in: R. WASSERSTROM (Ed.) (1979, 1975) *To-day's Moral Problems* (New York, Macmillan).

[9] See M. WOLLSTONECRAFT (1954) *The Rights of Woman* (London, Dent) (first published 1792).

[10] *J. S. Mill and Harriet Taylor: essays on sex equality*, (1970) A. S. ROSSI (Ed.) (Chicago, University of Chicago Press).

[11] A facsimile of Mill's letter on his marriage to Harriet Taylor, dated 6 March 1851, is reproduced in R.FLETCHER (Ed.) (1973, 1971) *John Stuart Mill: a logical critique of sociology*, pp. 44–45 (London: Nelson).

[12] See E. WIESEL *Night* (New York, Bantam Books), first published in Farrar, Straus & Giroux edition, 1960.

[13] See S. DE BEAUVOIR (1985) *The Prime of Life* (London, Penguin), (first published in France as *La Force de l'Age*, 1960), in particular her account of her reactions to Sartre's suggestion that they marry, pp. 75–78.

[14] Plato: *The Republic*, Book V.

[15] But for comment on some of the complexities of this, see B. BETTELHEIM (1969) *The Children of the Dream* (London, Thames & Hudson).

[16] A. SKOLNICK (1978, 1973) *The Intimate Environment: exploring marriage and the family*, p. 54 (Boston, Toronto, Little, Brown).

[17] T. S. ELIOT *The Family Reunion* in: T. S. ELIOT (1962) *Collected Plays* (London, Faber).

[18] C. PATEMAN (1980) 'The Disorder of Women': women, love and the sense of justice, *Ethics*, 91, p. 32.

[19] J. & C. MARGOLIS op. cit., p. 297. For similar proposals see also R. W. LIBBY & R. M. WHITEHURST (Eds) (1977) *Marriage and Alternatives: exploring intimate relationships* (Glenview, Illinois, Scott, Foresman).

[20] J. & C. MARGOLIS op. cit., p. 299.

[21] P. GREGORY (1984) Against couples, *Journal of Applied Philosophy*, 1, p. 267.

[22] The course of deliberate uncoupling by partners is illuminatingly charted in D. VAUGHAN (1986) *Uncoupling* (New York, Oxford University Press).

[23] See M. SCARFE (1981) *Unfinished Business: pressure-points in the lives of women* (London, Fontana).

[24] Quoted in J. GAYTHORNE-HARDY (1981) *Love, Sex, Marriage and Divorce*, p. 173 (London, Cape).

[25] Ibid., p. 164.

[26] This research is particularly associated with Carol Gilligan. For her account of it, and for her view that there is a distinctive 'women's voice' on morality, see C. GILLIGAN (1982) *In a Different Voice: psychological theory and women's development*, (Cambridge, Mass, Harvard University Press).
Her view, and the wider issue, is also discussed in B. ALMOND Women's right: reflections on ethics and gender, in: M. GRIFFITHS & M. WHITFORD (Eds) (1987) *Feminist Perspectives on Philosophy* (Basingstoke, Macmillan).

8

Parental Rights

EDGAR PAGE

ABSTRACT *This paper is concerned with the philosophical foundations of parental rights. Some commonly held accounts are rejected. The question of whether parental rights are property rights is examined. It is argued that there are useful analogies with property rights which help us to see that the ultimate justification of parental rights lies in the special value of parenthood in human life. It is further argued that the idea of generation is essential to our understanding of parenthood as having special value and that parental rights properly belong, in the first instance, to natural parents.*

It is generally acknowledged that in the past children had the legal status of property. In early Rome, along with their mothers and slaves, they were used, sold or disposed of at the will of the head of the family, even to the point of death. In other societies it was allegedly common for unwanted infants to be 'exposed'—left to die. In England, long after the practice of exposure of infants ceased, children and their mothers remained the chattels of the father until comparatively recent times. Parental rights, then, were property rights residing in the father. The mother, being herself property, could have no such rights. Things have now changed. Because of the comparative emancipation of women and, in particular, the change in the legal status of a wife, a mother is now legally a parent and has the same parental rights as the father [1]. At the same time, no doubt because of these changes in the position of women but also, I suspect, because of changes in our general attitudes to human rights and to the ownership of people, and to slavery in particular, the position of the child has changed. Children are no longer legally the property of their parents, and we find it morally repugnant to think of them as property at all.

Clearly attitudes to children have changed. Whereas they were once to be seen and not heard, their voices cannot now be ignored. If they are unable or unwilling to assert their rights themselves there are others ready to do so on their behalf. The liberation of children from the tyranny of parents, schoolteachers and adults generally is well on the way. Their rights to decide where they live, who their friends shall be, when and with whom they shall have sex, for example, have yet to gain legal recognition, but there are signs that we shall not have too long to wait. In the meantime one consequence of both parents coming to have equal parental rights has been the emergence of the principle that the welfare of the child is paramount as the primary principle of equity in the courts [2], in cases involving disputes between parents, or between parents and the various authorities, over who shall have custody of the child, for example. (Under common law the wishes of the father would have been respected.) More questionably, those professionally concerned with children have taken the principle of the welfare of the child far beyond its legal origins, and many people not professionally concerned with children seem to accept without question that children must come first in matters of daily life. The result is that the moral if not the legal status of parents is being correspondingly diminished [3].

The picture emerging from this is one of conflict between parents and their children and between parents' rights and children's rights. This, I think, is a false picture. It focuses attention on parents in relation to their adolescent and developing children and suggests that parental rights are aimed at protecting parents in their desire to control or repress children, while children's rights are designed to protect children in their desire for freedom. With this picture it is little wonder that people, particularly young people, should question whether parents have any rights at all. Many who would not go this far accept that if parents do have rights, most if not all of these rights wane and disappear as the child develops into an adult person. I shall therefore confine my attention to the rights of parents in relation to infants, or babies, and this must be borne in mind throughout. This will exclude consideration of some traditional parental rights, e.g. rights to obedience, gratitude and special consideration, but there is no doubt that parents have other rights over young infants. These can have little to do with exercising control over wilful youngsters. What purpose or interest, then, do they serve?

Parental Rights and Parental Duty

A first response to this question might be that parents' rights must be designed to serve the interest of parents, because a right usually protects some actual or possible interest of the right holder. However, under the spell of the principle that the welfare of the child is paramount, people are loath to accept that parents could have any rights over the child designed to protect their own interests. For this reason it is often supposed that the purpose of parents' rights is to serve the interests of children, a view which can be developed in a variety of ways. For example, if the family is construed as an institution having the function or purpose of providing for the nurture and protection of children, parental rights will be seen as part of a system of rights and duties aimed at this purpose. Or, without reference to the family as an institution, it could be argued directly that parental rights are necessary for parents to carry out their duties and responsibilities to their children. I shall call this the argument from necessity [4].

This argument from necessity might appear to provide an adequate account of some of the commonly acknowledged parental rights, for example, the right to chastise, but it provides a poor account of others such as the right to determine the child's religion and the right to consent to medical treatment. In any case, it is doubtful how much freedom from external constraints and interference is really necessary for the fulfilment of parental duties. Foster parents have the duty to protect and provide nurture without having the benefit of the full range of parental rights. A foster-parent might be instructed to bring a child up to a particular religion or to speak a given language, to educate it in a given manner, to raise it as a vegetarian, and so on. It is conceivable that natural parents should have found themselves responsible for the nurture and protection of their children within a similar framework of constraints. (We already have compulsory education.) Could it be argued that such constraints would make it impossible for natural parents, but not for foster parents, to carry out their duties and responsibilities? Surely, such constraints would be resisted, not for this reason, but because they constitute an invasion of the natural parents' rights.

Another objection to the argument from necessity is that it cannot account for the right of natural parents to possess and raise their own children. It might be argued that natural parents have a duty to provide for their child, having brought it into the world, and that it is only because they have this duty that they have the right to possess and raise the child; and the right to possess the child, at least, does seem necessary if they are to fulfil their duty to protect and provide nuture. However, the right to possess and raise the child could be claimed by parents independently of any consideration of duty and even if they denied having a duty to look after the child, as they might if the child was grotesquely handicapped as a result of culpable negligence on the part of the doctor attending the mother during pregnancy, or if the child was conceived as a result of rape.

Parental Rights and the Welfare of the Child

Any account which bases parental rights on the need to protect and promote the welfare of the child will encounter difficulty in showing how those rights can be upheld when it is plain that denying them would be in the best interests of the child. Some people see no problem here and tend to regard parental rights as being subject always to the proviso that what parents do in the exercise of their special rights should be for the good of the child [5]. But no-one who takes parental rights seriously could accept such a proviso [6], for where rights exist it is a person's will that counts concerning the exercise of his rights, not whether there are reasons for or against [7]. We need to observe the distinction between what a person has a right to do and what he ought to do, or what it would be right for him to do. Sometimes people say that we have no right to do things because they feel strongly that we ought not to do them; for example, that a parent has no right, which he clearly has, to refuse consent to medical treatment for the child because they think the parent ought not to refuse it. Whether certain actions by parents will benefit or harm their child is certainly relevant to whether they ought to perform those actions, but not necessarily to the question whether, as parents, they have a right to perform them. Here we must remember that parental rights are those rights which people have simply *as parents*, not as *good* parents. Parents cannot properly be called on to justify the possession of the special rights they have, as parents, by showing that they act in the interests of their children when they exercise those rights.

But, it might be argued, parents are not normally required to justify the possession of their special rights, in the manner suggested, because there is a natural parental affection which makes it reasonable to presume that they will generally act in the best interests of their children [8]. So it will be a matter only of showing when parents forfeit their normal rights by not acting in the interests of the child. Some cases will be clear cases of forfeiture. In others, were there is doubt, it being a matter of speculation how the child's interests are affected or even where its interests lie, it will be argued that the matter must be left with the parents, this policy being best for the child, by and large. Proponents of this kind of argument will be inclined to refer to agreed cases where parental rights are overridden (often extreme cases such as child battering or serious neglect, involving grave harm or danger to the child) and say that the parents lose their rights because it is clear that they have acted contrary to the interests of the child.

However, this involves a misunderstanding of these cases where we agree that parental rights are overridden, or forfeited, and wrongly suggests that whenever it is *clear* that it would benefit the child, parental rights can be set aside. In those extreme cases where we do agree that parental rights are lost, it is surely the *severity* of the harm, or the *seriousness* of the danger, that sways us, not the fact that it is *clear* that some harm is done or that some danger exists. Parents must not seriously damage or endanger the wellbeing of their children and if they do, their special rights as parents will be overridden or otherwise rendered of no account. In general both morality and the law forbid us to do any significant harm to others, no matter what rights we have, and no-one has the right to assault, or to be cruel to, another person. All individual rights are subject to these limitations and parental rights are no exception. There are, of course, special grounds on which parental rights can be overruled. This is largely because children are peculiarly vulnerable to harm through neglect, incompetence and illtreatment. However, to say that parents lose their normal rights if they seriously harm or endanger their children is one thing. It is quite another to hold that these rights are lost whenever parents fail to act in the interests of their children, or that they can be set aside on the basis of general benefit to the child [9].

Giving general priority to the welfare of the child would have far-reaching consequences. Many infants could benefit from being removed from their natural parents and placed with suitable adoptive parents. Adoptions of this sort occur, but normally only with the consent of the natural parents. Yet such consent would not be necessary if the paramount consideration was the welfare of the child. On that principle a child could be removed against the explicit wishes of its parents, if it was clear that it would benefit from being removed, but few of us could countenance that. The legal requirement of parental consent for adoption is sometimes waived by the courts—that is, the parental right is overruled—most commonly when parents are in serious breach of their duties, but not on the ground of general benefit to the child. An interesting legal qualification is that consent must not be withheld by parents *unreasonably*. It is worth asking what unreasonable withholding of consent would be. In one such case that came before the courts a father who was in prison for the murder of his child's mother was ruled to have withheld his consent unreasonably [10]. This ruling might have been influenced by a moral attitude to the parent, but it is possible that the outlook for the child was considered so bleak that any *reasonable* parent would have given consent. This would fit the criterion of severe harm or serious danger to the child.

A widely acknowledged parental right is the right of parents to consent to medical treatment of their child, but it is difficult to see why parents should have this right if the welfare of the child is of first importance. Frequently doctors or others are in a better position than parents to judge what will benefit the child, yet they cannot ignore or overrule the parents' wishes. Parents often recognise their own limitations in this respect yet accept and insist that the decision is properly theirs, as parents. If general priority were given to the welfare of the child the decision would be the doctor's. Why then should it not rest with doctors, or medical authorities, or with those best equipped to judge the interests of the child? Surely the cynical view that parental consent here is a device to protect doctors cannot be the whole story [11].

Neither the idea that parental rights are necessary for the performance of parental duties nor the principle that the welfare of the child is paramount is of much help in explaining the right of parents to consent to medical treatment or in setting limits to this right [12]. It is interesting, however, to see how the principle of the welfare of the child might apply in the case of a parent deciding whether to consent to her child being vaccinated in a programme where it is known that some of the children vaccinated will suffer serious consequences from it. If the parent is guided by consideration for her own child's welfare she might rationally decide against vaccination (while hoping that the programme will be generally successful as that will reduce the risk of infection for her own child). On the other hand, if she is guided by the welfare of children generally, she might decide to consent to vaccination for her child even though this involves some risk of serious harm to it. It is her right to decide either way, of course, notwithstanding her duty as a parent to protect her own child.

This highlights a general difficulty involved in taking the principle of the welfare of the child beyond its legal setting in the courts where a particular child is involved and the principle holds that *that* child's welfare is to be put before the interests of other parties. Once we move out of the courtroom it is not so clear what could be meant by the principle. If we attend only to extreme cases, like those considered above, it may seem clear, but the example of the vaccination programme shows that there will sometimes be a question whether a particular child's welfare or the welfare of children generally should be put first. If we take the case where parents put their own child first and decide not to consent to vaccination, as is their right, should the parents be overruled on the ground that the welfare of children generally is paramount? It is difficult to see how we could resist this if we first allow the welfare of the parents' own child to override their parental rights. But now, why should we stop at the welfare of children? Why not the welfare of people? And if we move to the welfare of people generally, presumably the interests and wellbeing of the parents can be taken into account as well! It looks as if allowing general benefit to the child to override parental rights leads to the view that consideration of general utility can override these rights, which I presume was not the intention.

It is instructive to compare the parental right to consent to medical treatment for the child with the right of an adult person to consent to medical treatment for himself. Often adults are unable to judge whether they will benefit from a particular treatment, so why should it be for them rather than doctors or medical authorities to decide whether they should have the treatment or not? Here the explanation is plainly that the individual's right is grounded in a respect for persons as autonomous beings. The same regard for the autonomy of the individual lies behind the right of hunger strikers to refuse food. A person has a moral right to refuse treatment or nutrition even if his refusal will result in damage to his health, or in his death, so it would be implausible to suggest that this right is designed to protect his health or wellbeing. When someone is unable to consent for himself, for example, when he is unconscious, his next of kin has the right to consent to treatment for him. We respect his standing as a person by allowing his kin to decide his destiny for him, to take his place when he is unable to decide for himself. Again there is a parallel with comatose hunger strikers and the right of the next of kin to give or withhold consent to intravenous feeding.

However, we cannot argue that the parental right to consent to treatment for the child is founded on respect for the person and autonomy of the child. An infant is not yet an autonomous person. Furthermore, parents could not be said to decide for their child, in the sense of taking the child's place, which is the sense in which the next of kin can be said to decide for incapacitated adults. So it is difficult to see how the parental right to consent to treatment for the child could be based on respect or regard for the child itself. I shall argue that the rationale of his right and of parental rights generally is to be located in our respect, or regard, for parents themselves, or more correctly for parenthood and the characteristic interests and concerns of parents. This fits more satisfactorily than other accounts with the powerful intuitive idea that parents, rather than their children, are wronged when parental rights are invaded. No account would be satisfactory unless it could do justice to this idea.

Personal Rights

There is a strong temptation to account for parental rights as extensions of the personal rights of parents [13]. From the parents' point of view, an invasion of their parental rights will often seem to be a direct invasion of their individual privacy and liberty—for example, if they are denied the freedom to determine the religious education of their children. Religion inevitably bears on and includes the upbringing of children as an integral part of religious practice, so parents who are religious naturally think of their right to determine the religious education of their children as an aspect of their own freedom to practise the religion of their choice. Religion aside, the values and preferences of parents and their life-styles are bound to enter into the way they raise their children and to be passed on to them. Consequently, criticism of the way parents raise their children will often constitute criticism of their personal values and preferences and will amount to an invasion of their own private space.

However, personal rights do not give one the right to control the lives of other adults, nor does any extension of them give a right to control the lives of children generally, so if parental rights were to be accounted for as extensions of personal rights, a special explanation would be required of why these rights should give parents control over their own children [14]. Sometimes it is suggested that children are parts, or extensions, of their natural parents and that this is the reason why the personal rights of parents give them rights of control over their offspring. But this would be satisfactory only if children were literally parts, or extensions, of their parents, which they obviously are not. We must therefore reject the suggestion, in the spirit of J. S. Mill when he says, "One would almost think that a man's children were supposed to be literally, and not metaphorically, a part of himself, so jealous is opinion of the smallest interference with his absolute and exclusive control over them" [15]. But, although we cannot explain parental rights as extensions of personal rights, we must try to preserve what is of particular value in this suggestion—that is, the idea that a violation of parental rights is an injustice against the parent. We can preserve this feature by developing an account which shows that, just as personal rights have the point of protecting vital aspects of human existence, so parental rights have the point of protecting something of comparable value in parenthood. I shall offer such an account, but first we must examine the relation between parental rights and property rights.

Parental Rights and Property Rights

Most people jib at the idea that parental rights are property rights and even think it is self-evident that they are not—as if there were some kind of contradiction involved in the idea of it [16]. Yet it is widely accepted that in the past children were property. Part of the difficulty is that there is no agreed set of rights that define property [17], but traditionally property is said to carry the right of absolute control—the exclusive right of the owner to use, sell (or transfer) or dispose of his property as he wishes. With this in mind, let us ask what would justify saying children were property in the past, but are not now? We could expect an answer in terms of the difference between parental rights as they used to be and parental rights as they presently are. If, in ancient times, parents had exclusive rights to use, sell or dispose of their children even to the point of death (as with slaves), we would tend to agree that children (and slaves) were then property. Can we be as confident that presently acknowledged parental rights are not property rights? (We must remember that children are used—for example, as models—for gain, transferred in adoption, and possibly even sold.) Such rights still give parents a fundamental control over their children. It is not *absolute* control, but the so-called absolute control traditionally associated with property rights was never quite absolute. It was always subject to general limitations, e.g. on uses of property which were harmful to others, and in any case, more specific constraints are commonly imposed on what may be done with certain kinds of property. For example, cruelty to animals is forbidden, even if the animals are one's own property, and a prohibition on killing them would be possible without it affecting their status as property. There are restrictions on uses of land, bans on exporting or destroying works of art, and limits on the number of people who may live in a house of a given size, and so on. So even though parents may not now use, sell or dispose of their children as they wish, and therefore have less than absolute control over them, that alone will not show that parental rights are not property rights. The rights they have give them considerable control and arguably as much as owners have over some other forms of property.

We see the importance of control as an element of property in the now almost universal condemnation of slavery. The evil of slavery is more complex than is often supposed [18], but given no more than the excessive control or power that slave owners have over their slaves, no-one could rationally choose to be a slave, unless driven to it by the most unbearable circumstances, and the vast majority, by far, of humankind would strive to avoid such a fate. This lies at the root of the moral objection to slavery. However, there could be no similar objection to treating infants as property. There could be no question of a conflict between parental control and a rational, responsible will in the child. We cannot say of young children (or babies) that they would not or could not agree to their parents having control over them. Because they are not yet rational, autonomous beings—not yet fully persons—there is no question of them consenting or not consenting to anything.

Children as Ends in Themselves

Of course, infants are potentially rational, autonomous beings and our attitudes towards them are conditioned by this fact. We view infants as young persons who, every bit as much as adults, must, in Kant's phrase, be treated as ends, as having absolute value, and never simply as means [19]. Children have feelings and interests and the capacity for future development and well-being. They are not mere objects. This conception of babies or infants as having absolute value lies behind an argument that people sometimes want to bring—that parental rights are not property rights because infants are not property. There is a strong intuitive feeling that infants cannot be property because they have special worth or value, as people, and are not objects.

Kant suggested that if we are to treat people as ends, as having absolute value, we must ask whether they could agree to, or share in, the ends of our own actions [20]. This implies, at least, that we should have consideration, or regard, for the wishes and preferences, interests and well-being of others. Inanimate objects do not have wishes, preferences or interests, and it is plain that this notion of treating beings as ends could have no application to them. We can have consideration for the interests and well-being of animals so perhaps we could make sense of treating animals as ends; but it would be a restricted sense because animals could not be said to agree to or to share in the ends of our actions, and, at least with the animals most of us are likely to encounter, they could not be said to consent to what we might do. Whether adult people would or could rationally consent to the way we treat them is clearly important for whether we treat them as ends. But as we have noted, this cannot be a factor where we are concerned with infants. This is not to put children in the same position as animals, because in taking into account an infant's interests and well-being, we have regard for the fact that it will become an autonomous, rational being. However, it does mean that treating children as ends will not necessarily come to the same thing as treating adults as ends. Because infants are not yet rational, autonomous beings, parental control over them is not morally objectionable, as comparable control over adults would be, and is not incompatible with their having absolute value. Of course, the parental rights which give this control must be relinquished as the child approaches maturity. If they were *not*, there would be little doubt, I suggest, that parental rights in our society were property rights and that adult children were property (and without absolute value in the society), rather as adult children were allegedly the property of the *pater familias* in ancient Rome.

Be that as it may, the consideration that settles the matter for most people is that children cannot be bought and sold in our society. They would argue from this that children cannot be property. Children can be transferred, as in adoption, but they cannot legally be bought and sold. However, this prohibition on buying and selling children does not flow as a necessary consequence of children having absolute value, as ends in themselves. If adults could be bought and sold, as slaves used to be, this would be inconsistent with them having absolute value as ends, because it would constitute a denial of their individual autonomy. But this does not apply to infants because they are not autonomous beings. Consequently, there would not be the same inconsistency in holding, as we do, that children have special value as people and having laws which allowed children to be sold, say, during the first six weeks of life. No doubt there are good reasons why we do not have such laws. (For example, if we had such laws it might lead to the exploitation of women, who could be pressured into bearing children so that others might obtain financial rewards.) However, such reasons are extrinsic and give no support to the view that laws allowing the sale of children are excluded simply by the conception that children are people with absolute value. So it does not follow from the fact children have absolute worth in the society that they cannot be sold and are not property; nor does the mere fact that we do not allow children to be bought and sold, for extrinsic reasons, show that they are not property. A law forbidding, say, the sale of household pets would not affect the status of pets as property. (Such a law might have the point of protecting animals that have been made into pets.)

Despite the above considerations, we must recognise that people do not think of children as property and tend to resist all suggestion that they are. There are good practical reasons for this, stemming from the fact that there is no clear line separating children from adults. It is probably better to have a system under which the protection given to adults—e.g. the prohibition on buying and selling—is extended to infants, even though there is not the same direct reason for it, rather than risk uncertainty or inconsistency in our attitudes to developing children and young adults, and inadequate protection. I have no desire to persuade people to think of children as property, nor am I particularly concerned that we should call parental rights property rights. What is important is that if we do deny that parental rights are property rights, then the denial should not be taken to imply that parental rights are to be accounted for in some way quite other than the way in which we account for property rights. While there is perhaps little to be gained from assimilating parental rights to other property rights, there are certain analogies between them which repay attention. While it may be misguided, as I shall argue later, to say simply that parental rights are producers' rights, for example, it might yet be profitable to look for analogies between the rights that producers have and why they have them, on the one hand, and the rights that parents have and why they have them, on the other.

As we have noticed, there are no rights which are definitive of property. In practice, what property rights come to varies according to the kind of thing we are concerned with and, more importantly, the kind of interests that people have in that kind of thing. The owner of a house has the right to live in it, rent it or sell it; the owner of a donkey has the right to work it or make a pet of it; the owner of land has the right to cultivate it, to walk on it, to exclude others from it; and so on. These differences are to be accounted for by the fact that houses, donkeys and land feature in our lives in different ways. Here I do not have in mind differences arising from the fact that individuals differ in the interests they have, but rather that different kinds of objects elicit different ranges of interests. By and large, we can expect the specific rights that people have in a given kind of property to reflect the interests characteristically taken in that kind of object. Similarly we can expect parental rights to reflect the characteristic interests of parents in having children. Also, we can hope to make sense of the diversity of the special rights that parents have by reference to these parental interests.

The Motive of Parenthood

How then do infants feature in our lives? It is traditionally held that parents have a natural affection for their children—a general concern for their welfare and well-being. Now if we attend solely to this aspect of the parental interest we shall be inclined to look for an account of parental rights in terms of what rights are required if parents are to attend to the welfare of their children. In other words it will tend toward the kind of account that I was concerned to reject above, so we need to go beyond that. We need an account that shows how parenthood can enhance the lives of people more directly than is suggested by natural affection. Parenthood surely has a point and a value beyond responding to the needs of children, however satisfying that might be. So we need to identify a positive interest that shows parenthood to be desired for its own sake. As well as natural affection, parents have a positive desire to influence the course of a child's life, to guide the child from infancy to maturity, a desire to mould it, to shape its life, to fix its basic values and broad attitudes, to lay the foundations of its lifestyle, its priorities, its most general beliefs and convictions, and in general to determine, to whatever degree is reasonable and possible, the kind of person the child will become. It would not be going too far to say that parents have a general propensity to try to send their children forward in their own image, not in every detail, but in broad outline. It would be unusual for parents to be entirely indifferent to whether their children would come to share any of their most cherished values and ideals. There are people who have a conscious aim to avoid imposing their own attitudes and values on their children and there are those who would like their children to grow up to be different from themselves. But paradoxically, despite the desire not to direct the child's life, there is still a concern about the kind of person the child will become, a conception of what is to be preferred and a policy of a general kind for bringing this about or making it more likely.

The desire to shape the child and set it on a course is not a selfish interest of the parent. Clearly it is closely bound up with the parents' natural affection for the child and their concern for its good. We can normally expect parents to pursue their interest in shaping the child's future with a clear regard for its good. But this does not mean that the parental interest in shaping the child can be reduced to this affection. It must be recognised as a positive and natural interest of parents which exists in its own right. The propensity of parents to exercise control and guidance over their children, the propensity to determine the development of the child, far from being aimed simply or primarily at the child's good, is the manifestation of a fundamental and unique interest which lies at the heart of human parenthood and at the foundation of parental rights.

Given this characteristic parental interest, there is no difficulty in accounting for the range of rights that parents have—for example, the right to determine the religion and education of the child, to determine its values and lifestyle, the right to consent to medical treatment, the right of possession, and so on. These rights clearly reflect the natural parental interest, just as the specific property rights of the owners of animals, land, buildings and the like reflect the characteristic interests of people in those things. Here, then, is one analogy between parental rights and property rights. However, we can go further than this. Paradigmatic property rights are often taken to be self-evident, but there is a point where we need to look behind the alleged self-evidence to see what kind of foundations even these rights have. If we take producers' rights, for example, it is far from self-evident that producers in modern industrial society should have the rights commonly accorded to them. However, the primitive concept of producers is of people making things for themselves or for their immediate neighbours. Producing and consuming at this level constitutes a fundamental dimension of human life, the importance of which will be evident to anyone who tries to imagine what it would be like without it. I do not mean the life of an individual person, but human life in general. It enters into our conception of what it is to be a human being. Clearly, this aspect of human life is protected by the producers' rights we generally recognise and this, I suggest, constitutes the main part of the justification for them, although equally clearly it is a justification that could not be given for the rights enjoyed by the large scale producers of modern industrial society.

The Justification of Parental Rights

This brief argument for the justification of primitive producers' rights aims to show that they are necessary for the protection of a form of human activity that, in a very general way, is of fundamental importance for human life. Now it would be absurd to argue that parental rights are simply a particular instance of producers' rights. This would suggest that their justification lies in the fact that together with other producers' rights they protect the general range of activity referred to above. Rather, the justification of parental rights is that they are needed for the protection of parenthood and that parenthood is to be protected in this way as a distinctive form of activity with a special place in human life and among our basic values. It is essential to my argument that parenthood is seen to have special value *in itself* and not simply as a means to the care and protection of children and the continuation of the human race. This special value attaching to parenthood constitutes the ultimate foundation of parental rights.

Parenthood characteristically embraces a range of activities. (So I refer to it as a form of activity rather than as the state of standing in a certain relation to children.) Parenthood also has a characteristic point which is to be understood in terms of the characteristic parental interest described above. Now the question is whether parenthood really is worthy of being protected by a system of parental rights, as I am suggesting it is. What makes it so worthy or valuable a form of human activity?

It would be tempting to argue that parenthood is of special value because it enriches and enhances our lives, but I do not want to find myself in the position of having to persuade people who do not already believe it, that this is true. Fortunately, it is not necessary for me to do this. Ultimately, the proof that parenthood has a special place of value in human life is the fact that human beings have an overwhelming propensity to choose parenthood as a major ingredient in their lives. Of course, many people choose not to have children; some who bear children choose not to rear them, and some people have children not of their choosing and rear them because there is no alternative. Nonetheless, for the most part people choose parenthood. People characteristically want to have children and to bring them up, giving protection and providing for their needs, moulding and shaping their lives, laying the foundations of their attitudes, moral values, personal ideals, and so on. Furthermore, it is clear that this activity is characteristically desired for its own sake, as an end in itself. This is not to deny that people sometimes have children for external purposes. Obviously, people sometimes want children so that there will be someone to plough the land, or someone to inherit the family fortune; and for a monarch it may be urgent that there should be an heir to the throne. But although people can and do see other benefits and have children for external purposes, such external purposes and benefits are not necessary to make this common activity intelligible as something positively sought as a major ingredient in life.

It is evident that parenthood is generally thought to enhance human life and I am inclined to take it that it does. (This is not to assert or imply that people who do not become parents do not lead complete lives.) However, we must not think that parenthood has a special place in our basic values simply because it enhances the lives of those people who happen to be parents. If this were all we could say, there would be a question of why *their* interests should be specially protected. (We might all agree that artistic creation enriches the life of the artist, but we would not for that reason think that artists should be protected by special rights.) The reason why parents should have special rights is not to protect their individual interests, although of course their interests are involved, but to protect parenthood—and this means to protect parenthood as a condition of human existence, to protect the possibility of parenthood. It would be a severe deprivation if the possibility of parenthood as a general feature of life were lost. This is partly because the vast generality of people want to participate in parenthood. However, it is also because parenthood is a basic dimension of human existence which conditions and structures our perceptions and conceptions of ourselves and others, and thus affects all our lives whether or not we become parents.

We can draw an analogy between parenthood, as a common feature of human existence, and sexuality. Sexuality involves a certain characteristic range of activities, interests and experiences. It is something which enriches and enhances life and the vast majority of people have a propensity to choose a life which includes sexually rewarding relationships, although it is also plain that some people choose not to have such relationships and regard life without sex as preferable. Characteristically, sexual activity is sought for its own sake, rather than as a means to some further end, although of course it is often desired also as a means to parenthood, and no doubt sometimes for other purposes. However, not only does sexuality tend to enrich the lives of people through sexual relationships, it also conditions and structures our perceptions and our conceptions of ourselves and others. Clearly, sexuality is a basic aspect of human existence and human sexuality has a special place in our basic values. By and large it is not in need of protection by the recognition of special rights, although there are occasions when it is necessary to recognise and defend people's right to sexual relations of their own choosing.

Natural Parents

Something needs to be said on the question of why children belong to their natural parents. It is difficult to see why the fact of generation is of importance here. Some philosophers discount it altogether. Hobbes pays lip-service to it when he says that "in the condition of mere nature . . . it cannot be known who is the father, unless it be declared by the mother; and therefore the right of dominion over the child dependeth on her will, and is consequently hers". But his main theory is that the right rests with "him in whose power it is to save, or destroy [the child]" and not necessarily with the natural parent [21]. Locke thought the blood relation was of only sociological significance and that, so far as they are deemed to attach to *natural* parents, parental rights have no proper foundation [22]. Sometimes it is argued that parental rights are granted to natural parents because they are best able to provide for the interests of children, parental rights then being contingent on the fulfillment of parental duties [23]. Sometimes it is argued that the natural parent's claim is something to be explained in terms of the (contingent) facts of human reproduction, with the suggestion that if these facts were different or were to change the natural parent wold have no special claim [24]. On such views there is no *necessary* connection between parental rights and natural parents, which seems to me to be mistaken. On my own account, parental rights have their justification in the protection they give to parenthood as a distinctive form of human activity and, ultimately, in the special value of parenthood. So, if natural parents enjoy a special position with respect to parental rights, we can expect it to be because the biological relation is somehow vital to parenthood, or to the special value of parenthood. I am inclined to think this is the case and that if the right of natural parents to possess and raise their own children were seriously threatened, this would undermine the possibility of parenthood as the valued activity that it is. (This is quite apart from the special form of suffering that would be inflicted on natural parents whose children were taken from them.)

Many people find this difficult to accept. They may be willing to concede a special value of parenthood but think of it as an activity which need not be founded on a biological relation between parent and child. Adoptive parents, they would argue, are parents in the only sense that matters, at least, and they can be as caring and involved in the upbringing of their children as natural parents are, often more so. What difference does it make then, that they are not the biological parents of the child? What difference would it make if they were the biological parents? These questions are difficult to answer. Certainly adoptive parents can develop the same affection for the child, and they can want to mould and shape its life and set its values and life style as much as any natural parent might. So it looks as if it is perfectly possible for people who are not natural parents, or not the natural parents of the child, to experience and enjoy parenthood and to have full access to whatever value it holds. And it could be argued further that we can conceive of possible worlds—'science fiction' worlds—in which *in vitro* technology has severed the connection between parenthood and physical generation altogether.

It cannot be formally demonstrated that the biological relation is an essential or important element of parenthood. It would be pointless, for example, to argue that the physical relation is implied in the very notion of parenthood, or that the word 'parent', taken strictly, means 'biological father or mother', because we are not concerned with the meanings of words, but rather with the nature of parenthood as a valued feature of the world. A more promising approach would be to argue from certain general principles such as the following:

> *P1.* Property owners own or otherwise have rights of control over whatever issues from their property, or over any parts which might become detached from it
>
> *P2.* People own or are otherwise entitled to the benefits of what they make, produce or create.
>
> *P3.* People are responsible for and are entitled to the benefits of what flows from their own voluntary acts.

I shall not discuss these principles and their application to our question in detail. P1 and P2 have certainly been used in attempts to show that natural parents have a right to possess and raise their offspring. P3, perhaps, is more often drawn on to argue that natural parents have responsibilities, obligations and duties to the child, but I see no reason why it should not also be used to argue for the existence of their rights. Something needs to be said about P1 because any argument for parental rights based on it would require the premiss that people own their own bodies. Although philosophers [25] sometimes take this premiss for granted, it is far from unproblematic, if only for the conceptual reason that we cannot independently identify the owners (ourselves) and that which is owned (our bodies.) However, there seems to be wide agreement that parts of the body like hair, teeth, blood, organs, and even sperm and ova, are owned by those from whose bodies they are taken. If it is not accepted that these parts are owned as property, it is certainly recognised that those from whom they are taken have important rights over them. Consequently, a general unifying principle something like P1 sems to be involved. If it is, there is no obvious reason why it should not be applied to natural parents and their progeny. A reason that will be given—that here we are concerned with children—would not iself be a good reason, as our earlier discussion showed.

These principles and possibly others like them carry some weight but they are far from conclusive and they are unlikely to persuade those opposed to the view that natural parents have a special claim over their offspring. The reason they fail is not that they have no application, but that they do not take us to the heart of the matter. They are external principles and therefore do not and could not show what it is about parenthood that results in natural parents having special rights, which is what is required. For this we must attend to the nature of parenthood itself. However, I have argued above that parenthood is an activity which is characteristically desired for its own sake and has intrinsic value. In that argument I was at pains to reveal the internal motive of parenthood as being a positive desire of parents to mould and shape the child and set it forth in their own image. This errs, possibly, in suggesting that the motive of parenthood relates to parents only when they already have children. To correct this, the motive of parents in their procreative role must be brought to the fore. We need to consider the motive *to* parenthood, or the desire *for* it. The desire for parenthood is not a desire simply to *have* children, in the sense of acquiring and possessing them, procreation being the most usual means to this end. It is a positive desire to *produce* children—a desire which reaches beyond mere physical reproduction. But really this does not go far enough. The motive, or the end, of parenthood is surely the creation of a whole person [26], and this takes within its grasp both the begetting and the raising of the child. Obviously, it includes the motive as previously described.

The parental aim is not simply the creation of a person, but rather the creation of a person in the parents' own image. There are two aspects to this. One aspect is that in raising their child parents do much to shape the person it will become. This they would do in any case, even if it were not part of their design, but I have argued that parents characteristically have a positive desire to determine the kind of person their child becomes. The other aspect is that natural parents produce from their own bodies the material to be shaped, the organism that is to become a person. Now it would be impossible to do justice to the importance of this latter aspect without taking into account heredity and our common knowledge and belief that a child inherits characteristics from its parents. In one way or another this has been a part of the common understanding throughout the ages. It enters into our general understanding of what parenthood is and into our understanding of the relation that exists between parents and their children. It enters, also, into the way individual parents perceive their children in relation to themselves—seeing in them the continuity of something of themselves [27]. This is a vitally important aspect of the intentionality of parenthood. Unfortunately, it smacks of the ideology of blood, much of which is rightly dimissed as superstition and misguided folklore. However, we must not allow this to turn us away from the plain fact that nature contributes to the shape of succeeding generations through genetic inheritance. Of course, this does not mean that parents can take credit for a felicitous genetic inheritance in their offspring or be held responsible for an infelicitous one. Nor can this physical relation alone constitute a basis for parental rights over the child. But it is clearly important for how parents perceive themselves and are perceived by others, as producers, in their procreative role, and it is bound to affect the way they understand and interpret the subsequent mental and physical development of their child. Now this is important for two different reasons. On the one hand it forms an important part of the characterisation of parenthood under which it is desired and, therefore, under which it has special value in human life. On the other hand, it has an important place in the distinctive relation that exists between parents and their children.

Perhaps the most important aspect of this relation is the special bond between parents and their children and an account of parenthood would be incomplete if it failed to say something about the nature of this bond. It is widely acknowledged that one of the most powerful and deeply felt of human sentiments is the protective affection of parents for their offspring. This suggests that the parental bond with the child is to be distinguished from other relations by the strength of the feelings involved. No doubt this strength of feeling is a factor, but it is a factor to be accounted for, not one in terms of which the relation can be explained. These powerful emotions cannot be regarded as spontaneous eruptions or as instinctive responses of the kind manifest in the behaviour of many animals. Human parents have a commitment to their children and an acceptance of them, for better or for worse, as the children that they produced or created. It is the nature of this commitment that is distinctive in the special relation of parents to their children.

We might be inclined to think of it as an emotional commitment or as a commitment of the will and, certainly, both of these are likely to be involved in the normal parent/child relationship. But a commitment of this kind could be sorely tested by an infant that proves to be less than the perfect child that was expected. If the child turns out to be less intelligent, less beautiful or less healthy than could have been expected, or defective, or if it has an unpleasant disposition, the parents might understandably become resentful and less committed to the child. I say 'understandably' because emotional commitments and commitments of the will are inherently likely to be eroded, or weakened, when subjected to this kind of strain. Of course, a commitment would not be worthy of the name if it could not withstand some test of this kind, but a commitment founded on a decision of the will or on affection will have its breaking point. Now one of the most important facts about the parent/child relation is precisely that, characteristically, the parents' commitment to the child, their acceptance of it for what it is, the bond between them and it, does not yield under this kind of strain. This is part of what was meant when I said it was a commitment and acceptance *for better or worse.*

If we consider the position of adoptive parents who, as we have acknowledged, commonly have an emotional attachment to their child equal to that of natural parents, it is difficult to see how their commitment to the child can be accounted for except in terms of a commitment of the will, reinforced by an emotional commitment probably developed over a period of time. As we have seen, this kind of commitment has an inherent vulnerability. However, more importantly, in their thoughts if not in their deeds, adoptive parents could turn to returning or replacing the child, for this is in principle a possibility for them. It is not a possibility for natural parents, not even in principle, for their child is not one 'off the shelf'. It is ineluctably theirs. The difference is not a difference of emotional responses, nor is it simply that in the one case but not in the other there is a physical, genetic relation, although that is an essential part of it. It is rather that, built around the physical relation, is a framework of thought within which natural parents are conceived of as having a positive creative role which sees the begetting and rearing of children as parts of a single process. And, as I have argued, their creative role is directed to the production of a child or person in their own likeness in whom they see the continuity of 'something of themselves'. It is this conceptual framework that contains the aspect under which parenthood is desired and has special value in human life. And it is through this framework that the distinctive parental bond with the child and acceptance of it, for better or worse, is to be understood. If all parents were in the position of adoptive parents, i.e. if there were no connection between parenthood and generation, as might be imagined in 'science fiction' worlds, parenthood would not have a place of special value in human life, or not the place it now has. Adoptive parenthood is modelled on natural parenthood and the commitment of adoptive parents to the child is parasitic on the special bond characteristic of natural parents. Without this model there would be a question as to the intelligibility of a commitment by adoptive parents' to young babies, particularly in conditions which severely test them, and indeed as to the intelligibility of their desire for parenthood. (Would it be comparable to the desire for pets?) For most people, I suspect, adopting a child falls short of being a perfect substitute for natural parenthood, but when they undertake it they can at least borrow from and follow the established patterns and practice and attitudes of parenthood grounded on the physical relation. It is difficult to know what adoptive parenthood would be without this.

In conclusion, then, the begetting and rearing of children must be taken as forming a single process and therefore must both be included in whatever understanding of parenthood is invoked to explain the nature and foundations of parental rights. Earlier in the paper I argued that parenthood is something that is valued for its own sake, and that it is because of its special value that it is protected by a system of parental rights. An important part of the argument was the recognition of the positive desire, characteristic of parents, to influence the child's development and fashion the person it will become. I argued that the range of specific rights that are generally accorded to parents can be made intelligible through recognition of this motive to parenthood and only in this way. We now see that the parental motive, or desire, was incompletely described at the earlier stage, in that it did not give a sufficient place to the procreative role of parents, although it did not exclude it. Having now put this role of parents firmly at the centre of the account we have in fact strengthened it. The two parts—begetting and rearing—are clearly complementary to each other and neither is entirely intelligible, as a form of human activity, without the other. Taken together they form a whole, *parenthood*, which is immediately intelligible as something to be desired for its own sake, as something having a special place in human values and as something to be protected by a system of parental rights.

Finally, I would like to note that much of the above will make disagreeable reading to radical feminists to whom it will seem that, far from choosing parenthood, women have had it forced upon them over the ages. Far from seeing parenthood as something of value to be preserved and protected, they would tend to regard it, along with the institution of the family, as a vehicle for the oppression of women [28]. There is also a long tradition of socialist thought that calls for the dissolution of the family as a necessary means to achieving equality for women and children [29]. Radical socialists tend to see the nuclear family as an institution designed to serve the interests of capitalism and to regard family values, including parental rights, as mere products of the dominant capitalist ideology. These views raise important issues which I could not hope to deal with here, although I would like to think that I am not merely bolstering up the capitalist system in this paper. Perhaps the key questions are:

(a) Could parenthood and a system of parental rights exist in a socialist society?

(b) Is parenthood as described in this paper compatible with equality for women (and children)?

I am strongly inclined to say it would be a sad outlook for socialism and feminism, both of which I support, if the achievement of their aims were dependent on the abolition of parenthood and the dissolution of the family. I cannot envisage a time when people generally will not choose to beget and rear children in the normal, natural way. So it seems to me that parenthood and the family in some form are here to stay. However, a radical change in the family is possible without this necessarily undermining parenthood. The ideal family need not remain the self-sufficient, economically independent social unit that is so well suited to capitalist interests. It is also important to take into account the fact that the precise form that the system of parental rights takes, and the detailed content of those rights, will depend on the social and political context in which they exist. The wider interest of society and the existence of other rights may legitimately place some limits on the extent of parental rights. We see this already with compulsory education for children.

Edgar Page, Department of Philosophy. University of Hull, Hull HU6 7RX, United Kingdom.

NOTES

[1] Since 1925, in England. *Vide* BROMLEY, T.M. (1981) *Family Law*, 6th edn (London, Butterworth), pp. 340f.

[2] The Guardianship of Infants Act (1886) and a further Act of 1925 were significant in this development. Cf. Bromley op. cit., p. 340. On the principle of the welfare of the child, see ERKELAAR, J.M. (1973) *Law Quarterly Review*, 89, pp. 210–234.

[3] This is not an entirely new theme. H. G. Wells observed, in 1906, that "the old sentiment was that the parent owned the child, the new is that the child owns the parents". Wells, H.G. (1906) *Socialism and the Family* (London), p. 31.

[4] Cf. COHEN, BRENDA (1981) *Education and the Individual* (London, Allen & Unwin), p. 29. A claim that, in general, one has a right to do what is necessary for the fulfillment of one's duty is made by McCLOSKEY, H.J. (1965) Rights, *Philosophical Quarterly*, 15, p. 121.

[5] Cf. GUTMANN, AMY (1980) Children, paternalism and education, *Philosophy and Public Affairs*, 9, p. 344.

[6] Cf. Ronald Dworkin's general point that to allow rights to be overruled on grounds of general benefit is to annihilate those rights. DWORKIN, RONALD (1977) *Taking Rights Seriously* (London, Duckworth), ch. 7, p. 194.

[7] Here I borrow a phrase from Philippa Foot's 'Euthanasia', rpr. in FOOT, P. *Virtues and Vices* (Oxford, Blackwell), p. 47.

[8] Cf. Gutmann, op. cit., p. 344.

[9] Cf. Bromley, op. cit., p. 311.

[10] A case referred to by TEICHMAN, JENNY (1982) *Illegitimacy* (Cornell University Press), p. 37.

[11] Cf. WOOZLEY, A.D. Euthanasia and the principle of harm; rpr., RACHELS, J. (Ed.) *Moral Problems*, 3rd edn, p. 502.

[12] R. Wasserstrom suggests parents would have a "right to have their consent secured before any fetal experimentation occurs" on an aborted fetus. Neither duty to the child nor consideration for its welfare could account for this. WASSERSTROM, R. The status of the fetus, rpr. in Rachels, op. cit., p. 126.

[13] Cf. FRIED, CHARLES (1978) *Right and Wrong* (Cambridge, Mass.), pp. 152–154. Fried argues that parental rights are extensions of personal rights. His view is criticised by Gutmann, op. cit., pp. 345f.

[14] Substantially the same point is made by Gutmann, op. cit., pp. 345–346.

[15] MILL, JOHN STUART *On Liberty* (Bobbs-Merrill), ch. V. p. 128. Aristotle refers to parents loving their children as parts of themselves; *Nichomachean Ethics*, 1161ᵇ17.

[16] Gutmann takes it for granted that children are not property. She says "we know that parents do not own their children," but gives no indication of how we know it. Gutmann, op. cit., p. 34.

[17] Cf. BECKER, LAWRENCE (1977) *Property Rights* (Henley, Routledge & Kegan Paul), pp. 18–23.

[18] Cf. PATTERSON, ORLANDO (1982) *Slavery and Social Death* (Harvard University Press).

[19] Cf. KANT, IMMANUEL *Groundwork of the Metaphysic of Morals* in PATON, H.J. (Trans.) *The Moral Law* (New York, Barnes & Noble), p. 96.

[20] Ibid., p. 97.

[21] HOBBES, THOMAS (1947) *Leviathan* (Oxford), p. 131.

[22] LOCKE, JOHN *Second Treatise of Government*, ch. VI.

[23] Cf. Gutmann, op. cit., p. 344.

[24] Cf. Charles Fried, loc. cit.

[25] E.g. JARVIS THOMSON, JUDITH A defense of abortion, rpr. in Rachels, op. cit., pp. 136–137. The premiss is discussed by Becker (op. cit., pp. 36f.) in connection with Locke's theory of property. He considers the use of it to derive parental property rights in children. A. M. Honoré says we do not own our bodies: Ownership, in: GUEST, A.G. (Ed.) *Oxford Essays in Jurisprudence*, pp. 129–130.

[26] I have been helped here and in many other places by Dilys Page.

[27] Cf. MELDEN, A.I. *Rights and Persons* (Oxford, Blackwell), p. 75.

[28] Here I am indebted to Kathleen Lennon. She also referred me to the interesting book, BARRETT, MICHELE & McINTOSH, MARY (1982) *The Anti-Social Family* (Verso).

[29] Cf. H. G. Wells, op. cit., pp. 56f; MARX, KARL & ENGELS, FREDERICK *The Communist Manifesto* (New York, International), pp. 26–27. But note the target is often the *bourgeois* family.

9

Against Couples

PAUL GREGORY

ABSTRACT   *The essay attacks the convention that a person should at any period in their life have not more than one sexual partner. The issues of the care of children and the desirability of a shared household are here bracketed out. The main argument proceeds by seeing conflicts between the requirement of exclusivity in sexual life, authenticity, and the principle that sexual communion should be an expression of love. A general social inertia, defined by the possessive introversion of couples, means that individuals will inevitably sometimes have to choose between sexual solitude and cultivating a more or less artificial relationship. The ideal of a single, central relationship is criticised on the grounds that (i) in some respects it is not desirable and (ii) it is in any case unrealistic to suppose that we can choose to create such an ideal relationship at will.*

In which contexts is sexual interchange held to be appropriate? What are the reasons given for these restrictions and how good are those reasons? In the West there have been three broadly accepted requirements for the sanctioning of sexual activity. The relationship within which sex takes place has been required to be permanent, exclusive and loving. Of these, the requirement of permanence has now been considerably relaxed, but the other two remain strong. Casual sex is generally rejected, at least in the sense that few if any would see it as a satisfactory approach to the long-term shaping of their sexual lives. In the following I shall challenge the reasons variously given in defence of the principle of exclusivity and examine how this principle fits in with the demand that the sexual relationship be one of love. More specifically, I shall argue that insistence on the exclusive nature of sexual relationships will tend to militate against full and authentic friendships between persons of different sexes and even result in the one central sexual relationship losing out on the singularly personal love which is supposedly its *raison d'être*.

I By the requirement of exclusivity I mean the principle that as long as any given relationship lasts the two partners should not enter into sexual relations with third persons. When asked why they uphold this restriction, most people will either reply that they feel no desire to sleep with people other than their partner, or they will explain that there is a bond of trust between the two of them and that unfaithfulness would hurt the other, possibly endangering their relationship. This of course begs the question of why it should hurt the other. Usually reference is made here to the peculiar nature of sexuality. Now it may be that there is something about sexual experience such that certain restrictions are appropriate, but if it is to justify our conventions that something needs spelling out. After all, in other cultures people uphold sexual mores which are very different from our own.

Many of the reasons given for our traditional norms have to do with the need to provide a common household for the care of the children issuing from the relationship. But modern contraceptive methods mean that our sexual life is no longer inextricably bound to the need to plan for children. (Apart from this, it is not self-evident that conventional family structures provide the only satisfactory setting for children to grow up in.)

Once the procreative aspect of sexual life has been bracketed out, there are few arguments, as opposed to appeals to tradition and intuition, in favour of the requirement of exclusivity. The one coherent defence I have been able to isolate rests on the idea that individuals need a central personal relationship so as to give their lives a certain focus. The sexual act is then variously understood as a symbol, a sacrament, or even simply as a cohesive force for the union within which it takes place. On this view, additional sexual involvement would detract from the unique status of the privileged relationship and so deprive the sexual act of its special meaning. This argument tends to support the principle of permanence as well as that of exclusivity.

The most obvious doubts that can be raised here concern the nature and the desirability of the relationship involved. There is also a general question as to whether the alleged need is universal and what might be meant by maintaining that it is a need. Possibly it is thought that it should be a need, but that would be to beg the question. There would at any rate seem to be people who, whilst feeling no special need for a single, central relationship, nonetheless do experience sexual desires and needs. And even if everyone should come round at some point in their lives to the conventional perspective, this does not necessarily prove that it is right or best.

To what extent is an all-encompassing personal relationship actually desirable? It is not in dispute here that people have (or at least, should have) a need for close friendship and companionship. But if we accept that there are many facets to each personality, then it must seem appropriate that a person should seek out a number of close friends, of both sexes, whose various strengths and sensibilities accord with the diverse aspects of his or her personality. Too great an attachment to a single relationship must normally involve the neglect of some and maybe of many of these facets. In any life there is of course neglect of some possibilities for the sake of others. But any consequent gain must be weighed against what is lost. (We are forced to measure things that seem incommensurable.) If we accord real respect to the many-sidedness of the human personality, then people would seem to have a need for a number of intimate friendships. Where this need is to a greater or lesser extent ignored, certain resonances will be lacking; the relationship for whose sake others are left untended can for its part turn into a routine. The security offered by constant companionship might be bought at the price of inertia and mediocrity. This does not have to happen, but the danger is not slight.

Nevertheless, it may seem that people have need of a unifying focus in their lives, and even of the feeling that they are for some other this focus. But are we free to choose whether our lives provide us with any such centre of gravity? And granted that we find a person who can be this focus, and whom we therefore claim to need unconditionally, do we not thereby accord to loss or rejection extreme dimensions such that they can hit at our very sense of meaning in life?

Perhaps, however, it is less an all-encompassing relationship that people need than a central friendship to whose continuing growth they make a special commitment. But what is the nature of that commitment? Why should it imply a monopoly over their sexual lives? Are there other areas of their lives over which it claims a monopoly? If the commitment means that the partners live together and share their possessions, then a limited case can be made for their restricting their sexual lives to this relationship, although even here there remains ample room for viewing the matter differently. But how is it when those involved choose a different life-style and live separately, whether alone or in a household together with others, i.e. third persons? The specialness of the central relationship begins to look artificial. The sexual act does not seem (does not tend) to be limited to the privileged union because that friendship is, for those involved, uniquely central at that moment in their lives; but the relationship is unique because it is their one friendship with a sexual dimension. Yet if the sexual act is to be understood as expressive, there must be something (other than itself) for it to be expressive of. Now if it is to be expressive of intimate friendship there is no reason why it should not be extended to other relationships where there is intimate friendship. Or is it to be maintained that further friendships of comparable intimacy are not possible? But how might this be so? Is it a matter of the proportion of time that can then be devoted to any one of the relationships? Or is it that people are psychologically incapable of devoting such affection to more than one of their fellow beings? The received wisdom will probably reply both. But it is surely wrong to suppose that one worthwhile relationship requires so vast a proportion of our time and energy that little is left over for others. And it would be naive to assume that those who cultivate a number of friendships thereby necessarily lose out on quality. Such crude calculations have no place here. After all, parents do not decide against having more than one child on the grounds that this would diminish the share of affection each child would receive.

This said, it does nevertheless occur that people are so in love with each other that there really is no room for a second relationship of comparable intensity and intimacy. This state of extreme passion is, however, virtually always temporary. If the relationship persists there is a change in the quality of the friendship; the jealous intensity which people experience when in love mellows as what was exceptional becomes normality. It is important we distinguish between ordinary affection and intimacy, on the one hand, and, in contrast to this, the extreme fascination by another that occurs when in love. Not everybody experiences love as an all-consuming passion, and, even for those who have experienced love in this way, such erotic passion (as I prefer to call the experience of being in love) generally remains an exception.

II I come now to the ways in which the prevailing norms tend to work against the free play of the personality. These norms generate a basic inertia which results in what we might call failures of distribution and redistribution. It is inevitable that many people will often find themselves badly matched or without a partner. The extent of this will reflect the measure in which individuals set real store by the specialness of the person they choose as a companion for their sexual and emotional life. How exactly does this come about?

I assume that it is in general important that a person should enjoy some sexual fulfillment and that there should be a high degree of compatibility and natural sympathy between sexual partners. Now in a society where people are paired off into exclusive couples, the more people commit themselves in this way, so the more restricted is the choice of those who remain uncommitted. In order to find some sexual fulfillment and emotional security people must settle for the best person they find (and are accepted by) rather than wait. Some are now bound to find themselves in a relationship they are less than happy about, and others will be alone. These imbalances can be partly overcome if people are able to meet others who are unattached fairly easily and naturally; and, of course, they must see that the demands they make of a prospective companion are sufficiently modest. But in fact it is not always easy to meet people one knows to be unattached in settings which allow for real spontaneity; and meeting and getting to know person after person must take up time and much emotional energy.

Still, provided that a person is not too demanding in what he or she seeks in a prospective partner, they can, given perseverence, find someone. But is it good that people should be constrained to reduce their demands in respect of the person with whom they are to have so very special a relationship? Is there not something artificial about cultivating a relationship simply because one needs someone to fulfill a certain role? And we should not close our eyes here to the extent to which this role is at least initially a sexual and a social one. (There is for the satisfaction of purely emotional needs comparatively wide scope within our social structures. But our society also creates, or at least encourages, a need to belong to and possess another exclusively. This is not necessarily a sexual need, although that is the subject of the present essay. It can be primarily a social and psychological need involving the desire to think of oneself and be seen as integrated within what is society's standard unit amongst adults, i.e. to be a member of a couple.)

In a world which was as if prearranged for us, where as in a fairy tale each person eventually found the other (or an other) he or she was ideally suited to, the value conflict outlined above would not arise. In any other world it must arise, although not for everyone. Generally it will be those who are most sensitised towards the central values of our culture who will both be subject to and feel the conflict most acutely. They will be forced either to jettison one value or another, or else to engage in a pretence or self-deceit. For example, in order to maintain a relationship, it may be necessary to pretend to harbour a sentiment of love when in fact what one feels is something much less intense and exceptional than love.

Apart from the compromise it implies for the authentic self, the ethic of exclusivity suffers from the more tangible failing that it must militate against new friendships. One way in which this can happen is that people are understandably reluctant to venture on any new relationship when this immediately puts in danger their current one. This hesitation need not indicate that they are happy about their present companion; it might mean merely that they do not wish to risk the insecurities and uncertainties which a fresh commitment must involve when this also means abandoning all that is good in their old relationship. There may also be moral reasons for their reluctance: the partner they are tempted to leave might suffer real hurt. The obvious solution to the dilemma—the pursuit of a fresh friendship whilst retaining the old—is ruled out precisely because of the prevailing norms. (These norms make themselves manifest in the jealousy which is provoked when someone has two sexual partners. The requirement of exclusivity is, of course, often defended by reference to this danger of jealousy. But is it not nearer the truth to say that the traditional norms encourage and justify jealousy? As has already been indicated, a person has in our culture good reason to fear sexual loneliness. Apart from this, people feel themselves to be morally in the right to feel jealousy: the ethic of exclusivity tells them that they have a right to an exclusive claim on their partner.)

A further cause for the hesitation which typically precedes fresh sexual involvements, and therefore inhibits the development of new friendships, is the fear people understandably have about making a commitment which can only be gone back on with difficulty.

The dominant ethic also militates against new friendships in that a person can hesitate to form a friendship with someone they know to be attached on account of the distress which might ensue if they should develop real affection for the person concerned, in consequence want to give sexual expression to their feelings, and subsequently face rejection and frustration. (Much of the sexual rejection that takes place is not a result of authentic disinclination but a consequence of complex anxieties born of the dominant ethic. There is here also the factor of individuals coming to desire of themselves the fidelity that society expects of them.) It is an indictment of traditional conventions that close friendships between people of opposite sex are comparatively rare.

Do not see these problems as inherent in the human condition. They are a direct consequence of an inflexible approach to a certain kind of friendship. In a society where people formed friendships with a sexual dimension in the same sort of way in which they now form other friendships these problems would not arise. As things stand, however, our sexual lives fail to go hand in hand with our friendships, our love and the alchemy of erotic attraction.

III In the preceding, I have placed great emphasis on the value of the individual personality and argued that this is often incompatible with the commitment to a single person which is prescribed by the traditional ethic. Against this, it is sometimes maintained that what counts is not the personality of the chosen person but the decision which is made to cultivate a special relationship with this person. (Note that here again the argument for an exclusive relationship cannot be readily distinguished from the argument for a permanent relationship.)

There is certainly an element of truth in this emphasis on the fact of making a commitment rather than on the object of the commitment. We can perhaps see this point at its clearest if we consider how things stand when someone is urged to choose a profession. It is sometimes incidental which profession they choose; what is important is that a choice is made. Some of the personal relationships which we cherish most are those which we have not, properly speaking, freely chosen, but which we have found ourselves living and relating in—think here of the ties between brothers and sisters. What can be important in a friendship is that those involved have spent a lot of time together. But obviously this is not always the case; and time and companionship are not the whole story. These things do not lend themselves to calculation, and devotion to a formula is neither a sufficient nor a necessary condition for the meeting of minds and lives which we seek in personal love.

IV Our society (our culture) has relaxed the requirement of permanence, but not that of exclusivity. It is indeed by reference to the principle of exclusivity that that of permanence is waived; (divorce is legal; polyandry and polygyny are not). Where other friendships die gently over time and distance, those with a sexual dimension tend to end more or less abruptly: when sexual interchange ceases, so too does the whole relationship. Yet it is not that the emotional ties have vanished overnight. They may, however, be too tightly interwoven with sexual desires for the one or the other partner to bear willingly the encounter where such desires must be suppressed. And one possible reason why they must be suppressed is that a new relationship, with its own exclusive demands, has made its entry. (In other cases, the total collapse of a relationship might simply reflect the fact that for one or both of the partners it was all along only a sexual relationship.)

The logic of the preference our culture gives the principle of exclusivity is that it is better to abandon a person with whom one has built up an intimate relationship than it is to have and express feelings of love and erotic attachment to two persons. Yet in the first case love is withdrawn completely, whereas in the second there is exactly no withholding of love.

V We have seen that the justifications available for the principle of exclusivity do not hold good. This is in part because certain biological, material and social factors have changed, and in part because the values implicit in the conventional way of thinking involve contradictions. Some people will inevitably find themselves trapped by this conflict of values, although they may well not see clearly what is happening. There is a vicious circle of sexual loneliness and possessive claims.

Possessiveness and jealousy are aroused when one person's (exclusive) claim on another is threatened or thought to be threatened. This kind of response is sometimes seen as a proof of love; it is in fact a sign of fear. In so far as it is allowed to overrule other values (of openness, authenticity, love), the principle of exclusivity aims at containing anxiety: where people are sure that their partner will be 'faithful' they can tolerate a degree of freedom which they might otherwise find unbearable. But this artificial exclusion of certain sexual developments has two negative consequences. Certain friendships with a high promise of emotional attachment must be avoided. And there must for some people be a problem of the availability of sexual partners with whom more than a superficial emotional involvement is possible.

The sum of these two consequences is that the individual is prevented from relating to certain others fully and authentically. An individual rebellion is not possible because it would take the guise of deceit or of disregard for the feelings of one's sexual partners. The conflict can, however, be lessened (albeit by no means resolved) where partners agree not to insist on each other's adhering to the principle of exclusivity.

Such a decision only becomes effective, of course, when it is shared by others. And not all who are persuaded of the logic of the case against exclusivity will be inclined to try to give up the sort of claims they have previously made: patterns of feeling and relating cannot be unlearnt by the work of reason alone. As long as people are happy with their situation they will quite naturally and understandably stay put. It is where individuals are faced in their emotional and sexual relationships with a crisis or a questioning that a clear appreciation of what is happening can help; and, perhaps, liberate.

Paul Gregory, Reichsbahnstr. 27, D–2000 Hamburg 54, West Germany.

10

Love and Lust Revisited: intentionality, homosexuality and moral education

J. MARTIN STAFFORD

ABSTRACT   *In his book* Sexual Desire, *Roger Scruton wrongly maintains that human sexual experience is essentially intentional. His thesis depends on his highly revisionary definitions of 'sexual arousal' and 'sexual desire', the artificial nature of which I expose and criticise.*

He admits that homosexual desire is capable of the same kind of intentionality as heterosexual desire, and is therefore not intrinsically obscene or perverted, but he advances reasons why homosexuality is morally different from heterosexuality and is therefore an object of disapproval. His arguments presuppose 'an impassable moral divide' between the sexes and are, on his own admission, not very cogent.

Since he allows that homosexual desire is a natural and spontaneous phenomenon and also proposes that moral education should guide us towards a state in which our sexuality is entirely integrated within a life of personal affection and responsibility, consistency requires that he adopt a sexual ideology which does not discriminate against homosexuality. For homosexuals are unlikely to achieve the 'sexual integrity' which Scruton advocates (and which I endorse) if they are constantly encouraged to disparage their own sexual nature and if social institutions make no positive provision for them.

> For such is the power of words, that if we can be brought to the habit of calling two things which are connected, by the same name, we are more easily led to believe them to be one and the same thing [1]. Thomas Reid

Ten years ago I published a paper entitled 'On distinguishing between love and lust' [2], in which I enumerated some of the distinctions between sexual love, which only human beings are capable of experiencing, and lust, an appetite which we share with other animals. What has impelled me to return to this issue after more than a decade is the appearance of Roger Scruton's recent book *Sexual Desire* [3]. I propose to deal here with three issues: (i) the intentionality of our sexual feelings; (ii) the moral status of homosexuality—an issue which Scruton ultimately evades; and (iii) the treatment of homosexuality in moral education and its accommodation within the ideology of sexuality. Notwithstanding the many criticisms I shall make of Scruton's book, it contains much that I agree with. I share his concern "to rescue sexual morality from the morass into which modern ways of thinking have enticed it" (SD 196), and, like Scruton, I write from a philosophical perspective which is conservative rather than revolutionary.

1 Intentionality

> We have to deal with Man as a product of evolution, with Society as a
> product of evolution, and with Moral Phenomena as products of evolution
> [4]. Herbert Spencer

In my earlier paper I maintained that whereas the higher manifestations of human
sexuality are characterised by their intentionality (which is to say that they are
accompanied by mental states which have a clearly focused directedness towards
particular objects) our more basic and primary sexual urges are not. Scruton, on the
other hand, contends that human sexuality is essentially intentional. I shall endeavour
to show that in this he is mistaken: that his thesis depends on a highly revisionary and
stipulative definition of 'sexual desire'; and that it entails an account of human
sexuality which accords ill with an evolutionary theory of human nature. Right at the
outset, Scruton declares his high-minded aim to "argue against the moral and
philosophical impulse that leads us to assign sexual desire to the animal part of our
nature" (SD 2). Human sexuality, he contends, is essentially characterised by its
intentionality. Sexual arousal is always directed towards a particular person (SD 29),
and is "not transferable to another, who 'might do just as well' " (SD 30). It can occur
only between persons, being an artefact of their social condition (SD 33). Accordingly,
"animals are never sexually aroused; they do not feel sexual desire, nor do they have
sexual fulfilment" (SD 36).

As Scruton admits, "to put the thesis so starkly is to invite scepticism". Indeed,
rather than merely inviting scepticism, Scruton's bold assertions should prompt us very
early in his book to realise—his failure to make any candid declaration notwithstanding—that he is using the terms 'sexual arousal' and 'sexual desire' in a radically
revisionary way. For anyone who has more than the most superficial acquaintance with
animals knows that they, no less than human beings, *are* capable of sexual arousal.
Similarly, his characterisation of sexual desire not as an appetitive instinct but as an
intentional mental state which is object-directed to a high degree seems to run counter
to so much experience of everyday life. Scruton contrasts sexual desire in which we
"... attribute an irreplaceable value to those with whom we are brought into relation"
(SD 78) with the appetite for food, which is satisfied by any sample of the appropriate
type. But many philosophers, not just Kant, whom Scruton mentions (SD 83), have
believed that sexual desire, in some of its manifestations at least, is a non-specific
appetite analogous to hunger. Francis Hutcheson explicitly says as much [5] as does his
contemporary (and on many issues his antagonist) the worldly Bernard Mandeville. In
a quaint though somewhat coarse passage, Mandeville appears expressly to deny
Scruton's thesis:

> A vicious young Fellow, after having been an Hour or two at Church, a Ball,
> or any other Assembly, where there is a great parcel of handsome Women
> dress'd to the best Advantage, will have his Imagination more fired than if he
> had the same time been Poling at *Guildhall*, or walking in the Country
> among a Flock of Sheep. The consequence of this is, that he'll strive to
> satisfy the Appetite that is raised in him; and when he finds honest Women
> obstinate and uncomatable, 'tis very natural to think, that he'll hasten to
> others that are more compliable [6].

A case which is discussed by both Scruton and Mandeville is that of sailors returning ashore after a long period of confinement at sea. The ways in which they describe the situation differ markedly.

Whatever the peculiarities of orgiastic desire, it is no exception to the rule that the other person enters essentially into the aim of desire. Likewise with randiness, the state of the sailor who storms ashore, with the one thought 'woman' in his body. His condition might be described as desire for a woman, but for no particular woman. Such a description, however, seriously misrepresents the transition that occurs when the woman is found and he is set on the path of satisfaction. For now he has found the woman whom he wants, whom he seeks to arouse and upon whom his thoughts and energies are focused. It would be better to say that until that moment, he desired *no* woman. His condition was one of desiring to desire. And such was his need that he took an early opportunity to gratify his longing: to exchange the desire to desire for desire. It is an important feature of sexual desire that it should arise in this way from a generalised impulse. Nevertheless, desire is as distinct from the impulse that compels it as is anger from the excess of adrenalin. One should think of 'sexual hunger' as one thinks of the hunger for conversation, not as an appetite, but as a predisposition towards an individualising response (SD 90).

Where six or seven Thousand sailors arrive at once, as it often happens at *Amsterdam*, that have seen none but their own Sex for many Months together, how is it to be suppos'd that honest Women should walk the Streets unmolested, if there were no Harlots to be had at reasonable Prices? For which Reason the Wise Rulers of that well-order'd City always tolerate an uncertain number of Houses, in which Women are hired as publickly as Horses at a Livery-Stable [7].

Plainly, Mandeville does not appear to think that the gross kind of sexual desire which finds its outlet in whoring stands in need of the individuating conceptualisation which Scruton thinks is characteristic of human sexual encounters: one hires a woman just as one hires a horse—more or less any woman or any horse would do.

I do not see how the controversy could ever be definitively resolved, since the only sexual feelings of which anyone has immediate experience are his own. But I cannot help thinking that Mandeville is closer to the truth that Scruton. Mandeville's view of human nature is—notoriously—much more debased than is Scruton's; yet he is able to render a straightforward account of a whole range of seamy sexual aspiration and activity, while Scruton's account seems fanciful and strained. Are we to believe that a man who goes curb-crawling in a city's red light district or a homosexual who loiters in a public lavatory seeks anything higher than sexual gratification of an impersonal kind? Neither resembles Prince Charming in his quest for a particular Cinderella. Pornography, striptease clubs, cinemas which show sleazy films: all pander to—and, I suspect, help to encourage—sexual cravings of the lowest kind. In crediting such activities with the kind of intentionality which characterises the higher emotions Scruton is looking at them through rose-tinted spectacles and paying them a tribute to which they have no proper claim. If he were right, prostitutes, strippers and pornographers would be as out of tune with human nature as gas mantles are unfit for use with electricity, and their services would be as little in demand.

That the senses in which he uses the terms 'sexual arousal' and 'sexual desire' are revisionary is implicitly conceded by Scruton as he progresses through the book: firstly, by the introduction of defining adjectives. What he originally denominates 'sexual arousal' and 'sexual desire' *tout court*, he later calls 'true sexual arousal' (SD 31) and 'true sexual desire' (SD 89) or 'developed' forms of sexual desire (SD 93). In this respect Scruton's enunciation of his doctrine savours of the claim made by Marxists that only communism allows mankind to become 'truly human': what is set out ostensibly as a description is in fact a prescription since it incorporates a value-laden element which cannot be derived from the ordinary empirical denotation of its terms. Secondly, by using the term 'sexual desire' in contexts where its meaning is inconsistent with his original characterisation: if desire is specific and non-transferable, it is self-contradictory to speak of "desire roaming freely" (SD 309) and of "the element of generality in desire which tempts us to experiment" (SD 339; see also 359). Only 18 lines later on the same page this is explicitly contradicted by the claim that "sexual desire is inherently 'nuptial': it involves concentration upon the embodied existence of the other..." Clearly, Scruton is talking about two sets of phenomena, one less extensive than the other and included within it. Perhaps he should have called the first 'sexual desire' and the second (that is, the more refined forms of the first) 'Sexual Desire'; for philosophers often resort to upper case initials when they fancy they are proclaiming something portentous! I would maintain, then, that the term 'sexual desire' as it is ordinarily used and understood may incorporate intentionality and conceptualisation, but it need not do so.

In his discussion, Scruton fails to distinguish between *three* levels of awareness: sensation, perception, and conception.

> ... the pleasures of sight are not pleasures of sensation, but pleasures of perception. They have precisely that epistemic dimension which belongs to sexual arousal. To think that pleasure at the sight of a desirable person is 'in the eye'... is to commit a grave philosophical mistake. It is to confuse perception with sensation, and the pleasures of the understanding with the pleasures of the flesh... The eye is the vehicle of sexual arousal, precisely because arousal is an epistemic condition: it is a state of alertness toward the other, based on the perception of his embodied form. But the eye is not, as the vehicle of arousal, a 'zone of pleasure'. It is, rather, a 'channel of communication' through which the intentionality of arousal may begin to flow (SD 206).

Scruton appears here to be conflating perception and *con*ception. Now if this distinction collapses, so also must that between material and intentional objects; for everything that we perceive would be an intentional object. But that an experience is one of perception and has an epistemic dimension surely does not imply that its object is intentional. The chair that I sit on, the painting I look at, and the person I see are—in the first instance—*material* not *intentional* objects; whereas the chair that I remember, the painting I imagine, and the person whom I love *are* intentional objects, though they may also exist materially. Consider a man ogling the picture on page three of a popular daily tabloid: what is before him is really nothing more than a configuration of tiny dots suggesting a certain shape and outline. It is perceived, however, as a picture of a girl posing seductively, and it evokes in our imaginary onlooker lascivious thoughts. Surely his interest is excited merely by the prospect of her appearance. Perceiving a 'body' which you fancy is a more immediate and epistemically less complex procedure than conceiving a person whom you might love [8]. It is, of course, possible that someone might be obsessed by such a picture and attribute to it a fictitious personality, in which case—but only then—his mental state will involve the conceptualising intentionality which Scruton thinks is essential to human sexual experience.

Apart from the incompatibility of Scruton's essentialistic characterisation of sexual desire with ordinary ways of thinking and the contradictions into which he therefore sometimes lapses, it has a further serious disadvantage: it tempts him to invert the natural history of human sexuality, though again, this is not done consistently. Many of his remarks accord perfectly with the sort of naturalistic, evolutionary account of human sexuality which I should favour. For example:

> ... we cannot doubt that desire is rooted in instincts which we share with the animals (SD 179).
> ... we develop from animals into social beings (SD 212).

And even:

> ... we are animals, governed by the implacable requirements of the flesh (SD 233).

These remarks seem dubiously consistent with his expressed intention to resist "the impulse that leads us to assign sexual desire to the animal part of our nature" (SD 2). It is, of course, fair to maintain that even though our sexual feelings have grown out of our animality, yet they ".. are not reducible to any aspect of human conduct that is shared with the 'lower' animals" (SD 182-3). For my own part, I cannot see why Scruton should find it so problematical that "one and the same thing [can] be both a person and an animal" (SD 253). To undertake so complete and precise a demarcation of the several features of human nature, denominating some 'animal' and others 'personal' or 'rational' may well be an enterprise which is grossly misconceived. In Scruton's case, it certainly gives rise to much needless agonising. He seems at times anxious expressly to dissociate desire from our animal nature, as when he speaks of "the introduction of sex into desire" (SD 278), rather than—as seems to me more plausible—the converse; as if the intentional features might have had a genesis and evolution quite divorced from anything so 'sordid' as our sexual instincts. Similarly, rather than defining desire (in his revisionary sense) as 'lust plus the intentional features', he defines lust as "genuine sexual desire from which the goal of erotic love has been excluded" (SD 344). If we were doing mathematical equations rather than philosophy, this would not matter, but Scruton's definition constitutes a deliberate suggestion that sexual desire (in his sense) is the primary category while lust is a derivative one. I would maintain that lust (our basic sexual appetite) is both temporally and logically prior to the higher sentiments which have grown out of it, and that Scruton's attempt to maintain otherwise is tantamount to turning natural history on its head. The analogy between the development of human sexuality and the growth of a tree (also employed by Herbert Spencer [9]) seems apposite, but Scruton too easily forgets that there are many people who appear content to rub their noses in the soil rather than contemplate the leaves.

> A tree grows in the soil, from which it takes its nourishment, and without which it would be nothing. And it would be almost nothing *to us* if it did not also spread itself in foliage, flower, and fruit. In a similar way, human sexuality grows from the soil of the reproductive urge, from which it takes its life, and without which it would be nothing. Furthermore, it would be almost nothing *for us*, if it did not flourish in personal form, clothing itself in the flower and foliage of desire. When we understand each other as sexual

beings, we see, not the soil which lies hidden beneath the leaves, but the leaves themselves, in which the matter of animality is intelligible, only because it has acquired a personal form (SD 254).

If one accepts an evolutionary account of the world and all that is therein, then our sexuality, rationality, and morality (all of which are inter-related) must have a natural history. Though the details are lost in the remoteness of the distant past, such an account is incongruous with any thesis which lays down what is essential to humanity as such; for in the course of time mankind has undergone changes and still continues to change, albeit imperceptibly. The capacity to conceptualise, on which intentionality depends, did not come about suddenly at a specific point in time. It is at least arguable that even now this capacity is not shared equally by all human beings or by all cultures—a possibility which I should expect to occasion no more distress or embarrassment to the editor of the *Salisbury Review* than it does to me, though one which Scruton could easily be suspected of having overlooked. For although the examples he cites bespeak a cultural awareness which is prodigiously wide-ranging, they are culled almost exclusively from the *belles lettres* and grand operas of the western world. One cannot, therefore, help wondering how applicable his speculations are to the sexual lives of primitive savages or of those who live in communities where women are owned in much the same way as horses or camels.

It is not entirely clear whether Scruton believes in evolution, since he says, "The difference between animality and selfhood is one of kind, and admits of no degrees... However, the transition... is built up of certain stages or 'moments'" (SD 331). The two halves of this quotation are to my mind glaringly inconsistent, the first part being difficult to reconcile to evolutionary theory, while the second half admits that the transition must have been accomplished gradually. Apart from its incompatibility with evolutionary theory, such essentialism also incorporates the risk of making our humanity seem more secure than it is; of blinding us to the precariousness and fragility of that thin veneer which civilisation has grafted onto our lower nature. However, I am in complete agreement with Scruton that intentionality is primary among the things which distinguish the more valuable from the less valuable sexual experiences; but the arguments I would use to support my evaluation are evolutionary rather than essentialist [10]. I would also agree that this factor is of paramount importance in the moral assessment of homosexuality, to which I shall now proceed.

2 Homosexuality

> It is surely one of the vital questions of sexual morality, whether homosexual is distinguishable from heterosexual intercourse (SD 254). Roger Scruton

Despite the admitted urgency and importance of this question, Scruton does not come up with any firm answer. In a book that runs to over four hundred pages, shortage of space could not be pleaded as an excuse for this conspicuous omission, which is due rather, I suspect, to the fact that while Scruton would like to conclude that homosexuality and heterosexuality should be differently appraised, much of what he says implies, or at least suggests, the contrary. The moral status of homosexual desire is broached at three or four points in the book, where Scruton tantalises his readers by holding out the prospect of a definitive—and hostile—conclusion. But no such pronouncement is ever made. In this respect, Scruton is like an exotic dancer, who by the deft manipulation of veils, ostrich feathers, or whatever, continually evokes in her audience the frenzied anticipation of what she never actually reveals.

As early as page 15 he promises an exploration of "the important differences between homosexual and heterosexual desire", but the first place where he actually examines the moral status of homosexual relationships is page 282, where there is a paragraph in which homosexual desire is discussed in relation to Kantian feminism—the doctrine that one's sex or gender is irrelevant to one's personality or 'personhood' since 'person' is a unitary category. He says:

> For the Kantian feminist, the *enracinement* of the person in the soil of animal activity is a single phenomenon, exemplified alike by man and woman. One and the same person might have taken root in either soil. If this were so, there can be no moral difference between homosexual and heterosexual desire. The body's sex would be irrelevant to the interpersonal emotions that are displayed in it; just *this* person might have had just *this* desire whatever his sex. Otherwise we must say that desire is not, after all, an interpersonal attitude, but simply a residue of bodily experience, indicating not the person but his biological destiny, in the manner of sensory pleasure and sensory pain. In other words, Kantian feminism has radical moral consequences. Either it denies the moral distinction between homosexual and heterosexual desire—and along with it the idea of a sexual 'normality' answerable to our nature as sexually reproducing beings. Or else it forces us to accept the Platonic view of desire as 'merely animal'. Neither view is acceptable (SD 282).

I am at a loss to know what this passage is intended to accomplish. Scruton is not (nor am I) a Kantian feminist: but from the falsity of Kantian feminism one cannot infer anything about the respective moral natures of heterosexual and homosexual desire—even if the truth of Kantian feminism would entail (as Scruton asserts) that they are equivalent. To derive the negative inference from the falsity of Kantian feminism would involve the fallacy of denying the antecedent [11]. I suppose Scruton may be arguing that since Kantian feminism would commit us either to the moral equivalence of homosexual and heterosexual desire or to the view that desire is 'merely animal', and neither of these alternatives is acceptable, then Kantian feminism must be false. Such an argument would indeed be valid, but would require an independent proof of the alleged distinction between homosexual and heterosexual desire. No such proof is offered.

A further issue raised by this passage is the putative connection between the moral propriety or impropriety of homosexual desire and concepts of sexual normality. The word 'norm' and its cognates are widely and correctly used both descriptively and prescriptively. Acknowledgement of the normality (in the descriptive sense) of heterosexuality is compatible with either approval or disapproval of homosexuality. It is only the *prescriptive* normality of heterosexuality which is undermined by an accommodating attitude to homosexuality; so it must be in this prescriptive sense that Scruton is using the term. In this case he can be called upon to explain how one is to bridge what has come to be called Hume's gap [12]: in particular, how can a description of our function as sexually reproducing beings imply a universal duty to perform heterosexually, especially when so many individuals have no spontaneous desire so to perform?

It is in this same section on 'Sex and Gender' that Scruton first adumbrates a further argument in support of his claim that homosexual and heterosexual desire are essentially different.

> The plain fact is that, because we live in a world structured by gender, the other sex is forever to some extent a mystery to us, with a dimension of experience which we can imagine but never inwardly know. In desiring to unite with it, we are desiring to mingle with something that is deeply—perhaps essentially—not ourselves, and which brings us to experience a character and inwardness that challenge us with their strangeness ...
>
> This might imply that there is a distinction between homosexual and heterosexual desire. The heterosexual ventures towards an individual whose gender confines him within another world. The homosexual unites with an individual who does not lie beyond the divide which separates the world of men from the world of women. Hence the homosexual has a peculiar inward familiarity with what his partner feels. His discovery of his partner's sexual nature is the discovery of what he knows (SD 283).

Is not the issue here raised a particular instance of the problem of 'other minds'? How can I know that other people resemble me or that their experiences resemble my own? Now we might just as well argue that *all* other people—not only members of the opposite sex—are 'a mystery to us'; for if our mental states are essentially private, we have no way of knowing, nor any reason to suppose, that members of the opposite sex differ from us mentally more than do members of our own. Even if one accepts as an apposite description Scruton's extremely sexist assumptions (which issue I am content to leave open), I cannot see how speculations which by their very nature are necessarily precarious could be used to support a moral conclusion as contentious as he is trying to establish. It would surely be (to use Scruton's own analogy) to hang too complex a moral argument on too fragile a peg (SD 287–8).

This argument is repeated in the chapter entitled 'Perversion', which incorporates Scruton's most extended discussion (just over five pages) of homosexuality despite the fact that by his own criterion homosexuality does not in itself constitute a perversion.

> The masculine and feminine denote two distinct kinds of person, and the experience of gender plays a significant part in determining the intentional content of desire. Homosexual desire may retain the interpersonal intentionality that is normal to us; but there may yet be a moral difference between homosexual and heterosexual conduct. The correct position, I believe, is this: homosexuality is perhaps not in itself a perversion, although it may exist in perverted forms. But it is *significantly* different from heterosexuality, in a way that partly explains, even if it does not justify, the traditional judgement of homosexuality as a perversion. I say this with extreme tentativeness, and knowing that it may be received as an outrage (SD 305).

How right Scruton is to express these reservations! But again on the next page the prospect of a censorious conclusion is hinted at.

> The question is whether we can distinguish the intentional content of homosexual from that of heterosexual desire, so as to justify the judgement that the first has a distinct moral character, and perhaps also to justify the judgement that it diverges from the norm of interpersonal relations in the direction of obscenity (SD 306).

He once more asserts that there is an 'impassable moral divide' between the sexes, and contends that this gives rise to a morally significant difference between homosexual and heterosexual relationships. I do not propose to devote too much space to refuting an argument which even Scruton himself admits is not very cogent. Its essence is that in a heterosexual relationship, each party sees the other as essentially different. This can give rise to a respect which requires "a peculiar delicacy of negotiation" and "a preparedness to take responsibility for the effects of this unknown thing". This "opening of the self to the mystery of another gender" is "one of the fundamental motives tending towards commitment" (SD 307). But as Scruton concedes, "such an observation is [not] always and everywhere valid." The features he attributes to heterosexual liaisons are by no means a sufficient condition of commitment; nor are they a necessary one: for there are many heterosexual relationships in which such commitment is wanting, just as there are at least some homosexual ones in which it is present. One would never imagine this from the literary examples which he cites (SD 234–5; 307–8). These are—not to overstate the case—heavily biased towards an impression of homosexuality which few people of ordinary moral sensitivities could fail to find repellent. I cannot help feeling that they were chosen for the sake of polemical convenience, and with a wilful disregard for what might have been said on the other side of the argument. The carnal excesses of antiquity and the morbid effusions of Proust and Genet evoke an image of homosexual desire which is at best pathological and at worst downright depraved. But then since homosexuals have only recently begun to emerge from nearly twenty centuries of unremitting oppression, it is hardly to be expected that there should be an imposing corpus of fine literature which depicts homosexuals in a fair—let alone a favourable—light.

Although Scruton is ingenuous enough to admit that any conclusion which might be drawn from a comparison of the works of Proust and Sappho is vitiated by the extreme disparity of their style and meaning, he none the less maintains that the contrast thereby exemplified between male and female sexuality underscores the complementary nature of heterosexual liaisons, the absence of such 'complementarity' being a "*fault* in the content of homosexual desire—an imbalance which, if left uncorrected, threatens the course of love" (SD 310). Even so, he allows that "homosexuality could be shown to be perverted only if the homosexual act were shown to be intrinsically depersonalised or intrinsically obscene" (SD 310). There ensues an argument which purports to explain why people do in fact so perceive homosexual acts, but it seems to be at best a rationalisation and even to "turn out to have a peculiarly tautologous quality" (SD 205). For Scruton says: "the obscenity is seen in the arousal of the flesh by its own sexual kind" (SD 310), whereas...

> ... heterosexual arousal is arousal by something through and through other than oneself, and other as *flesh*. In the heterosexual act, it might be said, I move out *from* my body *towards* the other, whose flesh is unknown to me; while in the homosexual act I remain locked within my body, narcissistically contemplating in the other an excitement that is the mirror of my own (SD 310).

This argument's first contention is tautologous: homosexual acts are perceived as obscene because they are homosexual and not heterosexual. Its second claim depends on the unsupported assumption that they are essentially narcissistic. Clearly, they have such a capacity, while heterosexual acts never could; but this hardly implies that they are characteristically so. As Scruton allows, his suggestion is far from being a proof. I might add that if it did constitute a genuine reason why homosexual acts are thought to be obscene, then its operation would not be so narrowly circumscribed to the people of a few particular cultures. In *The Origin and Development of the Moral Ideas* Edward Westermarck points out that attitudes to homosexuality range from benevolent toleration to severe interdiction, the greatest hostility having been manifested by Zoroastrian, Judaic, and Christian cultures. He argues at some length, moreover, that Judaeo-Christian antipathy towards homosexuality is rooted not in any of its intrinsic features but rather in its association with foreign cults, unbelief, and heresy [13].

Throughout the book much is made of the intentional nature of sexual desire and of the potential of relationships which are so endowed. On Scruton's own admission, homosexuality is not inherently perverted or obscene, nor does he offer any sound justification for the antipathy with which it has until recently been widely regarded in western societies. The conclusion which his work therefore supports—though he himself resists it—is that homosexual and heterosexual desire are on an equal footing, and that whatever factors may be relevant to the moral assessment of sexual activity, its orientation is not. All this has inescapable implications of the first importance for the way in which homosexuality is treated by moral educators. Since none of these is so much as hinted at by Scruton, I shall proceed to supply the deficiencies in what I consider to be the best part of his book—the chapter on 'Sexual Morality'.

3 Moral Education

> The end of all moral speculations is to teach us our duty; and, by proper representations of the deformity of vice and beauty of virtue, beget corre-spondent habits, and engage us to avoid the one, and embrace the other [14].
> David Hume

The penultimate chapter of Scruton's book is concerned with the scope and purpose of sexual morality, and the objective of moral education in matters sexual. He begins by emphasising the importance of the subject and expresses the hope that those who disagree with his conclusions will find in his supporting arguments a procedure whereby to refute them. Although I have elsewhere deployed an argument of a different kind [10], I am sympathetic, not hostile, to the conclusions that Scruton reaches. I think it would be fair to say that for many practical purposes, he and I would agree. Indeed, I think that this chapter, and in particular its last 11 pages, should be studied with the most assiduous attention by all who are interested in sex education. In it he makes a number of points with which I entirely agree, and of which I here offer a brief summary, using Scruton's own words as much as possible.

Education is concerned not just with a child's actions but also with his feelings and character (SD 325). In trying to develop the potential to be happy, we are concerned not with the immediate gratification of impulses but with the development of dispositions which will bring long-term fulfilment (SD 326). Among these is the ability to control one's sexual impulses (SD 330). A further prerequisite is the adoption of a system of values, and the capacity to see as desirable only those things which are the occasion of true fulfilment (SD 336). Because sexual desire has the most far-reaching consequences for those affected by it, it cannot be morally neutral. Since the capacity to give and receive erotic love is of incomparable value in the process of self-fulfilment, we have reason to acquire this capacity. Some sexual habits are vicious precisely because they destroy it (SD 337–8). Because erotic love is prone to jealousy, which can entail catastrophic consequences for both parties, the occasions of jealousy must be forestalled by the habit of fidelity, which is fostered by a complex process of moral education (SD 339). The task of sexual morality is to unite the personal and the sexual, to sustain thereby the intentionality of desire, and prepare the individual for erotic love. Only by safeguarding the integrity of our embodiment can we inculcate either innocence in the young or fidelity in the adult. Perversion consists precisely in diverting the sexual impulse from its interpersonal goal, or towards some act which is intrinsically destructive of personal relations and the values that we find in them (SD 343). The ideal of virtue remains one of 'sexual integrity', of a sexuality which is entirely integrated into the life of personal affection, and in which the self and its responsibility are centrally involved and indissolubly linked to the pleasures and passions of the body (SD 346).

I shall now proceed to argue that these conclusions, which I am delighted to endorse, have corollaries of a kind which Scruton will almost certainly find alarmingly radical. As he himself admits, "... sexual desire does not occur only between people of different sex; any account of sexual desire that could not be extended to homosexuality would be ludicrous..." (SD 254). By the same token, any ideology of sexuality or programme of moral education which ignores the fact that a significant minority of the population is homosexual must be accounted inadequate. Since many young people will turn out to be so orientated, should not wise and benevolent educators, unfettered by superstition and prejudice, take all practicable care to assist them to have as fulfilled and complete a life as possible? I would emphasise that such a policy is one not of proselytisation but merely of facing squarely up to reality. Although Scruton makes no suggestions either hortatory or censorious about how homosexuality should be treated by moral educators, his discussions both of homosexuality and of the functions of moral education have positive implications. For since, on Scruton's own admission, homosexual desire is capable of the same interpersonal intentionality as heterosexual desire, homosexual relationships have in this respect precisely the same potential. However, homosexuals can hardly be prepared for erotic love and encouraged towards a life-style in which their sexuality is "entirely integrated into the life of personal affection" (SD 346) if, as has traditionally been the case, they are constantly admonished to depreciate themselves and their sexual nature and offered no support by social norms and institutions. For this reason such negative and disparaging pronouncements as the one recently delivered by the Catholic Church are particularly to be deplored [15].

The Catholic Church's teaching on homosexuality and the depravity of some homosexuals afford a striking instance of a paradox expounded by Bernard Mandeville in *The Fable of the Bees* (1714), namely that "Parties directly opposite/Assist each other, as 'twere for spight" [16]. For it is certain that nothing has been more instrumental in driving homosexuals towards a degraded life-style than the indiscriminate censure they have suffered from Christian moralists. At the same time, nothing appears to justify this condemnation more than the professed wantonness of those homosexual 'spokespersons' who are as undiscriminating in their approval as the Catholic Church is in its condemnation. Herbert Spencer once wrote, "The suppression of every error is commonly followed by a temporary ascendency of the contrary one" [17]. It was once thought that *all* homosexual acts were morally reprehensible: some homosexual organisations would have us think that *no* homosexual acts are. There has long been a need to establish between these two equally pernicious extremes a consensus in which homosexual relationships, like heterosexual ones, can be individually appraised on their merits.

One reason why homosexuals are less likely than heterosexuals to have enduring relationships must be that whereas the latter grow up in a cultural climate (what one might call a 'moral community') which even now still guides most of them into relationships which are both personally satisfying and socially useful, the former are not supported by any positive norms or institutions. On the contrary, they are admonished, directly or indirectly, to view negatively their own sexuality. Hitherto, there has been nothing in popular culture to foster in homosexuals the higher manifestations of amorous passion (tenderness, affection, loyalty) to which heterosexuals are encouraged to aspire. Those who gravitate towards the so-called 'gay scene' will find not only a facile endorsement of promiscuity which creates an ethos that is essentially dehumanising and impersonal, but an ideology which provides a spurious theoretical justification for the wanton and irresponsible conduct to which it gives licence. This so-called liberational ideology has been most baneful where its influence has been greatest, and has led in some American cities to such inordinate and brutalising excesses as make the inhabitants of Sodom seem like paradigms of chastity and restraint [18]. It has served badly those who have been foolish enough to espouse it, for it has proved to be a harbinger of debauchery, disease, and death. The ideology of 'sexual integrity' proposed by Scruton, or something closely akin to it, is equally applicable to both heterosexuals and homosexuals and could serve as an antidote to the virulent poison of anarchic liberationism which menaces society.

I have recently championed elsewhere [19] the policy of promoting before young people positive images of caring and humane homosexuals, who are confident and secure in their own sexuality and responsible in the relationships they form. These would both serve as positive rôle models to those who grow up to be homosexual and also help to dispel ignorance and prejudice among those who do not. But I wonder if this is enough. One of the features which vitiate so much radical thinking about sexual morality is the naive contention that because human institutions are in a sense artificial, they are therefore arbitrary. This thesis is countered by Scruton in his final chapter, 'The Politics of Sex', where he maintains (in a manner similar to Hume's account of justice [20]) that some social artifacts are natural and even necessary to human beings since they bring human nature into harmony with the requirements of social living. Scruton in fact goes further than Hume by maintaining that some artifacts actually make human nature what it is. He dismisses recent 'Rousseauist' attempts to create a 'higher' civilisation based on a Utopian state of nature in which people are divested of the restraints imposed by social institutions, arguing rather that "the fate of persons is inseparable from the history of the institutions which form and nurture them" (SD 350).

If this supposition is correct (as I believe it is), then it emphasises how serious is the lack of appropriate institutions as an obstacle to the establishment of stable homosexual relationships; for since such institutions are the products of time, they cannot be created from scratch at short notice, howsoever desirable they might be; which itself is a point of contention. It is possible that as homosexuals are able to live more openly, any stable relationships they form will become objects of public perception and recognition, and this may in time lead to a kind of institutionalisation comparable to marriage. We have, then, an archetypal chicken/egg paradox: for on the one hand such relationships are likely to flourish to a significant degree only if they are nurtured by institutions; and on the other, the necessary institutions will come into being only through the recognition of phenomena which *ex hypothesi* depend on them. Inasmuch as the positive treatment of homosexuality by moral educators will not produce striking results overnight, some might be inclined to dismiss this policy as unequal to the problem it confronts. But perhaps this is all that can be done, and at least it is a step in the right direction. It is also one which Roger Scruton is bound to applaud if he really believes all that he has written.

J. Martin Stafford, 3 Woodlands Bank, 67 Stockport Road, Altrincham, Cheshire WA15 7LH, United Kingdom.

NOTES

[1] THOMAS REID (1863) *Works...*, p. 228 (Ed. Sir William Hamilton) (Edinburgh, Maclachlan & Stewart).

[2] J. MARTIN STAFFORD (1977) On distinguishing between Love and Lust, *Journal of Value Inquiry*, 11, pp. 292–303.

[3] ROGER SCRUTON (1986) *Sexual Desire* (London, Weidenfeld & Nicolson). Hereafter references are contained within the text as SD + page number.

[4] HERBERT SPENCER (1897) *The Principles of Ethics*, Vol. I, p. 478 (London, Williams & Norgate).

[5] FRANCIS HUTCHESON (1728) *An Essay on the Nature and Conduct of the Passions and Affections...*, pp. 88–90 (London). The relevant passage is quoted by me on p. 299 of [2] above.

[6] BERNARD MANDEVILLE (1924) *The Fable of the Bees* (Ed. F. B. KAYE), 2 vols (Oxford, Clarendon Press), Vol. I, p. 95.(First published 1714.)

[7] Ibid., p. 96.

[8] For a fuller discussion see pages 299–300 of [2].

[9] H. SPENCER (see [4] above) p. 463.

[10] Sexual relationships incorporating intentionality are, by the prerequisites of their own nature, confined to the most highly evolved species, namely man, and seem therefore to be vindicated by the evolutionary process. I have discussed the merits and weaknesses of evolutionary theories of ethics in 'Hume, Spencer and the Standard of Morals', *Philosophy*, 58 (1983), pp. 39–55.

[11] From the propositions: 'If p then q' and 'p', we may validly derive 'q'. But to derive 'not q' from the conjunction of 'if p then q' and 'not p' is to argue fallaciously. It is known as the fallacy of denying the antecedent. Any elementary textbook on propositional logic will expound on this.

[12] DAVID HUME (1978) *A Treatise of Human Nature* revised by P. H. NIDDITCH (Oxford, Clarendon Press). In a famous passage on p. 469, Hume remarks on the problem of deriving normative propositions (such as are about what ought to be) from descriptive ones (such as are about what is). (First published 1739–40.)

[13] EDWARD WESTERMARCK (1917) *The Origin and Development of the Moral Ideas*, Vol. II, p. 486 (London, Macmillan).

[14] DAVID HUME (1975) *Enquiries...* revised by P. H. Nidditch (Oxford, Clarendon Press), p. 172 (First published 1748 and 1751.)

[15] The *Letter to the Bishops of the Catholic Church on the Pastoral Care of Homosexual Persons* (London, Catholic Truth Society, 1986) states unequivocally that all homosexual activity is 'an intrinsic moral evil' and the disposition to it 'an objective disorder'. Any contrary statements made by the 'pro-homosexual movement' are dismissed as 'deceitful propaganda'. Thus the Holy See not only thinks fit to reaffirm the full rigour of its traditional obdurate doctrine, but also does not scruple to impugn the good faith of all who dissent. Now surely, an institution which has in its time, and to suit its convenience, burned heretics, sold indulgences, condoned the persecution of Jews and the systematic pillaging of South America, and to this day discountenances the use of contraceptives even in countries where people are starving to death—surely, I say, such an institution cannot expect to command unquestioning allegiance as an arbiter of morals. Of course, all the usual passages from *Leviticus, Romans,* and *Corinthians* are paraded before us; and yet the authors conveniently overlook the fact that homosexuality is a phenomenon which pervades the whole of the animal creation, not one which is confined to postlapsian man. Perhaps, after all, the intentions of the Creator are more reliably manifest in His works than in the writings of those who lay claim to His inspiration.

[16] B. MANDEVILLE (see note [6]), p. 25.

[17] HERBERT SPENCER (1861) *Education: intellectual, moral, and physical*, p. 60 (London, Manwaring; subsequent editions, Williams & Norgate).

[18] The BBC 1 programme *Panorama* on 26 January 1987 included a report from San Francisco in which one man stated that prior to the AIDS epidemic there had been places to which homosexual men might resort and in the course of a single weekend have as many as *fifty* different sexual partners.

[19] J. MARTIN STAFFORD (1988) In Defence of Gay Lessons, *Journal of Moral Education*, 17, 1, pp. 11–20.

[20] See p. 484 of [12] above.

Part III

Terrorism, War and Conflict

11

Terrorism and Morality

HAIG KHATCHADOURIAN

ABSTRACT   *The paper addresses the fundamental issue of the morality of terrorism. It distinguishes four types of terrorism—'predatory,' 'retaliatory,' 'political' and 'moralistic' —and argues that in all of them terrorism (in a 'descriptive,' value-neutral sense of the word) is always wrong. After a short introductory section the paper considers in some detail the conceptual problem of defining 'terrorism'. Next it considers the possible application to terrorism, with the necessary modifications, of two main conditions of a 'just war'; viz. the Principles of Discrimination and of Proportion. It argues that these conditions support the paper's central contention. Additional support is then found in the concept and principles of human rights. In the final section the paper evaluates utilitarian arguments brought forth by Kai Nielsen in* Violence and Terrorism: its uses and abuses, *in support of so-called 'revolutionary terrorism'.*

Throughout the discussion is illustrated by some actual examples from the recent past.

I

Terrorism, in all its types and forms, is always wrong; that is the claim I shall try to establish in this paper. A sequel will deal with the question of deterring and, more importantly, addressing the root causes of political terrorism and moralistic terrorism—terrorism aiming at a moral end. Although the claim that terrorism is always wrong is very widely held in the world today, some practitioners of terrorism and those who support them or sympathise with their goals believe that it is morally justifiable, at least in the form in which they practise or support it. Other practitioners or supporters of terrorism vehemently deny that they are terrorists or supporters of terrorism; implying that they too believe that terrorism is morally wrong. They argue that they are 'freedom fighters' or supporters of 'freedom fighting'. What terrorism therefore is or how the word should be employed is a much vexed question, and adds greatly to the confusion and divergence of views on the morality of terrorism. The practical importance of what people understand by the word is never greater than in the case of heads of state and governments that either support terrorism or attempt to fight it. For instance, President Reagan's characterisation of terrorism as the deliberate maiming or killing of innocent people, and of terrorists as 'base criminals,' reflects and at the same time shapes his administration's avowed condemnation of terrorism, and the diplomatic and military steps it has so far taken to fight terrorism [1].

Some moral philosophers argue on ethical grounds that certain types or species of terrorism (e.g. revolutionary terrorism) are morally justifiable: a view I shall consider in this paper.

In the following section I shall deal with the problem of defining 'terrorism,' and in Section III I shall consider the possible application of 'just war' theory to it. I shall argue that the relevant conditions of a 'just war,' duly modified, support this paper's overall contention. A consideration of human rights will provide additional support for my thesis. In the final section I shall examine some consequentialist arguments in favour of, and some arguments against, terrorism.

II

An adequate description of any type, species or form of terrorism must minimally include a description of the following five aspects or elements of terrorism in general: (1) the socioeconomic or historical and cultural root causes of its incidence (e.g. homelessness); (2) its immediate, intermediate and long-range or ultimate goals, e.g. retaliation, publicity, and the regaining of a lost homeland, respectively and (3) the forms and methods of coercion and force [2] generally used to terrorise the immediate victims and those the terrorists coerce or hope to coerce as a result (the 'patients' or 'sufferers' [3]). The forms and methods of coercion and force used define the different *species* or *forms* of terrorism of any given *type*. Another aspect of terrorism is (4) the nature or kinds of organisations and institutions, or the political systems, supporting or sponsoring the terrorism. In 'international terrorism' and 'state terrorism' the support is provided by one or more nation states. The final aspect of terrorism that must be considered is (5) the social, political, economic or military circumstances in which the terrorism occurs; e.g. whether it occurs in time of peace or in wartime.

Defining 'Terrorism': what's in a name

For the purposes of this paper, an adequate definition of 'terrorism' in general, besides reflecting the preceding five aspects or dimensions of terrorism, must be neutral, non-evaluative. It must not beg the issue of the morality of any type or form of terrorism, or of terrorism in general; though as I noted, the word is generally if not universally used as a highly condemnatory term at present. Like 'murder' it is generally used to designate a highly reprehensible act or series of acts. The strongly negative connotations of the word are not only reflected in the characterisation of terrorism by heads of governments and other politicians, and by the average person, but also in some purportedly objective, philosophical definitions of the term. A good example occurs in Burton M. Leiser's *Liberty, Justice, and Morals* [4]. According to the latter,

> *Terrorism* is any organized set of acts of violence designed to create an atmosphere of despair or fear, to shake the faith of ordinary citizens in their government and its representatives, to destroy the structure of authority which normally stands for security, or to reinforce and perpetuate a governmental regime whose popular support is shaky. It is a policy of seemingly senseless, irrational, and arbitrary murder, assassination, sabotage, subversion, robbery and other forms of violence, all committed with dedicated indifference to existing legal and moral codes or with claims to special exemption from conventional social norms [5].

This characterisation too makes all terrorism morally unjustifiable by definition. The link between terrorism and murder in Reagan's or Leiser's conception is immediately established if we add Elizabeth Anscombe's proposition that the deliberate killing of the innocent is, by definition, murder [6]. Apart from morally dismissing terrorism out of hand, both Reagan's and Leiser's characterisations are too broad; while Reagan's characterisation is also woefully incomplete. Leiser's definition does incorporate several of the aspects of terrorism I have mentioned, but fails to spell out the various sorts of causes of terrorism and makes only passing mention of what it calls the terrorists' 'political ends' [7]. In short, it is too narrow as well as too broad.

The two aforementioned characterisations share a significant element; viz. that terrorism *always* involves the maiming, killing or coercion of innocent—and only innocent—persons; where 'innocent persons' is defined by Leiser as " . . . persons who have little or no direct connection with the causes to which the terrorists are dedicated . . . " [8]. Although his definition of 'terrorism' is not quite clear on this point, Leiser sharply distinguishes terrorism from political assassination later in the chapter on terrorism, and appears to equate terrorism with "the victimisation of defenseless, innocent persons" as opposed to " . . . the assassination of political and military leaders" [9]. His dismissal of all Palestinian armed resistance to Israel as terrorism, naturally follows [10].

The question of whether non-innocents can be included among the possible targets of terrorism, in the current uses of 'terrorism' in the media and in everyday discourse, e.g. in Europe and the United States, is an unsettled and moot question. The absence of clarity and fixity—indeed, the ambivalence and uncertainty in the current employ-ments of the word—reflect the particular users' stand on the morality of terrorism, and the more general morality of the use of force. It is also intimately connected with the distinction between terrorism and 'freedom fighting,' including 'guerilla warfare.' Those who consider the harming of innocents alone as an essential feature of terrorism would tend to define 'freedom fighting' as involving (together with other elements analogous to the elements of 'terrorism' I listed earlier) the maiming, killing or coercing of non-innocents. That would permit considering 'political assassination' as a species of 'freedom fighting.' Leiser states that 'guerilla warfare' is characterised by small-scale, unconventional, limited actions carried out by irregular forces "*against regular military forces, their supply lines, and communications*" [11]. That definition (which aptly characterises the Afghan rebels as they are commonly called) would be perfectly in order if we include in it the notion that all the targeted soldiers are in the army of their own free will.

The preceding discussion indicates that the current concepts of terrorism, like other evaluative concepts, are what W. B. Gallie calls 'essentially contested' [12], as well as open textured and vague. Yet like most or all vague and unsettled terms, 'terrorism' has a 'common core of meaning' in its different usages. This 'core of meaning' includes the notion that terrorist acts are acts of coercion or of force [13], aiming at monetary gain (*predatory terrorism*), revenge (*retaliatory terrorism*), a political end (*political terrorism*), or a moral end (*moralistic terrorism*) [14]. It also includes the notion that all terrorism involves a crucial distinction between 'immediate victims' and 'sufferers.'

The *causes* and the *goals* of terrorism differ with the differnt types of terrorism: predatory, retaliatory, etc. The *methods* used by the terrorists also vary depending on these and other factors.

So-called 'state protected,' 'state sponsored' or 'state' terrorism is not (*pace* Edel) a distinct type of terrorism but only a special form of political terrorism. Instances of state terrorism may therefore also be instances of moralistic terrorism. Political terrorism, including state terrorism, is often international in character—so-called 'international terrorism'—as defined by the U.S. House Resolution 2781, 99th Con-gress, 1st Session, pp. 1–3. Among other things the Resolution states that an act of terror is an act of international terror if it transcends the national boundaries of the perpetrators or is directed against foreign nationals within the perpetrators' national boundaries. The act also falls within this definition if it violates any of the provisions set under the *Convention for the Suppression of Unlawful Seizures of Aircraft* (The Hague, 16 December 1970) [15].

All types of terrorism may be terrorism either in time of peace or in wartime. In the latter moralistic terrorism may be in the service of a putatively legitimate cause such as national self-defence (in general, as part of a putatively just war). On the other hand predatory and retaliatory terrorism may thrive in time of war, revolution or civil war, as in many instances of Lebanese terrorism during the past decade. Terrorism in war involves special complexities whenever it is practised by or on behalf of one or more of the belligerents, who may or may not be fighting a just war.

The foregoing discussion of the current uses of 'terrorism' bears out Edel's observation that terrorism "... is an emerging concept rather than one endowed with an established essence, and what will emerge will be a quasi-technical usage on which will hang a variety of legal and moral consequences" [16]. The definitions of 'international terrorism' I noted are examples of emerging quasi-technical legal usages; though, understandably, they are or will be mainly concerned with political terrorism.

In light of the complexity, diversity and variability of the activities and actions currently covered by the term 'terrorism' and reflected in the five aspects of terrorism I noted, an adequate *essentialist* definition of what is now usually called terrorism appears to me to be undesirable as well as impossible. Rather, a 'range definition' expressing a certain kind of 'family resemblance' concept would avoid the two opposite problems that plague essentialist definitions or concepts in such cases: narrowness and over-inclusiveness. Leiser's definition has the merit of characterising terrorism in terms of a set of disjunctions reflecting the diversity of the goals, hence the different types, of terrorism. But since there exist some very general features *common* to all acts of terrorism as generally understood (the 'common core of meaning' noted earlier), though neither peculiar to them nor exhaustive of their features as acts of terrorism, *terrorism* as we now have it and as I hope it will continue to be, is a 'quasi-essentialist' concept. Such a concept is logically intermediate between an essentialist concept, defined in terms of a set of necessary and sufficient conditions or a set of common and peculiar features, and a 'pure' 'family resemblance' concept [17], wholly and solely delimited in terms of criss-crossing resemblances of different degrees of generality or specificity.

III

Terrorism and Just-war Theory

The traditional conditions of a just war are of two sorts: conditions of *jus ad bellum* or conditions of a morally justified launching of a war, and conditions of *jus in bello* or conditions of the just prosecution of a war in progress. One of the fundamental conditions of the latter sort is the Principle of Discrimination, which prohibits the deliberate harming—above all the killing—of innocent persons. In *Just-war Theory* William O'Brien defines it as the principle that "prohibits direct intentional attacks on non-combatants and nonmilitary targets" [18]. Another fundamental condition is the Principle of Proportion, as "applied to discrete military ends" [19]. That condition is defined by O'Brien as "requiring proportionality of means to political and military ends" [20]. My contention is that these two principles, duly modified or adapted to terrorism, are applicable to all the types of terrorism I distinguished in Section II, and that they are flagrantly violated by them.

The Principle of Discrimination and Terrorism

Let us start with the Principle of Discrimination. It is a patent fact that in many acts of terrorism some or all of the immediate victims and/or the sufferers are innocent persons, in no way—morally or even causally—connected with or responsible in any degree for the physical or mental harm inflicted on them. Indeed, in predatory terrorism the immediate victims and sufferers are, almost without exception, innocent persons. In all other types of terrorism, whether in peacetime or in time of war, some of the immediate victims or sufferers tend to be innocent persons; though some may be non-innocents, such as high-ranking members or representatives of the governments or the military morally responsible for the real or imagined wrong that triggers the terrorism.

The problem of distinguishing innocent and non-innocent persons in relation to the different types and forms of terrorism, except terrorism in war, is generally less difficult than the much-vexed corresponding problem in relation to war. My position here, as, *mutatis mutandis*, in relation to war, stated briefly and simply, is this. (a) 'Innocence' and 'non-innocence' consist in *moral* innocence and non-innocence respectively, relative to the particular acts, types or forms of terrorism T; (b) they are a matter of degree; and (c) a perfectly innocent person is one who has no share in the moral responsibility, *a fortiori*, no causal responsibility at all, for any wrong, if any, that gives or gave rise to T. A paradigmatically non-innocent person is someone who has an appreciable degree of moral (hence direct or indirect causal) responsibility [21] for some real wrong triggering T. Between that extreme and paradigmatic non-innocents we find possible cases of decreasing moral responsibility corresponding to decreasing degrees of causal responsibility. Here the targets are to some extent non-innocent but less so than in paradigmatic cases. (d) Moral responsibility may be direct or indirect by virtue of a person's direct or indirect role in T's causation—where T is caused by some real injustice or wrong. The degree of a person's innocence may therefore also vary in that way. A person whose actions are a proximate cause of the wrong is non-innocent in a higher degree than someone who has only indirect responsibility for it. *In principle* it is always possible to ascertain in particular cases whether a given individual is (causally) directly involved. Generally, it is also actually possible though often quite difficult to do so. Ascertaining who is indirectly involved and who is not involved at all is another matter. That is not too disquieting for our purposes, in so far as we are mainly concerned with the theoretical problem of the morality of terrorism. But it is of the essence from the would-be terrorists' as well as the law's point of view, unless the terrorists happen to be deranged, and target individuals or groups they imagine to be morally responsible for the grievances they are out to avenge, redress, etc. Further, the very life of some individuals may depend on the potential terrorists' ability to distinguish innocent from non-innocent persons or groups. Political, retaliatory or moralistic terrorists, driven by passion or paranoia, often baselessly enlarge, sometimes to a tragically absurd extent, the circle of alleged non-innocents. They sometimes target individuals, groups or whole nations having only a tenuous relation, often of a completely innocent kind, to those who have wronged their compatriots or ancestors, stolen their land, etc. The example I gave earlier of terrorists striking at the high-ranking officials of governments whose predecessors committed crimes against their people, illustrates this. Another example is the terrorists' targeting innocent persons they presume to be guilty by association;

because they happen to be of the same race, ethnic heritage, nationality or religion as those they deem responsible for their hurt.

An extreme and horrifying type of justification of the targeting of completely innocent persons was brought to my attention by Anthony O'Hear in a private communication. It involves the justification one sometimes hears, of the killing of holidaymakers, travellers and others, in Israel and other terrorist targets, in O'Hear's words, "on the ground that ... the very fact that they were contributing to the economy and morale of the targeted country [unwittingly] implicated them". As O'Hear commented, that defence is "a disgusting piece of casuistry". Its implications, I might add, are so far-reaching as to be positively frightening. If the travellers or holidaymakers were guilty of a crime against, say, the Palestinian people, as is claimed, then by parity of reasoning all individuals, institutions, groups or peoples, all countries or nations that have any kind of economic dealings with Israel and so contribute to its economy would likewise be guilty of a crime against the Palestinian people and so may be justifiably targeted! But then why exempt those *Arabs* who live in Israel and even those *Palestinians* residing on the West Bank or in the Gaza Strip who are employed in Israel—indeed, all those who spend any amount of money there—from guilt? The absurdity of all this needs no further elaboration.

Finally, law enforcement agencies as well as governments in general, to be able to protect individuals against terrorism, need to make reliable predictions about who is a likely target of known terrorist organisations. Yet in few other kinds of coercion or the use of force is the element of unpredictability and surprise greater or the strikes more impelled by emotion and passion than in terrorism.

The Principle of Proportion and Terrorism

In his discussion of the principle of proportion William O'Brien observes that "One of the criteria [of just war] requires that the good to be achieved by the realisation of the war aims be proportionate to the evil resulting from the war" [22]. And "the calculus of proportionality in just cause [that is, the political purpose, *raison d'état*, 'the high interests of the state'] is the total good to be expected if the war is successful balanced against the total evil the war is likely to cause" [23]. As in the case of war, formidable problems face the attempt to reach even the roughest estimates of the total expected good *vis-à-vis* the total evil likely to be caused by a particular act, and more so by a series of connected acts, of *political* or *moralistic* terrorism. The crudest estimates of the expected good of some political cause against the suffering or death of even one victim or patient of terrorism are exceedingly difficult. And if we turn from isolated acts of political terror to a whole series of such acts extending over a period of years or decades, as with Arab or IRA terrorism, the task becomes utterly hopeless. For how can we possibly measure the expected good resulting from the creation of e.g. an independent Catholic Northern Ireland or a Catholic Northern Ireland united with the Irish Republic, and compare it with the overall evil likely to be the lot of the Ulster Protestants in such an eventuality or on different scenarios of their eventual fate —then add the latter evil to the evils consisting in and consequent upon all the acts of terrorism that are supposed to help realise the desired good end? I see no possible way in which these factors can be quantified, hence added or subtracted [24].

The conclusion to which we are driven is that the Principle of Proportion in the present sense does not enable us to ascertain the rightness *or* wrongness of political or moralistic terrorism. The same conclusion can be similarly shown to follow from the

Principle of Proportion as understood by Donald Wells in *The 'Just War' Justifies Too Much* [25] or in my *Self-defense and the Just War* [26], respectively.

In addition to stipulating the proportionality of the *raison d'état* and the evil resulting from a war as a whole, O'Brien rightly stipulates that "a discrete military means . . . when viewed independently on the basis of its intermediate military end (*raison de guerre*), must . . . be proportionate . . . to that military end for which it was used, irrespective of the ultimate end of the war at the level of *raison d'état*" [27]. Barring that, it would be an immoral act. This principle, applied to discrete military means, O'Brien observes, is in line with the law of Nuremberg, which judged the "legitimacy of discrete acts of the German forces, . . . inter alia, in terms of their proportionality to intermediate military goals, *raison de guerre* . . . It was . . . a reasonable way to evaluate the substance of the allegations that war crimes had occurred" [28].

The present, second form of the Principle of Proportion *can* be applied, *mutatis mutandis*, to discrete acts of terrorism; provided that their probable intermediate results can be roughly assessed. For example, in evaluating the morality of the Achille Lauro seajacking, the short-term and intermediate "political" gains the terrorists expected to receive from it must be weighed, if possible, against the killing of an innocent passenger and the terrors visited on the other passengers on board. It can be safely said that wholly apart from the damage the seajacking did to the PLO and to the Middle East peace process as a whole, whatever short term and intermediate benefit the seajackers expected to reap from their acts [29], such as publicity and the dramatisation of the plight of the Palestinians under Israeli military rule in the occupied territories, was vastly outweighed by the evils the seajacking resulted in [30]. More important still, the actual and not (as in O'Brien's formulation of the Principle) merely the expected outcome of acts of terrorism, good and bad, must be weighed if possible, against each other. That is, actual proportionality must obtain if, in retrospect, the acts are to be objectively evaluated. But to do so is precisely to assess the consequences of the acts in terms of a consequentialist criterion, and so will be left for later consideration.

IV

Terrorism and Human Rights

If one believes that human beings have a (an equal) human right to life, one can argue that acts of terrorism are wrong whenever they threaten the lives of, and, especially, kill, their immediate victims; on the ground that acts that violate a human right are morally wrong. Unfortunately this way of making short shrift with terrorism in general is not open to those who, like myself, do not believe that a human right to life *as such* ought to be acknowledged [31]. Elsewhere I have argued that we must acknowledge that all human beings have a fundamental human right to be treated as moral persons. Further, that that right includes an equal right of all to be free to satisfy their needs and interests [32], and to actualise their potentials: that is, to seek to realise themselves and their wellbeing [33]. In addition to that right, I contended, human beings have an equal human right to equal opportunity and treatment to help them realize the aforementioned values, and that that right is either part of or is implied by the right to be treated as a moral person.

The rights in question do not entail a moral right to life. But his/her being alive is obviously necessary for an individual's having the possibility of realising the preceding and other values. Consequently the protective umbrella of these rights must be extended to it [34]; except when that protection is overridden by strong moral or other axiological claims. These may include the protection of the equal rights of others; or situations where taking a human life or letting nature take its course is (1) the lesser of two evils and (2) the action violates no one's equal human rights or other moral rights.

From the above it follows that acts of terrorism that cause the immediate or delayed death of their victims—unless they satisfy e.g. conditions (1) and (2)—are morally wrong. Condition (1) may perhaps be sometimes satisfied; but condition (2) cannot ever be satisfied. In fact all forms of terrorism I have distinguished seriously violate their immediate victims' and the sufferers' human rights as moral persons. Treating people as moral persons means treating them with consideration, in two closely related ways. First, it means respecting their autonomy. That autonomy is clearly violated if they are humiliated, coerced and terrorised, taken hostage or kidnapped, and, above all, killed. Second, consideration involves "a certain cluster of attitudes, hence certain ways of acting toward, reacting to and thinking about" [35] people. Part of that lies in sensitivity to and consideration of their feelings and desires, aspirations, projects and goals. That in turn is an integral part of treating their life as a whole—including their relationships and memories—as a thing of value. In fact, it also includes respecting their "culture or ethnic, religious or racial identity or heritage" [36]. These things are the very antithesis of what terrorism does to its victims and sufferers.

In sum, terrorism in general violates both aspects of its targets' right to be treated as moral persons. In retaliatory and moralistic terrorism that is no less true of those victims or those sufferers who are morally responsible, in some degree, for the wrong that precipitates the terrorist strike than of those who are completely innocent of that wrong. In predatory terrorism the terrorism violates the human right of everyone directly or indirectly hurt by it. For the terrorists the life of the immediate victims and their human rights matter not in the least. Similarly with the sufferers they terrorise. The terrorists use both groups, against their will, simply as instruments [37] for their own ends.

The matter can also be looked upon in terms of the ordinary concepts of *justice* and *injustice*. Terror directd against innocent persons is a grave injustice against them. In no case is this truer than when terrorists impute to their immediate victims or to the sufferers guilt by association. It is equally true when the victims are representatives of a government one or more of whose predecessors committed large-scale atrocities, such as attempted genocide, against the terrorists' compatriots or ancestors. True, the present government would be tainted by the original crimes if, to cite an actual case, it categorically refuses to acknowledge its predecessors' guilt and take any steps to redress the grievous wrongs. Similarly if it verbally acknowledges its predecessors' guilt but washes its hands of all moral or legal responsibility to make amends to the survivors of the atrocities or to their families, on the ground that it is a new government, existing decades later than the perpetrators. Yet only if the targeted representatives of the present government themselves are in some way responsible for their government's stand would they be non-innocent in some degree. Otherwise targeting them from a desire for revenge would be sheer murder or attempted murder.

Whenever the victims or sufferers are innocent persons terrorism directed against them constitutes a very grave injustice, just like 'punishing' an innocent person for a crime he or she has not committed. For in the present sense justice consists in one's receiving what one merits or deserves, determined by what one has done or refrained from doing.

It may be argued that some terrorist acts *may* be just punishment for wrongs committed by the immediate victims or the sufferers themselves, against the terrorists or persons close to them. But first, punishment cannot be just if founded on a denial of the wrongdoer's human rights. Second, a vast difference exists between terrorist 'punishment' and just legal punishment, which presupposes the establishment of guilt by a preponderance of the evidence. By definition terrorists do not and cannot respect the victims' and the sufferers' legal protections and rights, but erect themselves both as judges and jury—and executioners—giving the 'accused' no opportunity to defend themselves or be defended by counsel against the terrorists' allegations; let alone the possibility of defending themselves physically against their assailants [38]. This is a further corollary of the terrorists' denial of the moral and legal rights of the victims and sufferers.

V

Terrorism and Consequences

In Section IV I attempted to establish that terrorism in general always violates the immediate victims' and the sufferers' human right to be treated as moral persons. But an act cannot be morally right if it violates anyone's human rights, or at least cannot be right except in those extreme and rather rare cases where, e.g. overriding consequentialist considerations may justify the violation. It is therefore important to inquire whether any type or form of terrorism can be morally justified on purely utilitarian, consequentialist criteria of rightness.

(A) *Predatory and retaliatory terrorism.* Predatory and retaliatory terrorism can be easily disposed of on consequentialist grounds: it is extremely doubtful that such terrorism can result in overall good consequences—indeed, the greatest overall good possible in the circumstances. However, there are special considerations in the case of retaliatory terrorism, at least in relation to political-moralistic terrorism, which must be noted. Retaliatory terrorism is purely negative; merely a reaction to a putative evil visited on the terrorist, his organisation or compatriots, etc. It is not itself a positive objective and may or may not be part of an ultimate political or moralistic objective. Terrorist retaliation by bombings or by killing victims or sufferers, even if immediately successful, backfires on the terrorists and their supporters, organisations, etc. by e.g. provoking counter-terrorism; as we see e.g. in Lebanon, in the unending rounds of retaliation and counter-retaliation by Israeli forces and the Palestinian resistance. However, events during 1986 have shown that retaliatory terrorism involving hostages can be more effective from the terrorists' point of view; since, as happened in 1986, it can result in considerable concessions by targeted countries. The swapping of arms or hostages for jailed terrorists is one actual example that comes to mind. Nevertheless, the terrorists' *ultimate* goals are not thereby appreciably advanced. One consequence may be the hardening of world opinion against negotiation with terrorists or with states that support them. Another may be stepped-up counter-terrorism.

It is noteworthy that even if some individual acts of predatory or retaliatory terrorism are justifiable on *act*-utilitarian grounds, a *rule*-utilitarian justification is scarcely possible. A rule permitting predatory or retaliatory terrorism as a class would be anything but useful, considering the dire consequences of its general application for society as a whole. In fact the prevalence of these two types of terrorism can lead to a

Hobbesian State of Nature; where fear, widespread distrust and insecurity, both physical and psychological, would make the majority's life utterly miserable. The situation in Lebanon since 1975 is again a major example. Where they obtain these conditions would dwarf the current fear and uncertainty of travellers and others in large parts of the world.

(B) *'Revolutionary terrorism'*. Kai Nielsen, in *Violence and Terrorism: its uses and abuses* [39], presents a spirited defence of what he calls 'revolutionary terrorism', which is a species of political terrorism and may be a species of moralistic terrorism as well. His general thesis is that "...we cannot, unless we can make the case for pacifism [40],... categorically rule out in all circumstances its [terrorism's] justifiable use even in what are formally and procedurally speaking democracies" [41].

The two kinds of 'revolutionary violence' Nielsen defends are: "(1) revolutionary violence—the violence necessary to overthrow the state and to bring into being a new and better or at least putatively better social order—and (2) violence within a state when revolution is not an end but violence is only used as a key instrument of social change within a social system that as a whole is accepted as legitimate" [42]. Nielsen adds that "...it is often argued that, in the latter type of circumstances, a resort to violence is *never* justified when the state in question is a democracy" [43].

Nielsen's 'revolutionary violence' logically includes (1') 'revolutionary terrorism,' defined by parity as "terrorism deemed necessary by the terrorists to overthrow the state and to bring into being a new and better or at least putatively better social order"; while his 'violence within a state...' includes (2') "terrorism within a state where terrorism is used as a key instrument of putative desirable social change within a social system that as a whole is accepted as legitimate" [44].

I shall begin, as he does, with Nielsen's second kind of socialist revolutionary terrorism. It is noteworthy that he limits himself to the attempt to justify individual acts of terrorism of that kind rather than the class of such acts; i.e. he adopts an act-utilitarian criterion of right and wrong action.

The two conditions which, according to him, justified acts of revolutionary violence satisfy, are (1) that the revolutionaries "had good reason to believe" that their violent acts "might be effective," and (2) "they had good reason to believe that their... violence would not cause more injury and suffering all round than would simple submission or non-violent resistance to the violence directed against them by the state." His first example is of a democratically constituted government engaged in 'institutional violence' against blacks in black ghettoes, whose riots occasioned by their long-standing condition spill into white middle-class neighbourhoods. The riots cause the destruction of some property but not lives. The authorities respond by hauling blacks "to concentration camps (more mildly 'detention centers') for long periods of incarceration ('preventive detention') without attempting to distinguish the guilty from the innocent" [46]. Nielsen thinks that blacks "would plainly be justified in resorting to violence to resist being so detained in such circumstances" [47], if conditions (1) and (2) are satisfied. My response to this is as follows.

Nielsen couches conditions (1) and (2) not in terms of the *actual* success of the blacks' putative moral purpose and the overall good's actually outweighing the injury and suffering caused by the counter-violence, but in terms of 'good reasons,' hence the *likelihood* of the preceding in terms of the facts available to the blacks at the time. As far as prospective action is concerned 'good reasons' are obviously all that we can rationally go by. As Bertrand Russell somewhere says, probability is the guide of life;

and, clearly, rationality with respect to action consists in being guided by probabilities. Since the example assumes that blacks have good reasons for their expectation and hope that they will succeed, their actions will be *rational*. But suppose the results turn out to be otherwise than expected: would their counter-violence be morally *right* on act-utilitarian grounds? Or would they be wrong although the agents themselves would not be morally blameworthy? Nielsen does not confront these crucial questions.

Similar remarks apply to Nielsen's second and third examples; namely, that of [(2)] concerned citizens of a democratic superpower turning to violence, as a last resort, to disrupt "in some small measure" and "thus to weaken the 'institutional violence'" of their government as it wages "... genocidal war of imperialist aggression against a small, poor, underdeveloped nation" [48]. And [(3)] the violence of a small ethnic minority in defence of its members' human rights, against their treatment as second-class citizens. It is unclear from Nielsen's description of example (2) whether the violence includes acts of terror; but (3) is clearly not an example of terrorism. In fact the same is true, *mutatis mutandis*, of example (1) considered earlier. In that example the blacks' use of force can be plausibly viewed as an act of self-defence, not terrorism. Further, Nielsen supposes without evidence—indeed, erroneously—that whatever moral considerations apply to 'revolutionary violence' in general, irrespective of the forms it takes, necessarily apply to 'revolutionary terrorism' as well.

Let us return to the question I raised earlier but left unanswered, as to whether the use of force in general should be morally judged in terms of its actual consequences or, instead, its rationally expected, hence probable consequences. The answer, it seems to me, is the following. (a) Actions are performed with a view to bringing certain effects or consequences into existence, and their overall value or worth, moral or other, lies, partly or wholly, in their *actual* production of the best consequences, i.e. the greatest value possible in the circumstances. However, (b) since, as Bertrand Russell some-where says, probability is the guide of life, an action that has the best *probable* consequences in the circumstances is not normally called wrong on the ordinary uses of 'right' and 'wrong,' even when its actual consequences turn out to be, on the whole, bad or much less good than expected. Instead, we regard that fact as merely regrettable or unfortunate, sometimes tragic.

In view of this we must accept Nielsen's condition (1) as a valid right-making condition. Moreover, I shall grant for the sake of argument his condition (2). Even then problems with his defence of the present kind of revolutionary violence remain. For one thing, although the scenario he imagines is theoretically possible, acts of terrorism of the kind he describes have in the past invariably failed to satisfy condition (1) or condition (2), or both; and there are good reasons, some of which I have detailed earlier, to believe that this will continue to be true.

The foregoing observations about self-defence versus terrorism are of general application and need some elaboration. There are obvious differences between terror-ism and the use of force in individual self-defence and in collective, e.g. national, defence, that may be noted. One such difference is that a defender's use of force is solely and wholly designed to prevent harm to himself or herself, etc., not to harm the assailant as such. This distinguishes self-defence from all types of terrorism considered in this paper; while the fact that the defender is a victim or would-be victim and not an aggressor clearly distinguishes him or her, etc. from a predatory or a retaliatory terrorist. Since this description of self-defence applies to his first two examples ((1) and (2)), Nielsen's discussion fails to show that 'revolutionary *terrorism*' is morally justified whenever his right-making conditions are met. A bona fide example of 'revolutionary terrorism' as Nielsen understands it would be the blacks' taking innocent whites as hostages to force the authorities to release the rioters and other detained blacks. Other, actual examples that come to mind include the skyjacking of the TWA flight 847 plane by Lebanese Shi'ite Moslems in 1984, in which several Americans were taken hostage, and the seajacking of the Achille Lauro cruise ship in 1985 and the killing of one American by Palestinian terrorists/freedom fighters.

Let us turn to Nielsen's defence of the use of violence "to obtain a [left] revolutionary transformation of society for establishing or promoting human freedom and happiness" [49]. To his earlier two conditions of the moral justifiability of such violence he now adds a third condition; viz. (3) " ... if there are equally adequate alternative nonviolent means, it [a revolutionary movement] must use them" [50]. He adds: " ... it is not enough to justify a revolution to establish that it produced desirable results; we must also show that without the revolution the desirable results would not have occurred as rapidly and with (everything considered) as little suffering and degradation" [51]. This is a valid consequentialist principle; but to put the matter mildly, anything like establishing the counterfactuals it requires in such complex and highly controversial historical phenomena as entire revolutions (or even parts of a revolution) is a very tall order. For example, can we say with any degree of assurance that either the English or the French Revolution satisfied that condition, as Nielsen supposes? Only in the case of individual acts or a limited series of acts, at best, does it sometimes appear possible to make plausible and perhaps verifiable though always contestable hypotheses concerning 'the roads not taken' [52].

But suppose again for the sake of argument that these or any other revolutions, whether socialist or no, did, or do in fact, satisfy condition (3): the question remains as to the role that *terrorism*, if any, played or plays in them, and whether *it* was or is morally justified. Determining the answer by appeal to empirical evidence is a very difficult and uncertain undertaking.

It follows that on Nielsen's own three conditions an empirical case for the moral justifiability of any instance of revolutionary terrorism of the second kind has not been and probably cannot be made. For instance, Nielsen merely speculates that "terrorism in conjunction with more conventional military tactics *might well be an effective tactic* to drive out an oppressor" [53].

A good example of the purely speculative character of that claim is the Rhodesian and Algerian resistance to an oppressive imperialist rule, which Nielsen himself mentions.

In addition to his failure to give historical support for his claim, Nielsen is unclear as to the:

extent to which such resistance was terrorism and to what extent it was 'freedom fighting' designed to defend the Rhodesians' or Algerians' human and other rights by attempting to end the oppressive rule. But as Nicholas Fotion rightly observes in 'The Burdens of Terrorism,' [54] terrorists must demonstrate that their acts satisfy the conditions for the justifiable use of force. Failing that, they bear 'a special burden of moral wrongdoing' [55]. For as he says, 'We do not ask people to justify their actions when they harm no one in the process of attempting to achieve a good or alleged good .... But the more their efforts harm others, the more we expect an accounting that makes sense' [56].

This paper is dedicated to the memory of my cousin Khatcho, an innocent victim of the terrorism in Lebanon.

Haig Khatchadourian, Department of Philosophy, The University of Wisconsin—Milwaukee, P.O. Box 413, Milwaukee, Wisconsin 53201, USA.

NOTES

[1] Cf. also Secretary of State GEORGE SCHULZ's characterisation of terrorism as "murderous adventures" ('Small Wins in a Long War,' *Newsweek*, May 26, 1986, p. 34). Israel's and the U.S.'s branding of the PLO as a terrorist organization is part of the grave and complex problem facing the quest for a negotiated settlement of the Palestine Problem.

It is noteworthy that up to this moment, in the aftermath of the Iran arms scandal, the Reagan administration continues to insist that there was no swap of arms for U.S. hostages of Lebanese terrorists; and that its policy toward terrorism and states that support it has not changed.

[2] I use 'force' rather than the more common 'violence' since it is morally neutral or near-neutral, unlike the latter expression.

[3] I borrow these terms as well as 'immediate victim' from Abraham Edel, 'Notes on terrorism,' *Values in Conflict*, edited by BURTON M. LEISER (New York, 1981), p. 458.

[4] Second Edition (New York, [1979]), 13, pp. 375–397.

[5] Ibid., p. 375. Italics in original.

[6] 'War and murder,' *War and Morality*, edited by RICHARD A. WASSERSTROM (Belmont, CA, 1970), p. 45.

[7] Op. cit., p. 375.

[8] Ibid., p. 375. For a more precise characterization see later.

[9] Ibid., p. 379. LEISER's view of terrorism is crystalized in the section on pp. 389–391, entitled 'Terrorists: enemies of mankind'.

[10] Ibid., pp. 386ff. LEISER's whole discussion of Palestinian armed resistance is conceived from a pro-Israeli, Zionist point of view.

[11] Ibid., p. 381. Italics in original.

[12] 'Essentially Contested Concepts,' *Proceedings of the Aristotelian Society*, N.S. vol. LVI (March, 1956), pp. 180ff. But Gallie maintains that a concept must have certain characteristics in addition to appraisiveness (enumerated in ibid., pp. 171–172; p. 180) in order to be 'essentially contested' in his sense.

[13] Those who use 'terrorism' in general as a condemnatory term would substitute 'violence' for 'force'; since the former is generally used to mean morally (or legally) unjustified use of force.

[14] I borrow the categories 'predatory' and 'moralistic' from EDEL LEISER (op. cit., p. 453). Some but not all moralistic terrorism is political terrorism, or vice versa.

[15] See also the CIA's definition, in: ALLAN S. NANES, *International Terrorism* (Congressional Research Service, 1985, p. 1), the *Convention for the Suppression of Unlawful Acts Against the Safety of Civil Aviation* (Montreal, 23 September 1971), and *Convention on the Prevention and Punishment of Crimes Against International Protected Persons, Including Diplomatic Agents*, adopted by the UN General Assembly, 14 December, 1973. See also Harriet Culley, *International Terrorism* (August 1985, Bureau of Public Affairs, Department of State).

I owe the material on U.S. Resolution 2781, 99th Congress, 1st Session, pp. 1–3, as well as the foregoing references, to the research of a former student of mine, Mr Thomas Kurzynski.

[16] In LEISER, op. cit., p. 458.

[17] The type of concept distinguished by LUDWIG WITTGENSTEIN in *Philosophical Investigations*.

[18] Op. cit., p. 39.

[19] Ibid., p. 30.

[20] Ibid., p. 37.

[21] What constitutes an appreciable degree of moral responsibility would of course be a matter of controversy.

[22] Ibid., p. 37.

[23] Ibid.

[24] For the special significance of this in relation to revolutionary terrorism, see Section V.

[25] *Philosophy For a New Generation* (New York, 1970), edited by A.K. BIERMAN & JAMES A. GOULD, pp.

218–230. WELLS, following JOSEPH MCKENNA ('Ethics and war: a Catholic view,' *American Political Science Review*, September 1960, pp. 647–658) states it as the condition that "... the seriousness of the injury inflicted on the enemy must be proportional to the damage suffered by the virtuous" (WELLS, op. cit., p. 220).

[26] As I stated the Principle in relation to morally justified collective self-defense, it stipulates that the defender's military response "must be measured and restrained. That is, as much as circumstances allow, not just the intended but the actual damage it inflicts on ... the aggressor, during the armed conflict, must be at most roughly proportional to the damage inflicted at the time by ... the aggressor" (Op. cit., p. 161).

[27] Op. cit., p. 37.

[28] Ibid., p. 38.

[29] One of the seajackers stated· after being captured that the seajackers' original objective was a suicidal mission in Israel. That objective, of course, was not realised.

[30] Note that the question whether the capture, trial and almost certain punishment of the seajackers and others implicated in the seajacking is to be judged a good or an evil to be added to the one or the other side of the balance sheet, partly depends for its answer on the evaluation of the seajacking itself as morally justified or unjustified. (I say "partly depends" because the legal implications of the act are also relevant.)

[31] See my 'Medical ethics and the value of human life,' *Philosophy in Context*, 14, 1984, pp. 42–50.

[32] 'Toward a foundation for human rights,' *Man and World*, 18, 1985, pp. 219–240.

[33] 'The human right to be treated as a person,' *The Journal of Value Inquiry*, 19, 1985, pp. 183–195.

[34] 'Medical ethics and the value of human life,' *passim.*

[35] 'The human right to be treated as a person,' p. 21.

[36] Ibid., p. 22.

[37] Cf. EDEL'S condemnation of terrorism on Kant's principle "... that people ought to be treated as ends in themselves and never as means only. Terrorists necessarily treat human beings as means to the achievement of their political, economic, or social goals" (from LEISER'S Introduction to the Section on Terrorism, in *Values in Conflict*, p. 343).

[38] See my 'Is political assassination ever morally justified?' in *Assassination* (Boston, [1975]), edited by HAROLD ZELLNER, pp. 41–55, for similar criticism of political assassination.

[39] In LEISER, op. cit., pp. 435–449.

[40] If my claims concerning the existence of human rights in general and the right to be treated as a moral person in particular are essentially correct, Nielsen is mistaken in claiming that only by making the case for pacifism can the moral justifiability of terrorism in all circumstances be ruled out.

For a consideration of some of the main difficulties in universal pacifism, see my 'Pacifism,' *World Futures*, 21, Nos. 3/4 (1985), pp. 263–278.

[41] Op. cit., p. 435.

[42] Ibid., p. 438.

[43] Ibid. Italics in original.

[44] Ibid. NIELSEN describes terrorism in the context of a socialist revolutionary activity as follows: "In this context we should view terrorism as a tactical weapon in achieving a socialist revolution .... A terrorist is one who attempts to further his or her political ends by means of coercive intimidation, and terrorism is a systematic policy designed to achieve that end" (Ibid., p. 445).

[45] Op. cit., pp. 438–9.

[46] Ibid., p. 438.

[47] Ibid.

[48] Ibid., p. 439.

[49] Op. cit., p. 442.

[50] Ibid., p. 445, footnote 15.

[51] Ibid., footnote 15. However, in his later discussion (ibid., p. 446) of the conditions of terrorism as a tactical weapon in achieving a socialist revolution, he makes that condition his *second* for justified revolutionary terrorism; either forgetting or consciously eliminating without explanation his original condition (2).

[52] An example from another quarter illustrates some of the complexities involved here. I refer to the recent U.S. raid on Libya. Apart from the question whether it was morally justified, or justified by international law, it is highly disputable whether, in the long run, it will be more effective in deterring terrorism (at least in its state-sponsored variety) than rigorous collective economic and diplomatic sanctions against Libya. One difficulty is the uncertainty of the raid's effects on Libya's future policy

toward terrorism, as well as its effects on Syria, Iran and other states that currently do support or are accused of supporting terrorism. Part of the difficulty of assessing the raid's own effects stems from the fact that after the raid the U.S. and its allies have begun imposing increasingly stringent economic and diplomatic sanctions against Libya. Hence if, for instance, Libyan or other state-sponsored terrorism decreases, it will be very hard to say what the share of the U.S. military action in the decrease has been.

[53] Ibid. My italics.
[54] In LEISER, op. cit., pp. 463–470.
[55] Ibid., p. 468.
[56] Ibid., pp. 468–469.

12

Area Bombing, Terrorism and the Death of Innocents

GERRY WALLACE

ABSTRACT *This paper is concerned with the view that, in so far as they involve the deliberate targeting of innocent people, neither terrorism nor area bombing is ever morally permissible. Four attempts to justify this view are considered, all of which are based on the intuition that deliberately killing innocent people is wrong. By means of a detailed examination of the introduction of area bombing by Britain in 1940–41, it is argued that in certain circumstances there are other equally powerful and accessible intuitions which support the opposite view. It is further argued that only moral theories which provide for the weighing of competing moral intuitions are capable of avoiding this kind of impasse and the biased selection of intuitions that this form of absolutism involves.*

Introduction

For the greater part of the Second World War, and certainly from 1941 onwards, the overwhelming majority of bombing raids carried out by the Allies consisted of 'area bombing' [1]. Prior to this, area bombing had occurred but strategic bombing was regarded as more important. Later still in the war, when Germany was a less powerful force, huge fleets of bombers destroyed German towns in daylight. Night or day, what was common to these raids was the deliberate targeting of towns, or areas of towns, hence 'area bombing', with the inevitable and enormous toll of civilian casualties. The death of these civilians was not incidental to the pursuit of some other strategic goal such as the destruction of factories or marshalling yards; the civilians themselves were the target.

The story of how area bombing came to be given priority over strategic bombing is an instructive one for anyone interested in the morality of conflict. It is also of great contemporary importance because there are striking parallels between area bombing and some terrorist activities: both being deliberately aimed at the deaths of people normally regarded as innocent. This suggests that it might prove useful to bear in mind the conviction that such terrorist acts are always wrong, alongside a consideration of the morality of area bombing. One of my concerns will be to consider whether a moral justification can be offered for the introduction of area bombing and, if so, what form such a justification might take. Given the similarities between area bombing and some terrorist acts, one would expect justifications in the former area to have some *prima facie* validity in the other. A. J. Coady in his excellent paper, *The Morality of Terrorism*, has argued that terrorist acts, inasmuch as they involve the deliberate killing of innocent people, are morally indefensible. Terrorist campaigns, even when they are in support of a 'just' revolution, must conform to the rules governing what is permissible in a just war. And since targeting innocent people in a just war is unjustifiable, terrorist acts which do this are indefensible [2].

Most of this paper is devoted to considering an absolutist approach to the killing of innocent people which I call Internalism [3]. According to the Internalist, when we focus on what is actually involved in killing innocent people—on, as it were, the 'internal' features of the action—we realise that it can never be morally justified. Internalism is thus a form of intuitionism. Consequentialists have rejected such intuitions both on general philosophical grounds and as adequate guides in war and other conflict situations. However although I reach the same conclusion as, for example, Hare and Brandt [4], I take a rather different route from them.

My methodology needs explanation. By adopting a similar intuitionist style of reasoning to the Internalist, I try to show that the intuition that killing innocent people is wrong is not uniquely relevant to the moral issues involved in area bombing. I argue that there are other moral intuitions, equally powerful and accessible, which are at odds with Internalism so the Internalist is in reality selecting—without explaining how or why—from a range of possible intuitions. This being the case, he/she needs to explain why they treat the intuition that killing innocent people is wrong as though it were unique or necessarily overriding. A method of weighing these competing intuitions against one another is required. Yet, as I try to show, it is far from clear that Internalism can offer such a principle because the Internalist is unable, in Hare's phrase [5], to think creatively at this point.

Consequentialism clearly provides *a* way of thinking about situations in which conflicts of moral intuitions arise; although my arguments do not show that it is the *only* possible way. It will be readily apparent, nevertheless, that the counter-intuitions I provide to the Internalist case are perfectly compatible with various forms of consequentialism and could be justified along consequentialist lines. In this sense, consequentialism can provide a rational foundation for the counter-intuitions I discuss whereas, if I am right, although Internalism needs some such foundations it is extremely difficult to see where they might be found.

As a final preliminary, I must say something about moral justification. I assume, without further argument, that if an agent is morally justified in doing X, or has a moral justification for doing X, then he/she is not morally blameworthy if he/she does X. I further assume that to deny that a person is morally blameworthy is not to imply that he/she is deserving of moral credit or praise. As I understand the term, and also I believe in ordinary speech, in order to have a justification for what you did, neither you nor your action need be praiseworthy. To have a justification implies only that it was permissible to do what you did. It is in this sense that we speak of justifiable homicide. I cannot make sense of the claim that a person who is morally justified in doing X might be morally blameworthy if he/she does X. To think otherwise, as Michael Walzer [6] appears to, I regard as a case of taking with one hand what you give with the other. Thus, I assume from the outset that if a justification can be given for the introduction of area bombing this will simply establish that the killing of innocent people in this way was permissible, not that it was good or praiseworthy or a moral duty.

I

The Introduction of Area Bombing

The Strategic Air Offensive against Germany 1939-45 is a cool, perhaps chilling, guide to the conversion to area bombing [7]. It does not, however, contain an explicit attempt to provide a moral justification for the decision to adopt a policy of targeting German civilians. Nevertheless, moral considerations surface occasionally along with strategic and prudential ones and it is not difficult to construct from the mass of memos, directives and reports we find there the beginnings of a moral defence that intuitively has considerable appeal.

It is necessary, however, before looking at the particular considerations which prompted the adoption of a policy of area bombing in 1940–41 to understand the strategic context in which this decision was reached. France had by this time suffered total military collapse. The British army had been forced to quit mainland Europe at Dunkirk. The invasion of Britain was still a possibility. It is true that the Battle of Britain had made this a less immediate threat but it certainly could not be discounted. Equally menacingly, at sea the Battle of the Atlantic, in which German submarines were destroying large numbers of Allied ships, threatened food and military supply lines. So acute were these difficulties at sea that Churchill thought the Navy might actually lose the war [8]. If Britain was to avoid defeat and eventually have a chance of winning the war, the onus was on the Air Force to play the leading role.

However, it was not well placed to do so. The number and types of bombers available to it were such that raids had to be undertaken at night; by day German fighters had little difficulty in destroying them. But such raids proved largely ineffective because of deficiencies in nocturnal navigation and bomb-aiming systems. Photographic evidence available at the time demonstrated their futility. In the course of night attacks on two oil installations one plant was attacked by 162 aircraft carrying 159 tons of bombs, the other by 134 aircraft carrying 103 tons of bombs. Neither plant suffered any major damage [9]. A policy of strategic bombing by night had little to recommend it. If Bomber Command was to hit its targets they would have to be very big targets. The Butt report to Bomber Command in 1941 underlined this: of all the planes *recorded as having attacked their targets* only one-third actually got within five miles of them. In the circumstances, if Bomber Command was to be relied on to do any damage the target would normally have to be a German town [10].

The decision to adopt a policy of area bombing was in part, therefore, the result of the very restricted range of military possibilities open to Britain in 1940–41. It was a last resort in desperate circumstances. There were also other important factors at work. At the time the Luftwaffe was causing considerable damage to British towns: London, Coventry, Hull, Birmingham and Liverpool being particularly badly hit. Retaliation was taken. One raid on Mannheim was explicitly in return for German raids on Coventry and Southampton. But retaliation eventually gave way to a less purely reactive stance and the targeting of German cities came to be seen as the best way of reducing the morale and will of the German people. Area bombing became Bomber Command's priority.

A moral argument. As far as I know, no explicitly moral justification for the introduction of area bombing was given at the time; which might suggest that no one thought it could be morally justified. But the truth is different; many people then and now did think Britain's action was justified, albeit as a last resort. It seems reasonable to suppose that their case would have been along the following lines.

Germany was the aggressor in World War II and aimed to establish Nazi control over large areas of the world. Our detailed knowledge of how the Nazis treated subject peoples was not available in 1940 but even by then it was clear that victory for its racist policies would be a moral catastrophe. In 1940–41, with its Navy on the defensive, its army withdrawn from mainland Europe, America on the sidelines and the rest of Europe defeated, Britain's survival was very much in doubt. Meanwhile its civilians were being killed and maimed in Luftwaffe raids which showed little regard for human life. Given the severely restricted range of options open to Bomber Command, if it was to make any contribution to the war effort it had to be a policy of area bombing. (I am not sure whether Germany had explicitly adopted a policy of area bombing by 1940. For the purposes of this paper, I shall assume that it had no scruples about targeting residential areas of British cities, with the inevitable civilian deaths. If I am wrong on this point, my argument will not be affected but my 'real' example will become an hypothetical one.)

Let us now suppose that these are the 'facts' which would have been advanced at the time to justify the introduction of area bombing. Notice that even if it is successful, the attempted justification is extremely limited in its scope. For instance, it needs to be remembered that the bombing of German cities in 1940–41 took place in a very different military climate to the mass daylight bombing raids of later in the war. The latter, including horrors such as the destruction of Dresden, cannot be justified, if they are justifiable at all, in the same way. By then many other military options were available: America had joined the war, daylight strategic bombing runs were technically feasible and Nazi Germany was in retreat on both its eastern and western fronts. The contrast between then and 1940–41 when Britain faced what Churchill called a 'supreme emergency' is obvious. Parallel arguments in defence of terrorist actions will be subject to similar severe restriction.

Nor does the attempted justification presuppose that nations, peoples or individuals have some absolute right to survive. Our attempted justification stresses the moral calamity that a Nazi invasion or victory would have brought and the responsibility Germany bore for starting the war for no good moral reason. An advocate of our justification could restrict the putative right to these exceptional circumstances. The best defence of area bombing is as a last resort method of collective self-defence in the face of similar raids from the Luftwaffe.

Nevertheless, despite its limitations and intuitive appeal, the argument is open to a number of objections which I shall now examine [11].

II

Some Absolute Objections to Area Bombing

A quick objection to the foregoing attempts at justification would simply rely on the definition of murder as the deliberate killing of an innocent person. Since both area bombing and many terrorist acts involve this, they involve murder and so are in principle incapable of justification. The recourse of Britain in 1940–41 to area bombing, and of oppressed peoples to terrorism, it may be said, is understandable but nevertheless *what* they have recourse to is murder.

This is perhaps too swift an objection because it is far from clear that a definition of murder can settle a moral issue such as this. Did Britain in 1940 *murder* German people when it espoused area bombing? I think many people would find it difficult to answer this question merely on the basis of a proposed definition of murder. To insist on this approach will simply lead a determined opponent to question either the definition of murder or whether murder in the proposed sense is always unjustifiable. Nor is it enough simply to describe killing innocent people as barbaric or grotesque. It is obviously a dreadful or terrible thing to do but this does not help us to decide whether it is ever a permissible thing to do.

A more profound kind of opposition, with which the rest of this paper will be concerned, comes from what I have called Internalism [12].

The Internalist tells us not to be seduced into consideration of consequences when we are making moral judgements about the killing of innocent people. Put in the most general terms, what we must do is focus on what is involved in deliberately killing an innocent person, on what one is actually doing in doing such a thing. Once we do so, he/she contends, the futility of attempted justification is apparent. Just reflect on what you are doing and you will see that it cannot be justified.

If we try to spell this out a little more, there would seem to be four important arguments which the Internalist might have in mind.

(1) When we reflect on what is involved in killing an innocent person, it is apparent there can be nothing about him/her—the victim—which can justify this treatment. Contrast this with killing in self-defence, judicial execution or shooting an enemy soldier; in all of these cases *if* the killing is justified there will be something about the person killed in virtue of which a justification is possible. But when a person is innocent there will be no such factor; if he/she is innocent he/she will not be a threat, nor will his/her past actions provide a justification. Thus, any attempted justification will rely not on facts about the victim but on facts about other people: how they will benefit from the death of innocent people, or how the misdeeds of others justify retaliation. In other words any attempted justification will rely on the assumption that the death of an innocent person can legitimately be used as a means to some purpose such as the good of others or as a reprisal for the deeds of others. But both ideas are morally repellent.

This is a powerful argument. It is hopeless and dishonest to respond to it by seeking to show that in modern war there are no innocents. If by innocents we have in mind those who are not involved in the organisation, manning or supplying of the war machine, a pretty broad understanding of the term, there will still be many non-combatants who are in this sense innocent. They will certainly include those who know nothing about the war, perhaps because they are too young or confused, and many of the aged and infirm.

It is surely more realistic to argue that although modern war does not obviate the distinction between innocent and non-innocent, it may sometimes be impossible to fight such wars without, as it were, putting the distinction on one side, and that it is sometimes permissible to do this. The Internalist may be inclined to reply that modern war can never be justified if this is what it involves. The trouble, I suggest, with this is that it takes no account whatsoever of the situation of those countries or states or communities which are the victims of unjustified attacks. Are we to say that their involvement in modern war, in their own defence, cannot be justified? Naturally, the Internalist will concede they have a right to defend themselves but only so long as they have no recourse to killing innocent people. But if the nature of modern warfare is such that on occasion it can only be successfully prosecuted by putting on one side the distinction between innocent and non-innocent, the Internalist will be allowing the aggrieved state or community the right to defend itself whilst denying it what conceivably may be its only means of doing so.

(2) Let us now turn to the second of the Internalist objections. This is to the effect that if it were possible to justify the deliberate killing of an innocent person in war, it would be possible to justify the action to the victim. But if one imagines oneself in the innocent victim-to-be's situation, one will readily appreciate that there can be no such justification. If I am to be killed for the misdeeds or good of others then this is

manifestly wrong. If my death is a means to the benefit of others what can possibly justify my losing totally while they gain?

Though it might be natural for the victim-to-be to think of his/her death as being for the misdeeds of others and therefore manifestly wrong, the ambiguity is obvious. If the introduction of area bombing in 1940–41 was justified, it was not as a punishment but as the only means to survival of a community suffering similar innocent deaths.

Nevertheless, it is true, as the Internalist contends, that there can be nothing about an individual victim, given that he/she is an innocent victim, which will justify his or her treatment. There is nothing about *him/her* which justifies anyone in taking *his/her* life so it seems reasonable to conclude that *his/her* death cannot be justified.

On the other hand, it is by no means self-evident that the Internalist requirement of justification to the victim—in terms of something about him/her—is a legitimate demand. If we take a parallel piece of reasoning: can a strike or piece of industrial action only be justified if there is something about each person adversely affected by the action which justifies the treating of *that* person in that way? Is it even possible to arrive at a reasonable or rational decision on issues like this without considering such things as the aims of the strike, the alternatives, the history of the conflict or the relationship between the workers and their employers: that is to say, factors which an 'Internalist' view of strikes would deem to be irrelevant? Strikes, like wars, are examples of collective conflicts, the nature of which may make it impossible to play by the rules that apply in conflicts between individuals. I suggest that just as the 'innocent' victims of a strike may not be prepared to condemn the strikers, it is at least conceivable that an innocent potential victim of area bombing, reflecting on the actions of his/her own government and military forces, and the options available to the enemy, might adopt the same approach.

This is by no means as strange a suggestion as it appears at first sight. Indeed, it is typically what happens when a moral rule is overridden. Take the example of keeping one's promises: when we acknowledge that an agent was justified in breaking a promise, must there be something about the *promisee* in virtue of which the breaking of the promise can be justified? Surely not. The considerations which justify the breaking of the promise may be totally unconnected with the promisee: if I had kept my promise something dreadful would have happened to a third party; therefore I was justified in breaking my promise to you. You lose out through no fault of your own. Similar examples could be constructed for other moral rules. Hence, if the requirement of justifiability to the victim applies in the case of killing, it must be because of something about killing as opposed to, say, promise keeping. I suggest that the onus is on the Internalist to explain what this difference is.

(3) The third Internalist objection applies specifically to examples of *retaliatory* killing of the innocent. There may have been an element of this in the conversion to area bombing, for many people at the time would have regarded it as relevant to point out that the Luftwaffe paid scant regard for innocent life when conducting their bombing raids on Britain. Similarly, many terrorist acts have been 'justified' on the ground that they are undertaken on behalf of communities which have themselves suffered murderous attacks from their oppressors. But, the Internalist objects: to retaliate in this way is simply to repeat the original deed whilst making the absurd claim that this time it is justified.

There are a number of things to notice about this important argument.

I accept that you cannot justify an action merely by establishing that it is in retaliation for what you have suffered. To this extent Internalism is correct. Obviously

retaliatory actions can be pointless; for instance revenge, which is necessarily retaliatory, may be aimed at, and achieve nothing more than, the satisfaction to be had from
the plight of others. It is difficult to see how that alone can provide a basis for moral
justification. Further, in extreme cases such as nuclear retaliation undertaken when
one's own country has been destroyed, it may have no point whatsoever. On the other
hand, some forms of retaliatory action, for example, taking reprisals, are not necessarily pointless; indeed, they may deter an enemy from repeating the original offence.
In situations of lawlessness, even the practice of taking revenge may make the overall
situation less perilous than might be otherwise be the case. Significantly, the distinction
between pointless and non-pointless retaliatory actions is of no importance for the
Internalist. Unlike the consequentialist, who can approach the morality of reactive
deeds in this way, the Internalist is committed to rejecting consideration of consequences as morally irrelevant. It follows that for the Internalist there is no moral
difference between killing innocent people as an act of (pointless) revenge and killing
innocent people as a reprisal designed to secure a de-escalation, or non-repetition, of
hostilities when there is a good chance of this succeeding. Retaliation in lawless
situations will be on a par with retaliation in law-governed situations. By ignoring the
variety of circumstances in which the action of killing an innocent person can occur,
the Internalist in effect *makes it true* that the retaliatory killing of innocent people is
merely a repetition of the original offence. Having deemed all possible distinguishing
features to be irrelevant, the Internalist concludes that any attempt to justify the
retaliatory killing of innocent people will be in breach of the principle that two wrongs
do not make a right (TWNMR from now on).

Intuitively the TWNMR seems to me to have some force. There are situations in
which to reply in kind is merely to behave in the same petty, stupid, rude or vicious
way as the person to whose behaviour one has taken exception. But, I suggest, the
Internalist goes wrong when he/she takes the TWNMR to be an infallible guide to
what is morally justifiable. One very important sphere in which I shall argue it is not a
good guide is that of self-defence.

If a person is physically attacked by another, it is agreed by all but pacifists, that
he/she is morally entitled to defend him/herself. In order to do so, he/she may need to
physically attack the aggressor. In recognising the legitimacy of this retaliatory
response, we would expect to be in breach of the TWNMR; but most people, I believe,
would judge that we are not, or that if we are, this has no bearing on the legitimacy of
the action. If the TWNMR has trouble in handling self-defence this is a serious fault
in it.

At this point something needs to be said about the connections between retaliation
and self-defence; after all, the Internalist argument we are considering is about
retaliation, not self-defence. Obviously there are important differences between the
two. A piece of retaliation may have nothing to do with self-defence; for instance,
when it is nothing more than a piece of revenge. Moreover, self-defence need not be
retaliatory; it may be anticipatory, as when one strikes first in the face of an imminent
threat. Nevertheless, despite these differences, actions undertaken in self-defence are
typically reactive in that they are normally in response to an attack which has already
occurred. Retaliatory actions, therefore, can be undertaken in self-defence, as well as
for other reasons such as revenge, retribution, reprisal or vengeance. When a retaliatory action, undertaken in self-defence, is justified the justification will derive from its
self-defensive rather than its retaliatory character. To this extent the Internalist is
correct in implying that retaliation alone never confers justification. But from what we

have said, it also follows that provided a retaliatory deed is a permissible piece of self-defence, there will be a potentially morally relevant difference between it (the reply) and the original attack. From which I conclude that the TWNMR principle cannot be used to establish that retaliation in kind can be no more justifiable than the attack to which it is a response.

We must now consider what I regard as the most plausible and attractive aspect of Internalism. By definition, innocent people are not aggressors, nor are they an imminent threat to anyone. So even if retaliatory actions can sometimes be justified in terms of self-defence, the retaliatory killing of innocent people cannot be so justified, for the simple reason that the victims of the response will not be aggressors. We might put this Internalist point as follows: you cannot defend yourself against an innocent person because there is nothing to defend yourself against; therefore killing innocent people can never be justified in terms of self-defence. So even if retaliatory killing is sometimes justifiable in terms of the right to self-defence this can never legitimise the deliberate killing of innocents.

It must be admitted that our defence of area bombing in terms of self-defence is paradoxical. If a person is innocent in the required sense then he/she is not a threat since he/she is neither a combatant nor involved in the organisation or supplying of the war machine. So how can that person's death ever be justified in terms of self-defence?

One might have two different points in mind here. First, if a person is not presently a threat how can that person's death contribute to the defence of anyone? The answer to this is that whether a death or class of deaths will lead to the cessation or decreased intensity of hostilities depends on the circumstances. The British in 1940–41 thought that the effects of area bombing on German morale would be considerable. Whether this belief was true or not cannot be decided by an appeal to a definition of innocence. Hence, whatever the morality of area bombing, there is no absurdity in the thought that a community might defend itself by killing innocent people on the other side.

On the other hand, the request for an explanation of how the death of an innocent person can be justified in terms of self-defence could be taken in another way. Granted, it might be said, that killing innocent people may stop or reduce the intensity of an attack: how can this be justified in terms of a right to self-defence? Unless the right of a country to defend itself licenses the killing of innocent people, we are no closer to a justification since it is surely common ground that there are both legitimate and illegitimate means of defence. If I am violently attacked by someone but can distract him and hence escape by shooting an innocent bystander this cannot be justified in terms of my right to self-defence. How is area bombing different?

What we have come face-to-face with is the strong temptation to analyse conflicts between states in the same terms as those which are appropriate for conflicts between individuals. If we give in, it becomes difficult to see how killing innocent people might ever be permissible. The innocent civilian in wartime comes to be represented by the innocent bystander in the dispute between individuals. Internalist methodology tends to reinforce this by ignoring context thus implying that there are no morally relevant differences between the two kinds of conflict. But if area bombing was justified, it was justified in terms of collective self-defence, a concept that has no place in the discussion of individual conflict. This is why we must not assume that the moral rules appropriate for conflicts between individuals can be applied without modification in group conflicts. Conflicts between individuals cannot generate the moral dilemmas which can arise in group conflicts. If killing innocent people is always wrong this will be so even when it is the only means of defence open to a community *that is itself suffering innocent deaths*; a state of affairs that cannot arise in conflicts between individuals. In these circumstances, Internalist morality will nevertheless require a country or community to accept innocent deaths in perilous circumstances without recourse to what may be its only form of defence, retaliation in kind. To make good this claim, the Internalist needs to show that the differences between individual and group conflict are of no moral significance.

I conclude that although Internalism is right to claim that in bombing innocent German civilians in 1940–41 the British could not have been defending themselves from those particular civilians, it does not follow that area bombing was not a justifiable means of collective defence.

(4) Finally, we must consider the important Internalist claim that once we make ourselves fully aware of what is involved in the action of deliberately killing an innocent person, we shall recognise that it is not an action a decent human being could bring him/herself to do. The ability to do such a thing demonstrates that one has a morally corrupt character and hence that the action can never be morally justified, still less morally required.

The Internalist, I believe, is right to this extent: there would appear to be some actions which no matter how good their consequences we would not require anyone to do. One such horror, discussed by Alan Gewirth, is that of a son who in order to avert a missile attack on a city by terrorists must torture his mother to death [13]. Ignoring questions about negative responsibility, the Internalist is surely correct: we would have the gravest possible doubts about the moral character of a son who was capable of this.

Nevertheless, whilst not denying that there are actions which appear to fit the Internalist case, I wonder whether the area bombing of German cities in 1940–41 is one. It is far from clear, I suggest, that those RAF personnel who carried out such raids must have been of defective moral character. Indeed, I think the suggestion only has to be made for its absurdity to be manifest. It is true and important that some personnel did object to such raids on conscientious grounds. But that is no reason for concluding that those who did not were morally corrupt. Nevertheless, in order to make good these assertions we must try to explain how a decent human being might be perfectly capable of deliberately killing innocent people.

To begin with, it needs to be emphasised that the Internalist's strategy is to arrive at a moral conclusion (that deliberately killing innocent people is always wrong) by reflecting on what an agent requires in terms of capacities in order to be able to do such a thing. Although I acknowledge that there may be a place for such arguments in moral philosophy, and reject the view that they necessarily put the cart before the horse, they obviously need to be handled with care because clearly some capacities for action will vary with circumstances. In particular these capacities are crucially affected by our beliefs and emotions. Internalism must therefore rest on a set of psychological assumptions about the unalterability of the decent person's incapacity to kill innocent people.

Let us first consider capacities and beliefs. Clearly, a person might believe—falsely, let us suppose for the moment—that he/she is morally justified in certain circumstances in participating in an area bombing raid. Anyone of a consequentialist outlook will take this view. Are we to conclude from this possibility that the Internalist account of what a decent human being can or cannot do is based on the assumption that such a person cannot have false moral beliefs? I accept that there are certain beliefs which no decent person could adopt, for example, that we have a moral duty to cause as much suffering as we possibly can. But unless we give 'decent' a bizarre meaning, this cannot be so for all false beliefs and without begging the question the Internalist cannot assume that it is so in the present case. Unfortunately, however, this does not get us very far because the Internalist need not be too troubled by an objection which presupposes the falsity of the view that the killing of innocent people can be morally justified.

So let us now consider how capacities for action vary with emotions and feelings. The Internalist must not arrive at what a decent or uncorrupted human being is capable of by writing in the psychological attitudes and emotions of peace time. We must not ignore the fact that RAF personnel were aware of what the Luftwaffe were doing to British cities, perhaps members of their families had been killed or injured. They were aware of the gravity of their country's situation in 1940. Is the Internalist assuming that a decent human being's capacities must remain untouched by these feelings and this knowledge? That is to say, is the decent human being incapable of being moved to retaliate when he/she thinks this is the only way to defend their country and save their family and fellow citizens from Nazi domination? If so, then surely psychological impossibility is bought at too high a price; for now the decent human being is beginning to sound decidedly saintly, and if we make what the saint would do in these circumstances the yardstick we are in danger of setting too high a standard. It is arguable that if Britain had endorsed Internalism in 1940–41 she would have behaved in a noble, if suicidal way. But this is not the point. There is no reason why we should accept this as a test of what a non-saintly but decent person could do. Note that this is a point about possible motivations, not justifications. It is not meant to justify area bombing but to rebut the Internalist claim about the capacities of a morally decent person. I conclude that there are no good reasons for asserting that service personnel, aware of the facts in 1940, would, as decent human beings, have found it impossible to implement a policy of area bombing.

III

Internalist Abstraction

The Internalist arrives at the conclusion that the deliberate killing of innocent people cannot be justified, by focusing on what this involves. In other words he/she abstracts from the many and various possible circumstances in which 'the' action can occur, thereby implying that no set of circumstances, actual or possible, can make a difference to the morality of the action in question. The action, abstracted in this way, is then deemed absolutely wrong: that is unjustifiable in any circumstances. Clearly the acceptability of this procedure depends on the legitimacy of the original abstraction. Provided this is justified, the conclusion appears to be correct, because once we have isolated the action in the required way we are left with nothing in terms of which it could possibly be justified and, given that the people involved are innocent, we have every reason for condemning the action.

On the other hand, how is the Internalist to justify such large-scale abstractionism? Our foregoing discussion suggests that it is at this point that Internalism needs foundations; it is far from self-evident that what Internalism treats as irrelevant really is so. As we have seen, Internalism simply ignores a number of factors out of which a possible and intuitively acceptable defence of area bombing might be constructed. But this is not the whole of the problem for Internalism. The main difficulty is in seeing where a defence of Internalist abstraction is to be found. After all, we are not dealing with a general theory about how moral decisions should be arrived at but with a very powerful, important and specific intuition. It follows that from an Internalist perspective there is no overall goal, point or purpose to morality in terms of which what is relevant can be decided or assessed. Hence, when acting in accordance with the Internalist prescription seems irrational or self-defeating or pointless, the Internalist can only agree and add that that is the way morality is. Similarly, when we find ourselves with a number of conflicting intuitions, as is the case I contend with area bombing, Internalism has run out of things to say.

It would be different if the Internalist could establish that it is a necessary truth that deliberately killing innocent people is morally unjustifiable. No further rationale would then be necessary. But it is not a necessary truth. In this paper, I have taken innocent people to be those who in time of war are not involved in manning, directing or supplying the war machine. Though by no means ideal, it is a fairly uncontentious definition and broadly in line with that to be found in Internalist writings. One might want to challenge it and clarify it in various ways but this will not make it a necessary truth that deliberately killing innocent people is morally unjustifiable. No contradiction will be involved in the denial of this statement unless 'innocent' is given a wholly new meaning.

But if it is not a necessary truth that deliberately killing innocent people is morally unjustifiable, and if from an Internalist perspective morality has no overall goal, point or purpose, it is difficult to see where a justification of Internalist abstraction can come from. We can see just how acute is this problem by quickly reviewing the different dimensions within which Internalist abstraction occurs.

Besides abstracting from the future, that is an action's conequences, Internalism also deems the past to be morally irrelevant. Accordingly, a nation is no more justified in introducing area bombing if it itself is being attacked in this way than if it is not. No matter how extreme the provocation, there is no right to reply in kind. As we have seen, Internalism is here relying on the principle that two wrongs do not make a right. But, of course, the effect of accepting this doctrine is that you must always fight clean no matter how dirty your opponent fights and no matter how desperate your plight. Thus, even when a nation's survival depends on its replying in kind against an unscrupulous aggressor, it may not do so. This is a possible view, but it is far from being a self-evidently correct one. Moreover, if morality requires one to fight clean, and thereby make one's own defeat certain, even when one is the victim of gratuitous and deadly attacks, it is surely in order to ask why one should act morally. The main problem for the Internalist is not just that the question has an extra bite when posed in these perilous circumstances but that in comparison with other moral outlooks Internalism seems to be particularly short of places to look for a plausible answer: a point that I hope will be reinforced if we look at another dimension of Internalist abstraction.

Internalism also abstracts from the future; in particular from an action's consequences. At this point it is relevant to distinguish between two elements in the consequences of an action which tend to be treated as though they were one. First, there are the general or global consequences: whether for instance the world is a better or worse place as a result of the action. And, secondly, contained within this there is what might be called the cost of compliance; that is to say the price the agent—individual or country, as the case may be—must pay for conforming to Internalist morality. In the present case this would have been the cost to Britain of not introducing area bombing which, we have supposed, would have been the greater likelihood of its defeat by a racist power committed to genocide, and hence the deaths of many innocent British people. The cost of complying with Internalist morality would have been enormous, without there being any compensating outcome. Internalism is unable to allow that too much is being demanded of an agent since whatever the price, global or individual, killing innocent people is absolutely ruled out. Consequentialists have often pointed out that there will be situations in which Internalism will lead to the world being overall a less good place than it could be, even when this is judged in terms of numbers of innocent deaths. In the light of our distinction, we can see that Internalism also involves a commitment to bringing about such an outcome no matter what the cost to the agent; even if that cost is total and self-sacrificial.

Conclusion

The Internalist arrives at the conclusion that deliberately killing people is always wrong by focusing on what is involved in such a deed. Past circumstances, future outcomes, the cost to an agent of complying with Internalist morality and the nature of the conflict within which the killing takes place are thereby deemed to be irrelevant. Yet, as we have seen, it is possible to offer an intuitively acceptable defence of area bombing in precisely these terms. Unless Internalism is provided with foundations, either by showing that it is a necessary truth that deliberately killing people is unjustifiable, or in some other way, it merely begs the question.

Gerry Wallace, Department of Philosophy, Hull University, Hull, North Humberside, HU6 7RX, United Kingdom.

NOTES

[1] SIR CHARLES WEBSTER & NOBLE FRANKLAND (1961) *The Strategic Air Offensive Against Germany 1939–45*, Vol. 1, p. 223 (London, HMSO).
[2] C. A. J. COADY (1985) The morality of terrorism, *Philosophy*, pp. 47–69.
[3] To avoid a possible confusion: it is the 'internal' features of an action—as opposed to, say, its consequences—that are to be considered, not the 'internal' features of the agent, for example, his motives, wishes or wants.
[4] R. M. HARE (1972) Rules of war and moral reasoning, and R. B. BRANDT (1972) Utilitarianism and the rules of war, both in *Philosophy and Public Affairs*, 1(2) and reprinted in (1974) *War and Moral Responsibility* (Princeton, N.J., Princeton University Press).
[5] For a detailed discussion of the notion see his (1981) *Moral Thinking* (Oxford, Clarendon Press).
[6] MICHAEL WALZER (1977, 1971, 1972, 1978) *Just and Unjust Wars* (London, Allen Lane), particularly Ch. 13 and 16. See also his Political action: the problem of dirty hands; and World War II: why was this war different? both reprinted in *War and Moral Responsibility* (1974), edited by M. COHEN, T. NAGEL & T. SCANLON (Princeton, N.J., Princeton University Press).
[7] WEBSTER & FRANKLAND, op. cit.
[8] Ibid., p. 155.
[9] Ibid., p. 164.
[10] Ibid., p. 178.
[11] I have ignored questions about the effectiveness of area bombing since in essence I am conducting an *argumentum ad hominem* against the 'Internalist' for whom consideration of consequences is irrelevant. As a matter of historical fact it does not seem to have been particularly effective but this is not an objection that the Internalist can make.

[12] I have in mind arguments of the kind offered or suggested by Walzer & Coady in the above-mentioned articles; also by THOMAS NAGEL (1972) in his War and massacre, *Philosophy and Public Affairs*, 1(2). But I do not wish to attribute the specific arguments I discuss here to them.

[13] ALAN GEWIRTH (1981) Are there any absolute rights?, *Philosophical Quarterly*, 31, pp. 1–16. Reprinted in JEREMY WALDRON (1984) *Theories of Rights*, pp. 91–110 (Oxford, Oxford University Press).

13

Extraordinary Evil or Common Malevolence? Evaluating the Jewish Holocaust

DOUGLAS P. LACKEY

ABSTRACT   *This essay considers and rejects the hypothesis of Fackenheim, Wiesel and others that the Jewish Holocaust contains some qualitatively or quantitatively distinct moral evil. The Holocaust was not qualitatively distinct because the intentions and vices of the mass murderer are qualitatively indistinguishable from the intentions and vices of the common murderer. The Holocaust was not quantitatively distinct either because the sum of the evils of the Holocaust is quantitatively indistinguishable from six million randomly selected individual murders or because the notion of a 'sum' of moral evils is conceptually incoherent.*

> Man was created as a single individual to teach us that anyone who destroys a single life is as though he destroyed an entire world. (*Mishnah*, tractate Sanhedrin 4/5)

The evils of the Jewish Holocaust are so numerous, so diverse, and so extreme that at first sight it seems presumptuous to attempt to judge them at all, much less to judge them by ordinary moral norms. Judgment requires comprehension and transcendence, and comprehension and transcendence of these events seems almost beyond human power. The ordinary moral categories feel too pale and narrow to do justice to our sense of condemnation; the facts seem to explode traditional standards and demand new categories and new moral principles, special to the character of what was done. Nevertheless, the invention of new moral principles to categorise these events has certain costs, not the least of which is that if the Holocaust is placed in a unique moral and historical setting it becomes impossible to learn from it or draw lessons from it. Furthermore, one cannot invent new moral categories at will; the new category must not only be described but justified, and arguments for the validity of a new moral category are hard to come by. Indeed, it is my own belief that the invention of new moral categories for the events of the Jewish holocaust is neither necessary nor desirable, and that the traditional categories of immorality and crime, principally the category of murder and the category of torture (and not a special kind of murder or a special kind of torture) are all that are needed to assess the Holocaust, if one is to be so bold as to make a moral assessment at all. In what follows, I concentrate exclusively on the category of murder. But what I assert about murder applies to Nazi torture as well.

Those who have claimed that the horrors of the Holocaust require new moral categories have defended this view in two different ways. Some have argued that most of the murders of the Holocaust, considered one by one, are murders of a special sort. Others have argued that *all* of the murders, considered as a single event, constitute a new and extraordinary moral evil, different in kind, and not merely in degree, from the six million individual murders that make it up [1]. On the first view, what makes the

Holocaust different is that it consists of many special murders. On the second view, what makes the Holocaust different is that it goes beyond murder to a new level of crime. Neither view withstands analysis.

(1) The Hypothesis of Special Murder

(a) Racial Murder

The Jews who perished at the hands of the Nazis were almost invariably selected for death because of their race, that is, because of a (putative) genetic characteristic [2]. The fact that the Holocaust killings were such racial killings explains the inflexible heartlessness of the Nazi murderers and the impossible predicament of the Judenrate as they sought grounds for negotiation with their tormentors. These were not murders like the murders of the Inquisition, from which a converted Jew could conceivably escape by demonstrations of fidelity. Heresy can be repudiated, but race cannot.

But if we recognise a *descriptive* difference between racial killing and non-racial killing, it does not follow that this descriptive difference implies a moral difference. If one person murders another because his victim is Jewish, that is immorality at a certain level of evil. If one person murders another because his victim has blue eyes, that is immorality at a certain level of evil. Are the levels of evil different? Is it a greater evil to kill someone because he is a Jew than to kill someone because he has blue eyes? We may feel, in our hearts, that racial killing is morally worse, but if we feel this way we might do so because we realise that statistically many more murders have been committed on grounds of race than have been committed on grounds of eye colour. This shows only that killing based on race is more common, not that it is morally worse. Or we might feel that racial killings are worse because racial killings are the sort of killings that we associate with Nazis, persons whom we judge to exhibit a special moral depravity. But if we do this we are assuming that racial killings are in a special moral category because they are perpetrated by Nazis and that Nazis are 'in a special moral category because they perpetrate racial killings.

What has been affirmed here about murder on the basis of eye colour holds as well for killing motivated by non-physical 'voluntary' characteristics, such as choice of religion. Consider the difference between a Jew immolated by the Inquisition because of his rejection of the hypocrisy of conversion and a Jew gassed by the Nazis because his maternal grandfather was Jewish. Is the fifteenth century murder at a different level of wickedness than the twentieth century murder? Certainly we should not feel tempted to say that the *converso* 'asked for it' by keeping up Jewish practices but that the twentieth century Jew was, by contrast, completely innocent, since both of them are completely innocent.

We might try to locate the difference between the moral objectionableness of religious murder and the moral objectionableness of racial murder in a differing moral quality discovered in the executioner's attitude towards his victim. Here, many have suggested, we find reasons for preferring the attitude of the Inquisitor to the attitude of the S.S. Commandant. The Inquisitor, in his effort to uproot heresy, exhibits concern for the soul of the victim, finds it worth the effort of saving; but the Commandant finds nothing of value in the Jew and regards even the effort of execution as a drain on resources [3]. For many, this suggests that the Commandant exhibits a greater perversion of spirit than the Inquisitor.

But we must think carefully before deciding that the Commandant is morally worse. Certainly, *before* he has resolved that the Jew in front of him is not going to give up

Jewish practices, the Inquisitor thinks that his soul can be saved and that his soul is worth saving. But *after* he has decided that the Jew is adamant, he concludes that his soul cannot be saved and that a despicable sinner has defied God's offer of grace through Christ. Likewise, *before* the Commandant determines that the person before him is Jewish, he thinks that the person before him possibly should be spared. Only after he makes the racial determination does he pronounce sentence. The process from arraignment to execution contains the same number of steps, one step involving a chance of reprieve, one step beyond all hope of reprieve.

The real difference between the attitude of the Inquisitor and the attitude of the Commandant lies not in the presence or absence of contempt or in its intensity, but in the fact that the contempt of the Inquisitor is individuated: it is this particular Jew who has rejected his God. The contempt of the Commandant is not directed at the particular Jew before him; his contempt is directed at Jews in general, and it is logically possible for him to feel sympathy for this particular Jew. It is perhaps this—rare, weak, ineffectual—tendency towards sympathy that incensed Himmler and provoked his 1943 remonstration before the S.S. Commanders, surely the low point in the history of human speech:

> I am referring to the evacuation of the Jews, the annihilation of the Jewish people. This is one of those things that are easily said. 'The Jewish people is going to be annihilated,' says every party member. 'Sure, it's in our program, elimination of the Jews, annihilation—so we'll take care of it.' And then they all come trudging, 80 million worthy Germans, and each one has his one decent Jew. Sure, the others are swine, but this one is an A-1 Jew. Of all those who talk this way, not one has seen it happen, not one has been through it. Most of you know what it means to see a hundred corpses lie side by side, or five hundred, or a thousand. To have stuck this out and—excepting cases of human weakness—to have kept our integrity, that is what has made us hard. In our history, this is an unwritten and never-to-be written page of glory. [4]

Is the Inquisitor who says, "I condemn you because of your despicable rejection of God's grace, not because you are a Jew", conspicuously less wicked than the Commandant who says "Personally, I do not despise you, but I condemn you because you happen to be a Jew"? (I do not say that there ever was such a Commandant, only that there could be one.) I find in the two a morally indistinguishable hardness of heart. And we should remember that the Inquisitor fully believed that the unrepenting Jew would suffer an eternity of torment after immolation, a torment from which he might be spared if given another day, or week, or month to repent.

(b) The Extermination of 'Inferior Beings'

If no moral difference can be found between religious killings and racial killings, perhaps one can be found between killings in which the victims are presumed to have rights and killings in which the victims are presumed to have no rights [5].

The Nazi sense that the killing of 'inferior' human beings is 'extermination' but not 'murder' because inferior human beings lack basic rights is certainly not unprecedented. But in this essay we are not concerned with whether or not the evils of the Holocaust are unprecedented (the problem of uniqueness) but with the question of whether these evils fall into a special moral category. Is there a moral difference between the slave trader who enslaves blacks, thinking that they are inferior beings without rights, and the slave trader who enslaves blacks, thinking that they are human beings with rights but that it is profitable to suppress those rights? Is there a moral difference between the non-vegetarian who eats meat and consents to the slaughter of non-human animals, thinking that non-human animals have no rights, and the non-vegetarian who eats meat and consents to the slaughter of non-human animals, believing that non-human animals have rights but that meat is too tasty to be given up? Many would place all these people at the same moral level; some might be inclined to judge that the slave trader who does not recognise that slaves have rights is less wicked than the slave trader who does recognise that they do, and that the meat eater who does not acknowledge that non-human animals have rights is less wicked than the meat eater who does recognise that they do: they, at least, do not violate the dictates of their consciences, such as they are. Why, then, should we reverse ourselves and say that the Nazi who does not recognise the rights of Jews when he kills Jews is more wicked than someone who kills Jews conceding full recognition of their human rights?

Consider and judge three different Nazis, each of whom orders the killing of one Jew. The first orders the killing, believing that Jews are inferior beings and that such killing violates no human rights. The second orders the killing, thinking that Jews have human rights but that it is his higher duty to carry forward Himmler's plans. The third orders the killing, believing that Jews have basic rights and that he has no higher duty to carry forward Himmler's plan, but because this is a propitious time to seize the Jew's property. The first is subject to a delusion about human rights. The second is subject to the delusion that the commands of morality are not overriding. The third is subject to moral weakness, unable to control his desires even when the fulfilment of those desires requires murder. Each has a different character flaw, but which flaw is worst?

Perhaps the reason why so many people feel that it is especially evil to believe that some people have no rights is that such a belief is a particularly dangerous belief. Certainly a person who believes that Jews are inferior beings without rights is more likely to kill a Jew than a person who may succumb to moral weakness if he comes to believe that murdering a Jew is in his interest. But the fact that a person is more likely to act immorally because he possesses a certain belief does not suffice to show that a person *is* more immoral than some other person who does not have this belief. Indeed, it does not seem to me that A is more immoral than B even if A possesses an *intention* which is more likely to emanate in an immoral action than the intention possessed by B. Suppose that A has formed an intention to murder all women whom he meets who are more than six feet tall, while B has formed an intention to murder all women whom he meets who are more than seven feet tall. A's intention is more dangerous than B's intention, since it is more likely that A will murder someone than it is likely that B will murder someone. But *morally* A and B are on the same level, and if each happens to murder someone, the crime of A is morally equal to the crime of B.

(c) The Demonisation of the Jew

To the hypothesis of racial inferiority and lack of moral rights the Nazis added the charge that Jews are a destructive presence in society. In *Mein Kampf*, in Streicher's pornographic cartoons, and in an avalanche of other publications, the Nazis characterised Jews as disease carriers, viruses, tumours, cancers, as lechers, rapists, child molesters and so forth [6]. Certainly the circulation of these obscene productions and the attitudes they fostered made the Final Solution more likely than it otherwise would have been. But, once again, we must not confuse the dangerousness of a belief or attitude with the degree of its moral wickedness. If Jews have no rights at all, killing Jews becomes morally permissible. If Jews are demons, killing Jews becomes morally obligatory, an even more dangerous attitude. But some additional moral argument is needed to show that a murder springing from *this* attitude is worse than a murder springing from less dangerous attitudes. If A kills B believing that B is a demon, is A morally worse than C, who kills D without believing that D is a demon? It is not obvious to me that what A has done is morally worse than what C has done, nor do I think that the victims will care much about the difference.

There is one abstract remark that one can make about murders resulting from the demonisation of the Jew. The person who kills a Jew thinking that Jews are demons believes that the eradication of the Jew is an intrinsic good, something that, considered by itself, increases the sum of value in the world. For many murderers, by contrast, the death of the victim is thought to be good because it produces some further good for the murderer. For the liberal tradition, each human life is an intrinsic good and each death is an intrinsic evil; for the believing Nazi, a Jewish life is intrinsically evil and a Jewish death is intrinsically good. It detracts little from the horror of the Nazi inversion to note that this attitude has precedents: "Better that the state should perish than rule over heretics" Philip II is said to have said, and indeed the Nazi inversion is found in any case in which murder is committed from hatred. But the fact that the Nazis dedicated themselves to murder as an end while many criminals permit themselves to murder only as a means does not show that the Nazis are morally different from professional hit men, felony murderers, and the like. From the standpoint of the victims and their feelings, there is little to distinguish murder-as-a-means from murder-as-an-end. In terms of terror, the thought that I am being killed because someone believes that I stand in the way of some further good is just as overwhelming as the thought that I am being killed because someone believes that the world would be better off without me [7]. My loss is the same either way.

(d) Impersonal Murder and Egoistic Murder

Many persons who have meditated on the evils of the Holocaust have commented that one extraordinary feature of the Final Solution can be discovered in the impersonal character of the good sought by slaughter. None of the murderers (at least in theory) was to profit personally by these killings; the effect to be obtained was a better world in the future, a racially purified Utopia. It is the impersonal character of the alleged good produced to which Himmler appeals in his speech in 1943; only future generations, Himmler says, will profit from the hard and dirty work that the S.S. must do in the present. The impersonal character of the goal sought in the Final Solution relates these murders to the other examples of large-scale political murder, such as Stalin's annihilation of the *kulaks*. But is killing for an impersonal apparent good—utilitarian killing—a morally worse sort of killing than killing for personal apparent good—egoistic killing? In comparing the two, it seems clear that utilitarian killing, once it starts rolling, is likely to claim more victims than egoistic killing, since the ability of one person to profit personally from murder is finite, while the capacity of 'the world' or 'future generations' to profit from murder can be believed to be infinite. But the fact that one kind of murder (type A) is more likely to claim more victims than another kind of murder (type B) does not prove that each murder of type A is morally worse than each murder of type B.

(e) The Banality of Evil

It is the impersonal, society-wide character of the alleged good aimed at by the Nazis that (partially) explains the bureaucratisation of the Nazi process of slaughter, and it is this bureacratisation of slaughter—the spectacle of civil servants painstakingly at work on a tedious job that must nevertheless be done for the presumed good of all—that led Arendt to her odd hypothesis that the murders of the Holocaust are different because they are banal.

In her controversial exposition, Arendt seems to argue that because Eichmann was a banal person, the evil that he did must be banal too [8]. But even if we ignore the extraordinary vigour with which Eichmann hunted down Jews in Budapest and accept Eichmann as Arendt describes him—a 'common mailman'—there is no reason to accept the logic of an argument that infers the banality of the evil done from the banality of the agent who did it. Indeed, from the standpoint of moral theory it seems more plausible to infer the character of the agent from the sort of thing he does than to judge the sort of thing a person does on the basis of the character he is presumed to have, before he performs the act in question. But I do not wish, in this essay, to enter into tangled questions of personal moral responsibility, of Eichmann's thoughtlessness, Hitler's insanity, and so forth. What is at issue is the character of what was done, and what was done was certainly not banal from the standpoint of the victims, which is what matters.

(2) The Holocaust as more than Murder

In the preceding sections, each murder of the Jewish Holocaust was considered separately, as if the other Holocaust murders had not occurred. But what if all the Holocaust murders are considered as a single group? Is there some supervenient evil in the six million murders of the Holocaust which we cannot discover in each murder separately? Is the difference betwen one Holocaust murder and six million a difference in quantity or a difference in kind?

One way of approaching this problem is to compare the evil of six million Holocaust murders with the evil of six million *other* murders, randomly selected from the roster of all the murders committed in human history, murders scattered among different times and different places. Are there features in the Holocaust Catalogue of murders which are not present in such a Random Catalogue? Many have thought so.

(a) The Crime of Genocide

One point that is true of the Holocaust murders and not about six million randomly selected murders is that the Holocaust murders satisfy the United Nations criteria of genocide while the randomly selected murders do not. The 1949 convention reads:

> In the present convention, genocide means any of the following acts committed with intent to destroy, in whole or in part, a national, ethnical, racial or religious group, as such:
>   (a) killing members of the group;
>   (b) causing serious bodily or mental harm to the members of the group;
>   (c) deliberately inflicting on the group conditions of life calculated to bring about its physical destruction in whole or in part;

(d) imposing measures intended to prevent births within the group;

(e) forcibly transferring children of the group to another group;

all conditions which the Nazi met to excess. From this one might infer that the Holocaust Murders constitute a special international crime while the Random Murders do not, and their special immorality is found in their criminal character.

There are, however, two difficulties with the argument that the Holocaust murders are different because they constitute the special crime of genocide. The first is that the Genocide Convention was not adopted until 1949 and cannot be retroactively applied to the perpetrators of the Holocaust [9]. Indeed, at Nuremberg the murders of the Holocaust were not judged as crimes because they were genocidal; they were judged as war crimes violative of the Hague Conventions. If Hitler had pursued the Final Solution in Germany alone, without declaring war on other nations, the Nuremberg judgments concerning crimes against humanity could not have been reached [9]. But by the Hague conventions, each Holocaust murder constitutes a distinct crime, and no supervenient crime is discovered in the sum of six million murders.

The second difficulty is that we cannot directly infer facts about morality from facts of international law, since there are many legal concepts, such as the concept of strict liability, which have standing in law but no standing in moral theory, and deserve none. If we have two immoral acts A and B, and A is a crime but B is not, it does not follow that A is morally worse than B for *that* reason, although we can say, of someone who does A, that he has committed the further immorality of breaking the law. The moral analysis of mass murder, then, must proceed independently of the detailed content of international law.

What the Genocide Convention encourages us to believe is that some special evil occurs when all the members of a (national, racial, ethnic, religious) group are annihilated that does not occur when the same number of (nationally, racially, ethnically, religiously heterogeneous) people are killed. Now the Nazis succeeded in annihilating some groups, the Jews of Poland, of Lithuania, of Germany, of Austria, and of Slovakia, so thoroughly that they effectively vanished from the stage of history. The problem is whether these annihilations constitute a worse evil than the murder of a same number of non-genocidally selected victims. Compare the genocidal annihilation of Polish Jewry with the political annihilation of the same number of *kulaks* and others during the great collectivisation drives. Is there a moral difference between these two mass murders? Is there a moral difference between the mass murder of Jews in the Ukraine and the annihilation of the same number of Soviet Party members wiped out in great purges of the late 1930s? Is there a moral difference between the non-genocidal mass murder of several hundred thousand real or suspected PKI members in Indonesia in 1965 and the genocidal mass murder of several hundred thousand Hutu in Burundi in 1972? Do we really want to say about the Indonesian massacre, "It was terrible, but at least it was not genocide?"

Now, in some classic analyses of genocide, for example, in Lemkin's pioneering study in 1944, the element of mass murder is incidental to genocide and what matters most is the destruction of the group, which need not be brought about by mass murder at all [10]. Lemkin does not address the question of what, precisely, is morally wrong about the annihilation of a group, if the annihilation is not achieved by mass murder, but it seems clear from his remarks that he thinks the destruction of groups involves the destruction of cultures, and that the destruction of cultures is the real evil of genocide as such. We need not accept the principle that every cultural destruction is morally evil—some might not regret the passing of the Old South—to agree that the

Nazi annihilation of East European Jewish culture was a great evil [11]. Furthermore, it seems that such an evil cannot be part of a Random Catalogue of six million murders. So it might appear that what makes the Holocaust a special and extraordinary evil is that it contains an unprecedented combination of evils, the evil of mass murder, the evil of cultural destruction, and so forth. Indeed, the combination makes the Holocaust different. But does it make it worse?

In the case of the Jewish Holocaust, the primary evil is mass murder, even though mass murder is not an essential part of genocide. The other genocidal aspects of the Holocaust, the cultural devastation and so forth, by and large emerged as side-effects of mass murder. So in comparing the Holocaust Catalogue with the Random Catalogue, we must compare all the evil side-effects in the Holocaust with all the evil side-effects in the Random Catalogue. The side-effects of the six million murders in the Random Catalogue will not be as visible or as categorisable as the side-effects of the Holocaust, since they are not bunched up in a small stretch of space and time, but they are there, usually in the form of grief and loss among the families of the murder victims. If such 'short range' losses do not, by themselves, weigh as much on the moral scales as the loss of a language or the destruction of a whole pattern of social relations, they will, when added together, make up a sum of evil roughly equal to the evil of the side-effects in the Holocaust. The reason that the sums should be roughly equal is that, in a genocidal mass murder, the cultural side-effects are greater but the short range side-effects are less, since those who would suffer them are usually victims as well.

(b) Preventability

One striking difference between the murders of the Holocaust and the murders of the Random Catalogue is that the Holocaust murders seem preventable in a way that the randomly selected murders do not. One can argue about historical determinism, but nothing can dispel the impression that the Holocaust would not have happened but for the actions of one man, and if that man had been killed in World War I, or hit by a bus in the 1920s, the Holocaust would never have occurred. We can fantasise going back in a time machine to 1925, killing Hitler, and saving those six million lives. We cannot imagine doing this in the case of six million randomly selected murders. Even if we had a time machine, we would have to stop the time machine six million times to prevent six million murders; we would never get the job done. Thus our feeling is that each of the six million randomly selected murders might have been prevented but that the whole ensemble is not preventable. In the case of the Holocaust, we feel that each of the murders is preventable *and* that the ensemble is preventable.

Doubtless our belief, true or false, that the Holocaust was preventable invests the Holocaust with a terrible poignancy that it otherwise would not have. Our sense of loss is compounded by the tragic perception that the loss was unnecessary. Conversely, our belief that the ensemble of six million randomly selected murders was not preventable reconciles us to the Random Catalogue: we bow before the inevitable and call it the way of the world. Whereas the last thing that anyone could say or should say about the Holocaust is that these things happen. This sense of preventability pervades our perception of Holocaust events. But this sensibility, this tragic feeling, should not affect our assessment of the evil that these events contain. We feel that the execution of an innocent man is more tragic if a reprieve arrives one minute too late than if there be no reprieve at all, but the amount of evil in the execution is the same whether or not there is a reprieve. The death of a soldier on the day of the Armistice seems more tragic than the death of a soldier in the middle of the war, but the evil of a soldier's death is the same regardless of the day on which it falls. We feel that the sum of six million deaths in the Holocaust is more tragic than the sum of six million randomly selected murders because it seems more preventable, and, indeed, it *is* more tragic. But this tragic sense, which is primarily aesthetic—involving perception and emotion but not moral intuition—is not relevant to the weighing of good and bad and right and wrong.

(c) The Character of the Mass Murderer

In comparing the six million Holocaust murders with six million murders scattered through space and time, let us assume that each of the six million murders in the Random Catalogue is perpetrated by a different murderer. On this assumption, another striking difference emerges between the Holocaust Catalogue and the Random Catalogue. In the Random Catalogue, each murderer is responsible for one murder only; in the Holocaust Catalogue, some people are responsible for many murders. Indeed, some are responsible for all six million. In the Random Catalogue, there are no mass murderers; in the Holocaust Catalogue, there are many. Perhaps the special moral evil of the Holocaust can be inferred from the special evil that distinguishes the character of the mass murderer from the character of the common murderer. But is there a special evil in the character of the mass murderer?

Certainly someone who murders two people has done something worse, *ceteris paribus*, than someone who has murdered one person only. But this difference in moral evil is discovered in the effects, not in the characters of the murderers. Consider two people, A and B, and suppose, as before, that A is set on murdering all women whom he meets who are over six feet tall and that B is set on murdering all women whom he meets who are over seven feet. A happens to meet quite a few women over six feet tall and murders them all. B happens to meet only one woman over seven feet, and murders her, but *had* he met more such women, he *would* have murdered them too. A is a mass murderer, and B is not, but between their moral characters there is little discernible difference. What has been said here about B can also be said about any murderer C who has killed only one person. Of C we can say that there occurred circumstances which, in his view, justified murder. If similar circumstances arise, he will kill again. At least there is nothing in his character which shows that he will not. There is no moral line which separates the soul of the murderer from the soul of the mass murderer.

This abstract argument for equality of character (not equality of deed) among murderers and mass murderers is reflected in our ordinary intuitions about murderers. We feel that the man who has murdered one person is morally much worse than the man who has murdered none, and that the man who has murdered 20 is morally much worse than the man who has murdered only one. But we also feel that the moral *gap* between the man who has murdered none and the man who has murdered one is greater than the moral gap between the man who has murdered 20 and the man who has murdered 21. Ordinary moral judgment accepts some principle of the diminishing marginal turpitude of murder, and when the number of victims is very great the difference at the margin becomes negligible. We would not think a whole lot better of Hitler if we discovered that he murdered five million Jews rather than six million.

For those who still persist in believing that the character of the mass murderer contains a special vice, far darker than the vices of the common murderer, consider this. Suppose that God has once again given the Devil the power of temptation, and the Devil sets out to corrupt human souls. Suppose that the Devil has sufficient power to get six men to murder one person each, that he has sufficient power to get one man to murder six people, but that he does not have the power to do both. It would seem that if the Devil wants to create as much sin as possible he will create six murderers rather than one mass murderer. And if his goal is really corruption, and not destruction, he will prefer tempting six non-murderers to become murderers to tempting one killer of five million to kill a million more. If this is right, then there is more sin in the Random Catalogue than in the Holocaust Catalogue.

(d) The Technology of Mass Murder

Some commentators on the Holocaust have discerned a special evil in the development of the machinery with which it was accomplished. Fackenheim, for example, writes:

> Where else and at what other time have executioners ever separated those to be murdered now from those to be murdered later to the strains of Vienna waltzes? Where else has human skin ever been made into lampshades, and human body-fat into soap—not by isolated perverts but under the direction of ordinary bureaucrats? [12]

Anyone reading Fackenheim's remarks cannot fail to respond; intellect reels and imagination falters when one tries to conceive of the discussions in planning conferences for the construction of death camps. No such killing apparatus is found in the six million murders of the Random Catalogue. Nevertheless it does not seem to me that there is in this respect greater moral perversity in the Holocaust than in six million randomly selected murders.

To begin with, the mere construction of a killing apparatus, considered in itself, apart from the intentions connected with prospective use, constitutes only a relatively minor evil. From 1945 to 1960 the United States constructed a killing apparatus—the Strategic Air Command—which dwarfed by an order of magnitude the Nazi killing apparatus of 1943. In late 1959 and 1960, the American Secretary of Defence, Thomas Gates, and a dedicated staff of 'common mailmen', organised the first Single Integrated Operational Plan for the use of American strategic forces, a plan which gave the President, in the event of a nuclear attack on the United States or some other form of Soviet aggression, the single option of a massive strategic strike against the Soviet Union, its satellite states, and China, a strike which, if executed, would have killed, by the Joints Chiefs' own estimates, at least three hundred million people. Yet we do not think about Gates and Eisenhower the way we think about Himmler and Heydrich (at least not yet), and we do not think about the Saandia Corporation the way we think about I. G. Farben (at least not yet), and one reason why we think differently about the American manufacturers and organisers of the instruments of mass murder is that the Americans think that there is little chance that the instruments will be used, and hope that they never will be used, while their German counterparts believed that they would be used, and intended that they would be [13].

Next, we must consider that in each of six million murders of the Random Catalogue some method of murder had to be chosen. Consider the darkness of spirit involved in six million murderers choosing six million murder weapons, the poisoner selecting his poison, the arsonist setting a homicidal fire, and so forth. Imagine all these murder devices in a single place (or imagine all six million random murders taking place in a confined area of space and time). Placed next to six million murder weapons, it is not obvious that the technology of the death camps represents a new and deeper perversion of the human spirit [14].

(e) The Quantitative Preeminence of the Holocaust

The fact that the events of the Holocaust have a common causal origin, that the Holocaust would not have happened if a few events occurring a short time before the Holocaust had not taken place, is what gives the Holocaust its unity and makes it a single historical event. By contrast, the Random Catalogue does not describe a single historical event, but six million different historical happenings. Among unified historical events, the Jewish Holocaust contains the greatest number of murders, far outdistancing the Cambodian, Bengali, and Armenian massacres which are its closest historical competitors. From this it seems to follow that the Holocaust contains more evil than any other historical event. The Holocaust, then, claims quantitative preeminence among evil events, even if the preceding arguments deny it qualitative preeminence. But the reasoning behind this judgment must be carefully scrutinised.

To begin with, one can find unified historical events that contain more deaths than the Jewish Holocaust: the Black Death, for example. Anyone who argues that the Jewish Holocaust was worse than the Armenian massacre because more people were killed in the Jewish Holocaust than in Turkey in 1915 must concede that the Black Death was worse than the Jewish Holocaust, since more people were killed in the Black Death than in the Jewish Holocaust. Certainly, if Mephistopheles presented us with an exclusive choice between preventing the Black Death or preventing the Jewish Holocaust, agents accepting some concept of the summation of evils would feel duty bound to prevent the Black Death.

I am sure that most people who assert that the Jewish Holocaust is history's supreme evil have in mind a sum of *moral* evil, not some sum of physical evil. They will remark that what makes the Jewish Holocaust worse is not that it contains more *deaths*, but that it contains more *murders*, than any event in history. But there are conceptual difficulties even with this seemingly simple claim. If we combine the fact that the Holocaust does not contain more deaths than any other historical event with the observation that the character of a mass murderer does not differ from the character of a common murderer, there is little left to support the claim that the Holocaust contains more moral evil than any other historical event: the act and the consequences are both within the range of common evil. Furthermore, those who would say that the Jewish Holocaust was a greater evil than the Armenian massacre because it contains more murders presume that the evils of the many murders that make up a mass murder can be summed together, and that these sums can be compared. But such summations are in fact unintelligible.

Some philosophers and many economists believe that it is impossible to sum together evils suffered by different persons. A typical argument against summation might go like this: It is self-evident that every evil is an evil for some individual. If I inflict an evil on someone (pain, for example) I make that person worse off, other things being equal, than he would have been if I had not inflicted pain on him. If I inflict pain on two people (A and B), I make each of them worse off. But if I inflict pain on A and B, there is no sum of evil which I inflict on both, since there is no single pain suffered by the two [15]. From this it follows that it is not worse to inflict ten pains on ten people that one pain on some other person; the ten cannot be summed to outweigh the one. The same holds for the evil of death. If I murder A and B, there is A's death and B's death, but no single death which the two have suffered. Thus if I murder A and B I have created two evils, but I have not created an evil which is the sum of the two. From this it follows that the deaths, and the murders, of the Jewish Holocaust cannot be summed so that they outweigh the sum of evils found in the Armenian massacre or any other mass murder.

Now I am far from accepting this argument against summation of evils in its entirety. For one thing, it yields counter-intuitive verdicts in matters of population policy [16]. For another, if it is not possible to sum the pains of different persons, it seems to me that it should not be possible to sum the pains experienced by one person at different times. But I do feel something of the force of this argument, particularly in matters of historical judgment and particularly when the evil involved is the evil of death. For if we ask each of the victims of the Holocaust, what is the evil, or at least the main evil, of the Holocaust *for him*, his answer must be that the evil for him is that he loses his life. This evil is an evil that exists *for him* independently of the evils of the Holocaust for others; so far as his loss is concerned, it does not matter if only he is killed or if six million others are killed along with him [17].

A mass murderer, then, is a person who creates many evils; he is not a person who creates some larger evil than the murderer who kills but once. Thus we should say that the Holocaust contains a greater number of evils than any other massacre, not that the Jewish Holocaust contains a greater evil than any other massacre. The historical unity of the Holocaust cannot synthesise its evils into a single immoral whole. The Holocaust is not the most evil event in history because there can be no such event, and the murderers who perpetrated the Holocaust are not the most evil murderers in history, because there can be no such people. But to say that the Holocaust is not the most evil event in history takes nothing away from the suffering of the Holocaust victims. Each of them lost everything. No one could have done them worse.

Acknowledgements

I am indebted to David Novak, James Rachels, and Michael Wyschogrod for comments on earlier drafts of this essay, which should not be taken to represent their views.

Douglas P. Lackey, Department of Philosophy, Baruch College and Graduate Center, City University of New York, 17 Lexington Avenue, New York, NY 10010, USA.

NOTES

[1] For the 'special murder' hypothesis see Emil Fackenheim (1978):

> Must [the Jew] say that the death of a Jewish child at Auschwitz is no more lamentable than the death of a German child at Dresden? He must say it. And in saying it, he must also refuse to dissolve Auschwitz into suffering-in-general... Must he distinguish between the mass-killing at Hiroshima and that at Auschwitz?... He must forever repeat that Eichmann was moved by no such rational objective as 'victory' when he diverted trains needed for military purposes in order to dispatch Jews to their death. He must add that there was no 'irrational' objective either. Torquemada burned bodies in order to save souls. Eichmann sought to destroy both bodies and souls.

The Jewish Return Into History, p. 27 (New York, Schocken). For the view that the Holocaust is more than a sum of murders consider:

> After Auschwitz many Jews did not need Nietzsche to tell them that that the old God of Jewish patriarchal monotheism was dead beyond all hope of resurrection.

RICHARD R. RUBENSTEIN (1966) *After Auschwitz*, p. 227 (New York, Bobbs-Merrill). (Note if Holocaust evils challenge belief in God's existence in a way that pre-Holocaust evils do not, it follows that they are qualitatively different.)

> I don't compare [Hiroshima and Auschwitz]. Auschwitz was a unique phenomenon, like the revelation at Sinai.

In Conversation with Elie Wiesel, HARRY JAMES CARGAS (Ed.) (1976), p. 8 (New York, Paulist Press).

> We [the Holocaust survivors] were too numb, too weak, and perhaps too timid to object to what was happening before our eyes. The Holocaust no longer evokes the mystery of the forbidden; it no longer arouses fear and trembling, or even outrage or compassion. For you, it is one calamity among so many others, slightly more morbid than the others. You thought yourselves capable of imagining the unimaginable; you have seen nothing. You thought yourselves capable of discussing the unspeakable; you have understood nothing, you have retained nothing. You have retained nothing of its blinding truth....
>
> You have not grasped it until now, and it is time you did: Auschwitz signifies death—total, absolute death—of man and of mankind, of reason and of the heart, of language and of the senses. Auschwitz is the death of time, the end of creation; its mystery is doomed to stay whole, inviolate.

ELIE WIESEL (1978) *A Jew Today*, pp. 186, 198 (New York, Random House).

> We are forbidden to turn present and future life into death, at the price of remembering death at Auschwitz. And we are equally forbidden to affirm present and future life, at the price of forgetting Auschwitz....
>
> After the events associated with the name of Auschwitz, everything is shaken; nothing is safe....
>
> Auschwitz is a unique descent into hell. It is an unprecedented celebration of evil. It is ... the scandal of evil for evil's sake, an eruption of demonism without analogy; and the singling out of Jews, ultimately, is an unparalleled expression of what the rabbis call groundless hate.

EMIL FACKENHEIM, op. cit., pp. 22, 27, 29.

> I am not persuaded that the Holocaust is just an instance of the ancient problem of evil. That would be true if Judaism were a philosophy dealing with abstract problems. Instead Judaism is an historic faith which pays very close attention to what happens in history. And the Holocaust actually happened. That is the whole point.

MICHAEL WYSCHOGROD (1975) Some theological reflections on the Holocaust, *Response: a contemporary Jewish review*, p. 68.

> The concept is that there is much evil in the world and that most evil, evil as it is, is not altogether abnormal evil. Ordinary evil is evil enough: crimes of private individuals against other individuals, economic injustices of various societies, and the limits put on individual freedom. But then there appear evils which are qualitatively different from all other evils. The paradigmatic case is the Holocaust.

MICHAEL WYSCHOGROD (1980) Religion and international human rights: a Jewish perspective, in: EUGENE J. FISHER & DANIEL F. POLISH (Eds) (1980) *Formation of Social Policy in the Catholic and Jewish Traditions*, p. 137 (South Bend, Ind., Notre Dame Press).

[2] I say 'putative' because there is a scientific problem as to whether the Jews form one, or two, or three races, or no race at all. See RAPHAEL PATAI & JENNIFER P. WING (1975) *The Myth of the Jewish Race* (New York, Charles Scribner's Sons).

[3] In the summer of 1944, the supply of Zyklon-B was running short at Auschwitz and the S.S. began throwing live Jewish children directly into the crematoria. Irving Greenberg has estimated that the Nazis saved .004 cents per victim by this change in methods of murder. See I. GREENBERG (1977) Some theological reflections on the Holocaust, in: EVA FLEISCHNER (Ed.) *Auschwitz: beginning of a new era?* (New York, KTAV).

[4] LUCY S. DAVIDOWICZ (1976) *A Holocaust Reader*, p. 133 (New York, Behrman House).

[5] This line of reasoning has been specially investigated by Helen Fein (1979) who notes that it is

characteristic of genocide that the victims are placed outside the 'sanctified universe'. *Accounting for Genocide*, pp. 3–30 (New York, Free Press).

[6] See, for example, the German Army propaganda leaflet, *The Jew in Human History*, quoted in Davidowicz (1976) *The War Against the Jews*, p. 115 (New York, Holt, Reinhardt & Winston).

> We Germans fight a twofold fight today. With regard to non-Jewish peoples we want only to accomplish our vital interests. We respect them, and conduct a chivalrous argument with them. But we fight World Jewry as one has to fight a poisonous parasite; we encounter in him not only the enemy of our people, but a plague of all peoples, the fight against Jewry is a moral fight for the purity and health of god-created humanity and for a new more just order in the world.

See also Hitler's 1942 speech, quoted in J. FEST (1974) *Hitler*, p. 212 (New York, Harcourt, Brace, Jovanovich). In Nazi ideology, the charge of 'disease carrier' is logically distinct from the charge of racial inferiority; it was apparently levelled only at Jews, not at gypsies, Slavs, and other 'racially inferior' groups. (See A. BEIN (1964) The Jewish parasite, *Yearbook of the Leo Baeck Institute*).

[7] This paragraph serves to rebut the oft-repeated claim that Nazi murders were special because they were *irrational*, diverting resources from the war effort. In 1941 and 1942, organisation of the Einsatzgruppen and implementation of the Final Solution was not irrational (relative to Nazi goals) since it did not diminish the chance of victory, which was thought certain. After El Alamein and Stalingrad, continuing the Final Solution was not irrational since it did not increase the chance of defeat, which was thought certain. Indeed, since annihilation of the Jews was the first goal of Nazi policy (after 1939), the strategic problem for 1943 and 1944 was to apportion resources in such a way that the Final Solution could be completed before the Wehrmacht collapsed. For the Jewish Community in Hungary, the tragedy was consummated when Himmler discovered in Eichmann a singularly obscene example of technical rationality.

[8] "To evacuate and deport Jews had become routine business" (p. 76) *and so*, "The lesson of this long course in human wickedness has taught us—the lesson of the fearsome, thought-and-word defying banality of evil". HANNAH ARENDT (1963) *Eichmann in Jerusalem: a report on the banality of evil* (New York, Viking Press). Even if one accepts this tortured reasoning, it applies only to Eichmann and others at the middle level, not to the top and the bottom of the S.S. killing machine.

[9] Though the indictments at Nuremberg listed 'crimes against humanity' as distinct from war crimes, in its final judgment the Tribunal gave legal standing to 'crimes against humanity' only as a species of war crime:

> The Tribunal cannot therefore make a general declaration that the acts before 1939 were crimes against humanity within the meaning of the charter, but from the beginning of the war in 1939 war crimes were committed on a vast scale, which were also crimes against humanity; and insofar as the inhumane acts charged in the indictment, and committed after the beginning of the war, did not constitute war crimes, they were all committed in execution of, or in connection with, the aggressive war, and therefore constituted crimes against humanity.

RICHARD FALK, GABRIEL KOLKO & ROBERT JAY LIFTON (Eds) *Crimes of War*, p. 106 (New York, Vintage Books).

[10] The term was introduced by RAPHAEL LEMKIN (1944) in *Axis Rule in Occupied Europe* (New York, Carnegie Endowment). Lemkin's discussion is in many ways superior to the 1949 genocide convention:

> By 'genocide' we mean the destruction of a nation or of an ethnic group ... Generally speaking, genocide does not necessarily mean the immediate destruction of a nation, except when accomplished by mass killings of all members of a nation. It is intended rather to signify a coordinated plan of different actions aiming at the destruction of essential foundations of the life of national groups, with the aim of annihilating the groups themselves. The objectives of such a plan would be disintegration of the political and social institutions, of culture, language, national feelings, religion ... Genocide is directed against the national group as an entity, and the actions are directed against individuals, not in their individual capacity, but as members of the national group. (p. 79)

[11] This argument assumes that the Nazis *did* destroy whole cultures, though the point might be raised that East European Jewry constituted a single culture but that the Nazis did not succeed in destroying it because it survived in the Ukraine, in Russia, and elsewhere. Obviously in many cases the dividing lines between cultures are hard to define. If all the Ashkenazim formed one culture, the Nazi crime by Lemkins's standards is 'attempted genocide'. Perhaps to avoid such inferences the U.N. convention

defines genocide as deliberately inflicting destruction on a group in whole or *in part*. One wants, of course, to convict the Nazis of genocide, but the 'in part' qualification in the genocide convention makes as much sense as saying that homicide consists in killing a person in whole or in part.

[12] FACKENHEIM, op. cit., p. 27.

[13] I am not trying to exonerate Truman, Eisenhower, Gates *et al.* Saying that they are not as bad as Himmler does not get them very far.

[14] Analogous remarks can be about the quantity of suffering produced in the Holocaust Catalogue and in the Random Catalogue. And if we consider quality of suffering, it is not clear that the moral perversity exhibited in Nazi technology represents a level of sadism not reached, say, by the racks and strappadoes of the Inquisition.

[15] This argument has been vigorously pressed by JOHN TAUREK (1977) in Do the numbers count? *Philosophy and Public Affairs.*

[16] The deviant cases are those where comparisons must be made between actions that determine the populations of the groups that they subsequently affect. In these cases, we can speak of group A as being made worse off (by act A) than group B, even though no individual in A is worse off than he would have been if A had not been done. (See D. PARFIT (1984)) *Reasons and Persons*, pp. 351–390 (Oxford, Oxford University Press). None of the problems of estimating the evils of the Holocaust are of this type.

[17] I owe this point to James Rachels (in correspondence).

14

Response to Douglas P. Lackey

M. KRIŽAN

I should like to make the following comment on Douglas P. Lackey's 'Extraordinary evil or common malevolence? Evaluating the Jewish Holocaust' (*Journal of Applied Philosophy*, Vol. 3, pp. 167–181).

Ethical systems are not separable from cultures of which they are a part. That means that ethical values and norms are always in a relation of interdependence with broader systems of values and norms that characterise (and define) a particular cultural system. Therefore, ethical assessments of human actions have to include both consequences concerning directly the particular (human or other) objects of action, and those concerning the wider social and cultural environment. On the other hand, the moral judge has to keep in mind that he is pronouncing his judgements always from the standpoint of a particular culture.

Since cultures are historical phenomena, so are ethical systems. Moreover, at every moment of the history of mankind, several different cultures existed simultaneously. Thus, actions and events can be judged from a rather large number of different cultural standpoints. It is a matter of self-respect for a practical philosopher to define his cultural and ethical standpoint.

The Holocaust became possible because the Nazi ideology gave up the highest cultural value of Enlightenment: reason. It gave it up both in its individualistic interpretation—the Nazis saw men not as actors endowed with reason, but as objects of mass manipulation controlled by instinct and emotion—and in some supra-individualistic, historical-philosophical (for instance Hegelian) interpretation- they replaced reason as the driving force of history by the (German) race.

These premises accepted, several arguments in connection with Lackey's ethical analysis can be formulated, leading to somewhat different conclusions. Their central idea is that the author analyses the Holocaust from a standpoint of moral values reduced to the categories of murder and torture.

Because of a different cultural background, even the classical forms of evil such as murder and torture did not have the same moral quality in sixteenth as they do in twentieth century Europe. This general statement is clearly confirmed by the comparison of crimes committed by the Inquisition and those committed by the Nazi regime. The Inquisitor was acting in accordance with his contemporary culture—his aim was to protect the (however distorted) absolute values of Christianity from the obstinate sinners. He had no other values at his disposal. As history has shown, Christianity was able to correct these distortions by reinterpreting its own system of values. The Nazis, on the contrary, did have other value-systems at their disposal, but they chose the one of destruction of modern European culture. In other words: the crime of the SS Commandant is worse not only because he *a priori* defines the Jew as a person deserving only contempt, but also because, by doing so, he participates in the destruction of the culture whose values he was given a chance to internalise. The destruction of life as an abstract, allegedly culturally independent value has in both cases the same moral status. The destruction of culture as a value hasn't.

The developed cultural perspective allows questioning of some other of Lackey's conclusions: the slave trader thinking that blacks are inferior beings is then morally worse than the cynical profiteer, because the former negates a fundamental value of (modern western) culture, whereas the latter inadequately solves a conflict of values (pp. 169–170); killing a Jew because he is considered to be a demon is worse than killing him without that belief, for a similar reason. All this amounts to the required "additional moral argument" (p. 171) demonstrating the "supervenient evil in the six million murders of the Holocaust" (p. 172): not that the killed persons are worse off, but the whole cultural environment. These "cultural side-effects", as the author euphemistically says (p. 174), *indeed are an evil of a different quality* in comparison to individual crimes, and therefore unsuitable for the arithmetic the author proposes.

To conclude: the question that really matters to all those who want to uphold the values and norms of western culture, developed in the wake of the European Enlightenment, is not whether the Holocaust was unique in some undefined general sense, because to answer such a question is almost impossible, nor whether its criminal acts, analysed individually and by stressing their aspect of damage caused to the victims, have a particular moral status, nor whether special moral categories have to be developed to assess it. The question to be answered is, what moral status can be ascribed to the Holocaust from the standpoint of that culture (the only one which we really know and positively evaluate)? The answer is: the whole culture was severely threatened. Probably such a threat is not historically unique when other cultures are taken into account. But up to the present it certainly has been the worst man-made challenge to Enlightenment.

Ironically enough, probably because of geographical reasons, the Ashkenazim concentrated their hopes for emancipation on the German Enlightenment.

Yours faithfully,

M. KRIŽAN
Stiegel 7
34–Göttingen
Federal Republic of Germany

15

Oskar Schindler and Moral Theory

M. W. JACKSON

ABSTRACT *Imagine Oskar Schindler before the bar of moral theory. Schindler, a minor industrialist, sheltered more than 1000 Jews during the Holocaust. This would seem to be a record of virtue. Or is it? The dominant consensus in moral theory stresses a rationality and universality of judgement and action that Oskar did not even consider. Efforts to interpret Schindler in universal terms by reference to human rights or to the tenet that ought implies can are entertained and denied. If Schindler's deeds are moral reality, the consensus in contemporary moral theory is the poorer for being unable to recognise them. Schindler's virtue is noteworthy in its own right and also as a limiting case for the mainline of contemporary moral theory.*

> He who saves a single life, saves the world entire.
>
> Talmud

Oskar Schindler was a minor industrialist in the 1930s, a member of the neo-Nazi Sudeten German Party. He was a colourful man, famed for drinking and whoring. Throughout the war he manufactured enamelware and, toward the end, shell casings for the German army. His works were in Poland, but as the war drew to a close he succeeded in moving his factory to Czechoslovakia. His enamelware business was successful even after the war began, but his effort at munitions manufacturing was a failure. He made little, if any profit from it, and his products were inferior. On top of this failure he also squandered the firm's assets from the enamelware on wine, women, and endless bribes and gifts to officials. All in all Schindler's Deutsche Emailwaren Fabrik was not a success story destined for the immortality of the *Harvard Business Review* or *Fortune*.

What the accountant's ledger does not show is that from the fall of 1943 to the bitter end of the war, Schindler devoted his firm and himself to recruiting and protecting Jews. Combining bravado in equal measure with bribery, Schindler managed to draw into his firm about 1000 Jews who were otherwise destined for the Final Solution. Once on his payroll each of them was classified by Berlin as a valuable war worker, thanks to Schindler's inventive chicanery. Schindler's adventure into the manufacture of munitions was not the search for profits in a war economy but the search for a good cover story for the protection of his workforce and himself for even the S.S. was chary about disrupting arms works. As Thomas Keneally makes clear in his novel based upon Oskar Schindler's exploits, *Schindler's Ark*, Schindler collected Jews quite literally as he came across them [1]. It is also quite clear that but for Schindler these thousand would have been swallowed up in the maw of the Holocaust. The personal risk that Schindler took and the financial losses that he suffered were real.

Though Keneally's book is a novel, it is based on thorough research and interviews with *Schindlerjuden* around the world that no scholar could hope to finance. Moreover, it is written in a straightforward chronology. Like Thucydides, Keneally may have invented the words said in the dialogue but he is faithful to the record of the action and intention. Indeed his novel is such a faithful narrative that it has been claimed that it is not a novel at all, but a work of non-fiction [2].

The millions of readers of Thomas Keneally's novel may be surprised to know that despite the good that Oskar did in saving that 1000 Jews, according to a strict interpretation of the dominant strain of contemporary moral theory, he cannot be said to have acted morally. Contemporary moral theory posits certain criteria of moral reasoning and behaviour. Schindler's intentions and actions do not meet these criteria. Consequently, his virtue cannot be recognised. That moral theory in its dominant contemporary form cannot recognise Schindler's virtue is not because Schindler had no virtue but because contemporary moral theory has little if any, place for virtue. Readers of Hegel may recall his aphorism that "no man is a hero to his valet; not because the man is not a hero, but because a valet—is a valet..." [3] Contemporary moral theory, like Hegel's valet, has insufficient perspective to understand moral practice in the case of someone like Oskar Schindler. Schindler's case is of interest in its own right as the record of a virtuous man *and* also as a limiting case for the dominant version of contemporary moral theory.

Moral theory has probably never been more vigorous. New books appear regularly; important books frequently. There are more and more journals that are receptive to it. Some specialise in it. Debates between different perspectives fill pages. Critiques follow every development. All in all the theory class is hard at work. But for all of the superficial differences among contributors to contemporary moral theory there is an underlying consensus that marks its in-built operating system. This consensus is the dominant characteristic of contemporary moral theory. This consensus has evolved from a focus on problems and decision-making.

The aim has been to make moral theory relevant to the kinds of problems we face. One celebrated moral theorist is Stephen Toulmin who put it this way:

> Ethics is everybody's concern...Everyone is faced with *moral problems* —problems about which, after more or less reflection, a decision must be reached [4].

In the effort to ensure that moral theory is not taken to be the history of what moral theorists have written, R. M. Hare began his book *Freedom and Reason* by asking "the reader to start by supposing that someone (himself perhaps) is faced with a serious moral *problem*..." [5] Contemporary "ethical theory must be about the *solution* to such [moral] problems" as we all have, R. M. Brandt has written [6].

Focusing on problems is the first, not the last, step in the analysis of contemporary moral theory. The purpose of focusing on problems is not to revel in them, but to solve them. Marcus Singer has written that his,

> ultimate aim is to determine...how moral judgements can *rationally* be supported, how moral perplexities can be *resolved*, and how moral disputes can rationally be settled [7].

The key words in this passage from Singer are 'solution' (resolved) and 'rational' (rationally). The programme of contemporary moral theory is nothing less than the *rational solution* of moral problems. This then is the dominant consensus that underlies the superficial disputes that mainly occupy contemporary moral theorists. It is, as Edmund Pincoffs has written, a consensus so pervasive that it would be tedious to document it [8]. From its foundation this consensus has expanded and become institutionalised, notably with the creation and prosperity of *Philosophy & Public*

Affairs, a learned journal devoted to the rational resolution of moral problems like abortion and war crimes [9].

If moral problems are the focus of moral theory, then Oskar Schindler would seem to come within the ambit of moral theory. He certainly had problems. But to win the palm from moral theory the criteria of rationality and solution must also be met. It is on these grounds that moral theory rules Oskar Schindler beyond the pale. Seen from the heights of moral theory Oskar's fault is not that he tried and failed to find a rational solution, but that he did not even try to be rational or to find a solution. Had he tried to follow the North Star of rationality, I suspect, he would not have been able to save many Jews. There will be more on this point presently. Admittedly, there are many who accept the dominant consensus of contemporary moral theory and yet recognise Schindler's virtue. Their human sympathy prevails over the gleaming logic of contemporary moral theory. A less sympathetic subscriber to the dominant strain of contemporary moral theory cannot even say of Schindler that he did what a moral person would do but that he did not do it as a moral person would do it. This Aristotelian concession does not apply, as I shall show, because Schindler did not act morally according to the criteria of contemporary moral theory.

If there is an Olympus in contemporary moral theory it is *A Theory of Justice*, published in 1971 by John Rawls [10]. In *A Theory of Justice* the kind of morality that would rationally solve our problems was spelt out. It was one based on what James Fishkin has since, appositely, termed 'transcultural criteria' [11]. It is a morality of rules and principles that are free of the "contamination of sex, age, race, class, socialisation" and the other impurities that putatively determine our moral judgment, according to Fishkin. Rules and principles free of such contaminations are, like Rawls's principles of justice, meant to apply anywhere and at any time. In short, they are universal. This is the received character of moral theory.

In a morality composed of universal rules and principles, the solution to problems lies in deciding which rules or principles apply to a particular case. This adjudication of application can be a difficult and complex procedure. It was the kind of decision that Immanuel Kant called a 'determinative judgement' [12]. One determines which rule or principle applies. Once that is decided the rule is applied.

Oskar Schindler would not recognise himself in this description. He certainly had no solutions. If he had been asked—by an all-seeing angel—whether he was doing the right thing, I doubt that he could or would have had an answer. Though I am sure he would have offered his heavenly interlocuter a cognac while they discussed the matter. A persistent acolyte of contemporary moral theory might insist that Oskar's actions were consistent with the principle of the human right to life, but the case cannot be sustained. First Schindler did not think, speak, or act in terms of rights. He simply responded to life, to the lives that came within his purview. Ergo, he did not try in any way to aid Jews or other victims of Naziism beyond his ken. Yet he was all too well aware of what was happening to the millions of Jews outside the twilight zone of Deutsch Emailwaren Fabrik. This knowledge did not make him guilty or make him feel guilty. He simply pressed on.

Nor did Oskar act in a way so as to be a maxim for all others *pace* Immanuel Kant. Not everyone else was placed to deal with, or experienced at dealing with, the German, Nazi, S.S. and Gestapo authorities that Schindler dealt with daily. For most, to try would have led to failure if not fatality, as it almost did for him. Indeed, Oskar did not even seem ever to ask himself if he had done the right thing. He never ignored the opportunity to recruit yet another Jew. It never occurred to him that the boat was full.

He did not rationally calculate. When some of his Jewish workers were mistakenly transported to Auschwitz while his factory was being re-located from East to West, a move he planned in order to put his Jews into American rather than Russian hands at the end of hostilities, he moved the earth to get them back, drawing the attention of numerous little Eichmanns to himself in the process. He did not hesitate in trying to rescue his workers from Auschwitz as a utilitarian would surely have hesitated, calculating the lives of *Schindlerjuden* in Auschwitz against the remainder who might be lost if his efforts aroused the notice of the S.S. Nor did he, as a deontologist would require, strive to save every Jew in Europe. Still less did he ask himself if he had done as much as he could.

The dominant consensus of contemporary moral theory represents a long development. Socrates held that no judgment of a particular case could be made before the (universal) criteria that determined it were clear. Thus when the discussion turned to instances of truth, beauty, or courage, Socrates would ask 'What is truth . . . beauty . . . or courage'? Before hearing the details of a particular truth, Socrates insisted that we establish the criteria assumed. Of course, if the criteria articulated were not trans-personal, trans-cultural, and timeless, Socrates would persist in his interrogation much to annoyance of many of his auditors. In the hands of Socrates the method of trans-cultural criteria in ethics was a critical technical pedagogy. Pompous and opinionated people were forced to think again or be shown up as ignorant fools unable to state their ground. Socrates himself did not attempt to use criteria to develop a positive doctrine. For him it was only a critical tool, but for many others it has been made the basis for a positive doctrine.

The drive to universal criteria enjoyed its hey-day during the historical epoch known as the Enlightenment. In morality Kant's categorical imperative answered the Socratic question: 'What is morality'? Kant defined a moral act as one that it would be right for everyone to do. Leaving aside the academic details of Kant's formulation of the categorical imperative, his test of morality is known as universalizability [13]. That is, if it would be right for the act to be performed anywhere at any time by anyone, it is the moral act.

If it is right for me to save a drowning swimmer by tossing in a life preserver, involving absolutely no risk and very little effort to myself, it would be right for anyone else so situated to do so. If I am a strong swimmer lolling on the beach, I cannot pick and choose whom I will save, assuming that the act of saving involves no risk or loss to myself. I cannot save one drowning swimmer, but later neglect another because the soccer match on the radio has reached its climax. To discriminate is to violate the universal rule, acting in a way that it would not be right for everyone to emulate. Where there are costs or risks to be borne by the saviour, as they were by Oskar, it is more complicated. It would not be wrong for me to refuse to risk my life to save another person. On the other hand to risk my life once to save another and to refuse to do it again is less obviously acceptable, though it is easy to imagine the explanation that could be given for the failure to act for the second time:

> I did it once, but never again!
> I was almost killed [14]!

However, these cases of supererogation do not fit Oskar's case. He was constantly at risk as soon as he sheltered the first Jew. Taking one refugee after another may have contributed to the probability of exposure in the calculus of a reasonable person, but it did not increase the penalty that would befall Oskar and his employees if they were found out [15]. According to Keneally's account, Schindler never ever turned away a Jew. Obviously he was not a reasonable person who calculated the probability of exoposure against the lives at risk. But then again he was not a deontologist who martyred himself the first time he saw something terrible or heard something worse. If it exists, he waived John Stuart Mill's right to a quite life [16].

The most astonishing thing about Schindler is that he became neither a martyr nor a paralytic. Frustration and confusion did not drive him to end it all in a death wish, say by provoking the S.S.'s suspicions or by suicide. Nor did he paralyse himself with doubts, as the characters of an early Woody Allen film would have done. Cast as Schindler, one of these Allen personae would have intellectualised the problem in the search for a rational solution exactly as contemporary moral theory requires. A solution would have to be a universal rule. "How can I save, for who knows how long, this one when there are thousands and thousands more suffering and dying while I'm drowning in cognac?" such a self-doubting character would say. I should think that this Woody Allen/Schindler would not be able to answer this question rationally. The answer, of course, is that he saved those that he could, but that is not a rational justification. After all, he could have tried harder or gone to one place rather than another where he might have recruited different people. The people he recruited were usually those who were lucky enough to cross his path, nothing more, nothing less. They came to him. For his part he never systematically searched for Jews. Nor was there any reason to end up with 1000. Why not 1200? The futility of saving one, but not all others is a common tenet in our intellectual life when self-styled revolutionaries decry the limited—in their view, pathetic—endeavours of reformers, as for example allegorically in Luis Bunuel's film *La Viridiana*.

The truth on Keneally's showing is that Schindler avoided Woody Allen's intellectual paralysis by not thinking too much. He operated on feelings, failing to respect the Enlightenment divide between thinking and feeling [17]. When he saw someone in need he responded. He did not think about all of those he was not helping. He concentrated on those he was helping.

If Schindler's instinctive reactions do not obtain the crown from contemporary moral philosophy, it may be just as well, as far as those whom he saved are concerned. It seems all too likely that many people throughout Europe before, during, and after the war were paralysed by the test of universality as much as by the fear of the risks. They could not help nor save all under threat; so they said to themselves, 'There is no point in helping even one'. It was all, or none. It is certainly a defence of inaction that many people have since given. One of the merits of Keneally's novel is that he makes clear that Schindler was not alone in his human sympathy for the suffering of others. He documents many instances of by-standers, officials, German soldiers, and others in small ways aiding individual Jews. These *kleinen* Schindlers did what they could. Schindler could do more, and he did it. Nowhere in Schindler's story is there a problem, a solution, or rationality defined as universality. Consequently, what he did fails to meet the criteria of contemporary moral theory.

I have made a number of related claims about Schindler. Before going on it is time to take stock. First, I have claimed that Schindler acted on feeling. He did not calculate or ratiocinate, as the dominant criteria of contemporary moral theory require. Secondly, I have noted in passing that Schindler was absolutely loyal to the Jews he chanced to recruit. This is a minor point. Thirdly, I emphasised that Schindler saved some, but not others. The dominant version of contemporary moral theory equates rationality with universality as defining characteristics of morality. Particular and partial acts do not meet the criteria of moral theory. This is my main point.

Against my third point immediately above, a defender of the consensus in contemporary moral theory might argue from the tenet that 'ought implies can'. Such a defender would see the rationality in Oskar's actions to be that he did what he could, as I have said earlier in this article. The defender would then conclude that contemporary moral theory can interpret the moral reality of Schindler and so is vindicated.

What the defender fails to appreciate is the force of my first point. Schindler acted as opportunities presented themselves. As I have stressed he did not set out to save Jews, search for Jews to save, or decide to save one kind of Jew rather than another (a young woman rather than an old woman). The punch line is that Schindler probably did not do all he could have done. Had he tried harder, been more systematic he might well have saved more Jews.

There is a second, more general weakness in the defender's argument that cannot pass in silence. Ought may imply can but the realm of the possible marked by the word 'can' is not determinant. Schindler had no foreknowledge of what he could do (i.e. succeed in doing) until 1945 (nor did he know the war would end in that year). He discovered what he could do by doing it, as do most of us.

If we realise Schindler's virtues today it is despite, not because of dominant character of moral theory. It is because we hear the voice still of an older tradition kept alive by a distinct minority of contemporary contributors to moral theory like Iris Murdoch, Peter Winch, Alasdair MacIntyre and Bernard Williams [18]. Recently Stanley G. Clarke has attempted to synthesize the older tradition into the newer tradition that I have described as dominant [19]. He does so by characterising the newer consensus as theoretical and the older as anti-theoretical. Predictably, he then argues that the anti-theory school has a theory and consequently is a part of the newer, dominant consensus. Clarke is to be congratulated on his ingenuity.

However, lost in the glare of this ingenuity is that the older, minority tradition recognises a different kind of morality. This other tradition concerns moral enlightenment, moral education, moral character, and, above all, virtue. It does not address problems, search for solutions, or aspire to universal rationality. This other tradition includes Socrates (with a foot in both camps), Aristotle, the Stoics, Augustine, Aquinas, Hume, and Hegel among others. A thinker like Aristotle does not proceed by the study of problems. He is not interested in rationally resolving problems, but in how we should live. On the few occasions when he produces an example, the purpose is to warn his auditors against falling into traps that will have undesirable effects on their character in the long run.

Morality for Aristotle was what a person did, not the rules, principles, and procedures flourished. The measure of morality for him was what a person does, not what the person demands of others in the way of uncontaminated rules and principles. One's actions are based on one's character. In turn, character is not formed by learning rules and principles, nor is it equipped for action by the possession of a set of rules, principles, and procedures. Character is formed throughout a lifetime. It starts as habit. We learn to do good deeds by doing good at the instruction of an adult, and gradually we learn to do this autonomously and gradually we learn why it is good, though we may never be able to articulate and define its goodness by universal criteria on a philosophy examination paper [20]. That silence only proves that the measure of the good life is not a philosophy examination paper, not that some things are not good.

No method of ethics (rules, principles, procedures) can guide us throughout life.

The evidence of our century indicates that the capacity to do evil outstrips the capacity to anticipate it. For that we need what, toward the end of her life, Hannah Arendt called reflective judgement [21]. While Kant's moral theory was based on universalisability and determinative judgement, his aesthetic theory was based on reflective judgement. Arendt thought reflective judgement would be the basis for moral judgement in our time. In the realm of ethics one judges a particular without reference to a universal rule or principle, and these judgements are valid for more than the judging subject, though they certainly are not universal as the truths of physics are.

A reflective judgement is made without a universal. Such a judgement is made when we find, say, an *objet d'art* beautiful or a taste at the table pleasing. This kind of judgement is reflective precisely because it is based on a direct experience. No one can judge the beauty of an unseen object, but one can judge the truth of a scientific proposition without direct experience of the phenomenon. Judgement requires the context of a narrative [22]. In Kant's words, "The judgement of taste is not based on concepts; for if it were, it would be open to dispute (decision by means of proofs)" [23]. For Arendt moral judgements in our time cannot be laid up in a heaven of universal rules and principles [24]. Instead they must arise in direct experience such as Schindler's. If universality is the criterion of rationality as Fishkin has said, then reflective judgement in the light of direct experience will be condemned as irrational. Arendt, however, argues in more detail than can be summarized here that universality is not the sole defining feature of morality. Universality is a kind of rationality that has proven itself successful in science, in one particular science, namely physics, and on the strength of that success it has been conflated with rationality itself. One particular kind of rationality (that of physics) has been universalised into rationality itself.

The limit of universality is easily shown in the case of Schindler. According to a precept of universality like Kant's categorical imperative an act is right if and only if it would be right for everyone so situated to do it. The standard example in textbooks, and one used by Kant himself, is lying. It would not be right for everyone to lie, so it is never right for anyone to lie. Hence, it is always right to tell the truth. But would it have been right for Oskar to have told the truth to the Gestapo officials who occasionally questioned him? Certainly not. Was it wrong for him to lie to them? Certainly not.

Lest it be supposed that the criterion of universality is not a general feature of contemporary moral theory, but only of Kantian deontological theory, the same limitation is to be found in the prime alternative, namely utilitarianism. Utilitarianism demands a universal point of view before which all pleasures, pains, and lives are equal. Schindler did not adopt this point of view. For all he knew the faulty munitions that Deutsch Emailwaren Fabrik despatched to the Wehrmacht may have contributed to more than a thousand deaths. Even if that were the case we could hardly convict him of immorality, though a strict utilitarian would have to do so. Oskar was not a rational person in the prescribed fashion of contemporary moral theory.

Oskar Schindler acted instinctively in the face of direct experience. At the moment of truth he discovered the kind of character he had. It probably surprised him as much as everyone who knew him. His wife, Emilie, whom he had treated badly, said in 1973 that before the war there was nothing special about Oskar, nor was there after [25]. Like Hector, he was fortunate that in a few short years of his life he had met a challenge that had found the angel within himself. The first soul that Oskar Schindler saved when he began to help Jews was his own. So, too, for all the little Schindlers who do some good.

M. W. *Jackson, Department of Government and Public Administration, The University of Sydney, N.S.W., Australia 2006.*

NOTES

The fellowship of participants at the Salzburg Seminar on 'Philosophy & Public Affairs' stimulated this work. I am grateful to my university, the Potter Foundation of Melbourne, and the Salzburg Seminar for the grants that made it possible for me to attend. The comments of Philip Pettit and Stephen Cohen are much appreciated.

[1] THOMAS KENEALLY (1983) *Schindler's Ark* (Sevenoaks, Hodder & Stoughton.

[2] See *Sunday Times* of 3 October, 1982, p. 20 and 31 October, 1982, p. 8.

[3] G. W. F. HEGEL (1977) *The Phenomenology of Mind* (trans. A. V. Miller) (Oxford, Oxford University Press), p. 404.

[4] STEPHEN TOULMIN (1964) *Reason in Ethics* (London, Cambridge University Press), p. 1, emphasis added.

[5] R. M. HARE (1963) *Freedom and Reason* (Oxford, Oxford University Press), p. 1, emphasis added.

[6] RICHARD BRANDT (1959) *Ethical Theory* (Englewood Cliffs, N.J., Prentice-Hall) p. 1 and see also his (1979) *A Theory of the Good and the Right* (New York, Oxford University Press), p. v.

[7] MARCUS SINGER (1961) *Generalization in Ethics* (New York, Knopf), p. 6, emphasis added. Cf. ALAN GERWIRTH (1978) *Reason and Morality* (Chicago, University of Chicago Press) or ROBERT NOZICK (1981) *Philosophical Explanations* (Cambridge, Mass., Harvard University Press) pp. 399–570.

[8] EDMUND PINCOFFS (1986) *Quandaries and Virtues* (Lawrence, University Press of Kansas), p. 32. Much of the impetus for this piece derives from this excellent book.

[9] See the Statement of purpose inside the front cover of any issue of *Philosophy & Public Affairs*.

[10] JOHN RAWLS (1971) *A Theory of Justice* (Cambridge, Harvard University Press).

[11] JAMES FISHKIN (1984) Defending equality, *Michigan Law Review*, 82, p. 760.

[12] IMMANUEL KANT (1978) *Critique of Aesthetic Judgement* (London, Oxford University Press), p. 198.

[13] The power of universalisability is evinced throughout the dozen papers in (1985) *Morality and Universality: Essays on Ethical Universalizability* (Ed. Nelson T. Potter & Mark Timmons) (Boston, Reidel).

[14] Contrast these points with the bloodless discussion of JONATHAN GLOVER (1975) 'It makes no difference whether or not I do it, *Aristotelian Society, Supp.* 49, pp. 171–190.

[15] See M. W. JACKSON (1986) *Matters of Justice* (Beckenham, Croom Helm).

[16] I refer to Mill's advocacy of what is known as negative utilitarianism in (1910) [1861] *Utilitarianism* (London, Everyman), p. 56.

[17] See SHERRY TURKLE (1984) *The Second Self: computers and the human spirit* (London, Granada), pp. 319–320.

[18] IRIS MURDOCH (1970) *The Sovereignty of Good* (London, Routledge & Kegan Paul), ALASDAIR MACINTYRE (1985) *After Virtue*, 2nd edn (London, Duckworth); and BERNARD WILLIAMS (1985) *Ethics and the Limits of Philosophy* (London, Fontana).

[19] S. G. CLARKE (1987) Anti-theory in ethics, *American Philosophical Quarterly*, 24, pp. 237–244.

[20] A recent literary example is Chuck from ALISON LURIE (1984) *Foreign Affairs* (New York, Random House).

[21] HANNAH ARENDT (1978) *Life of the Mind*, two volumes (London, Secker & Warburg).

[22] See ALISDAIR MACINTYRE (1977) Epistemological crises, narrative, and science, *Monist*, 60, pp. 453–456 or CAROL GILLIGAN (1982) *In a Different Voice* (Cambridge, Mass., Harvard University Press).

[23] KANT, p. 198.

[24] An invigorating recent example is DEREK PHILLIPS (1986) *Toward a Just Social Order* (Princeton, Princeton University Press).

[25] KENEALLY, p. 400.

16

The Case for Pacifism

RICHARD NORMAN

ABSTRACT   *I present the case for pacifism by formulating what I take to be the most plausible version of the idea of respect for human life. This generates a very strong, though not necessarily absolute, moral presumption against killing, in war or any other situation. I then show how difficult it is for this presumption to be overridden, either by the considerations invoked in 'just war' theory, or by consequentialist claims about what can be achieved through war.*

Despite the strength of the moral case against war, people sometimes say that they have no choice but to fight. In the concluding section of the paper I attempt to identify the relevant sense in which this could be said, and I discuss briefly how this affects the case for pacifism.

The conclusion of this paper will not be an unqualified endorsement of pacifism. I nevertheless want to present the case for pacifism as strongly as I can, for I do not think that the plausibility of that case has been adequately recognised in the philosophical literature. An unconditional rejection of, say, abortion, or euthanasia, or the death penalty, or even the killing of animals, has been treated as a standard position in philosophical discussions, and as an appropriate point of reference for other, more nuanced positions. When it comes to the morality of war, however, pacifism—the unconditional rejection of war—has typically been treated as an eccentric or marginal position, with the implication that the important issues and arguments are to be found elsewhere [1]. I want to maintain, on the contrary, that pacifism is central to the arguments, and that other positions ought to define themselves primarily in relation to pacifism. To describe the position which eventually emerges in this paper I am inclined to adopt a recent suggestion and call it 'pacificist' rather than 'pacifist' [2]. I believe that the case for pacifism is very strong indeed, and I shall set out that case, but I shall also suggest that there are situations where people can properly say that, in a sense which I shall try to explain, they have no choice but to resort to war. I am inclined to think that, at least at the theoretical level, there is no way of resolving the ethical dilemma posed by war and pacifism. Nevertheless, en route to that rather unsatisfactory conclusion, I shall argue that the case for pacifism is stronger, and the standard justifications for war are weaker, then they are generally taken to be.

I define 'pacifism' as the view that it is always wrong to go to war. As such it is addressed to governments, and to political movements, especially those which aspire to be governments, since these are the bodies which, by definition, are capable of waging wars and therefore have to decide whether or not to do so. Violence or killing engaged in by individuals solely as individuals would not be war, whatever else it might be. However, as individuals we can, to a greater or lesser extent, influence governments, and we can either support or oppose the decisions of governments and political movements to resort to war. Pacifism, therefore, would require us as individuals to oppose any resort to war. There remains the question what the individual should do if his or her government has in fact embarked on a war. Pacifism has normally been taken to require that even if one is unable to prevent one's own country going to war, one should still refuse to participate; this however raises further questions about the nature of political allegiance, which I shall not discuss. I shall focus on the initial, and logically primary, claim that it can never be right for governments or would-be governments to resort to war.

The absolutist formulation of that claim is crucial. The horrors of war are obvious, they increase with every advance in men's technical capacity to inflict death and destruction, and, reviewing the historical record, one might doubt whether any war could achieve sufficient good to counterbalance those horrors. One might then arrive at the position which Anne Seller has called 'unprincipled pacifism'. That phrase, however, is deliberately paradoxical. One thinks of pacifism as, par excellence, a principled position, not just a rule-of-thumb about probable consequences. The principle which underlies it is, I suggest, that of the wrongness of killing: war is morally unacceptable because it is the unjustified taking of human life. I am aware that pacifism is not always formulated in such terms. In particular, it is sometimes formulated as the view that it is always wrong to employ force, or to employ violence. These various formulations, in terms of force, or violence, or killing, will have importantly different implications, which I cannot explore here. I can only state dogmatically that the most plausible of the three versions seems to me to be that which is formulated in terms of the wrongness of killing. This does not mean that I want to dispense with the vocabulary of 'violence' and 'non-violence'. The phrase 'non-violent resistance' is well-entrenched as a way of referring to alternatives to war; it is the most convenient way of identifying an important tradition of thought and action, and in due course I shall myself use it in that way. Nevertheless I want to put the main weight of the ethical case for pacifism on the concept of 'killing' rather than the concept of 'violence'.

I do not want to maintain that the pacifist, as an absolutist about killing in war, needs to be an absolutist about the wrongness of killing in general, nor about the killing of human beings generally. That again would make pacifism less plausible than it needs to be. What I shall do is to offer an account of the wrongness of killing which is grounded in the attitude of respect for human life as such. I shall try to show how deeply rooted that attitude is in our moral thinking, and hence how difficult it is for the presumption against killing to be overridden. Although there are possible circumstances in which an exception could justifiably be made to the principle of not taking human life, the standard justifications for overriding that principle in war are, I shall suggest, inadequate; hence the strength of the case for pacifism.

Respect for Human Life

What is wrong with taking human life? Two obvious answers are that to kill someone against their will is to override their autonomy, and the utilitarian answer that to kill someone normally causes great suffering and deprives the victim of possible happiness. An account composed exclusively of these two elements, however, seems to rule out the attitude of respect for human life as such, and hence the idea that killing is wrong just because it is the taking of life. There are familiar difficulties with that idea. Respect for human life as such seems to attribute value to the mere fact of being alive, even if in an irreversible coma. And if we respect human life, are we not being arbitrarily 'speciesist' unless we extend the same respect to all life, including the bacteria which are killed by medicines, the weeds which are killed by any gardener, and the crops which are harvested for food?

To meet these difficulties, I want to defend the suggestion which has been made by James Rachels [3], that we should interpret the idea of respect for life as referring not to the merely biological condition of 'being alive', but to that of 'having a life'. We should think of human life as something which is *lived*, something in which a human being is actively engaged. Of course, in a weak sense any living thing 'lives' its own life, but I have in mind something stronger—the ability of a normal human being to give a distinctive shape to his or her life as a whole. We typically think of a human life as following a distinctive pattern, developing from birth, through childhood, youth and maturity to old age. These are the characteristic contours of human life. Within this framework, each person will live his or her own life in his or her own way, giving it a particular content and making something meaningful out of it. People do this in innumerable different ways: they may pursue a career, or devote themselves to a cause or a movement or a set of beliefs; their lives may revolve around a close relationship with another person, or around family relationships, around the process of growing up within a family and then raising the next generation. These possibilities are of course neither exclusive nor exhaustive, but I list them as typical ways in which people live their lives, shaping them and making something of them. They all illustrate what I mean when I speak of a human life as something which is actively lived.

I do not want to suggest that, to count as living his or her own life, a person must consciously think about his or her life as a whole in this sort of way. That would be an absurdly intellectualist understanding of what it is to live one's own life. Nevertheless my account does presuppose certain minimal abilities, those which are required if one is to be capable of acting in the sorts of ways which do, as a matter of fact, give a shape to a person's life. This means being able, at least to some extent, to reflect on one's past experiences, to feel satisfaction or regret concerning them and to act in the light of such reflections. Similarly it means being able to entertain hopes and aspirations for one's life which extend beyond the immediate future. These conditions remain exceedingly vague, and much more would need to be said about them. Nevertheless they serve to distinguish, for example, the muddled, the lazy, the unambitious, the bed-ridden, the neurotic or the psychotic, all of whom can (though their capacity for effective action is curtailed) uncontroversially be said to live their own lives, from the anencephalic or the permanently comatose, who cannot.

More worryingly, these conditions may seem to exclude infants. Here I want to say that the new-born child, though as yet it lacks a sense of its own past and future, has embarked on the process of learning, of interacting with its environment and forming relationships with others, and has thus taken its first steps in making a life. Again the idea of the shape of a life as a whole is important. A being whose activity remained always at the level of the new-born baby could not be said to live its own life in the sense I am proposing. The picture changes when we see those infant activities as the beginning of a process of development, as leading naturally into the more sophisticated activities which I have taken to be distinctive of 'living a life'. In a sense, then, I am employing a notion of 'potentiality'—but in a strong sense; I am referring not just to the baby's future capacities, but to what it is already doing, because 'what it is already doing' is the beginning of a continuing process, and it is in the light of the later stages in the process that we can see these initial stages also as 'the living of a life'.

This way of thinking about a human life leads us to a proper understanding of the act of killing. We should think of killing, correspondingly, not just as the destruction of a biological condition but as depriving someone of the opportunity actively to live his or her own life. Understanding the wrongness of killing in this way then enables us to see why it is ethically fundamental. In particular—and this will be important for later stages of my argument—it enables us to see why respect for human life is more fundamental than the value of freedom or autonomy, and more fundamental than a utilitarian evaluation of consequences. Take first the point about autonomy. It will be apparent that my interpretation of respect for human life brings it close to the Kantian notion of 'respect for persons'. This latter has, in turn, been assimilated by many recent philosophers to the idea of respect for people's autonomy. The problem is then that the capacity for autonomy, in the full sense of the ability to make conscious choices and decisions about one's own life, is a capacity which is not fully realised at birth but develops only slowly and gradually. Nevertheless, as I have indicated, even the new-born baby has embarked on the process of living its life, and as such is entitled to respect. Respect for persons, then, I take to mean respect for the uniqueness of each individual life and for the person who lives it. It will mean also respect for the conscious choices which the person makes in directing and shaping his or her own life, but this is derivative from the more general notion of respect for the life itself.

The same can be said of the relation between respect for life and utilitarian ethics. One of the notorious problems at the heart of utilitarianism is: why should we be concerned to promote the general happiness at all? Why does it matter? Utilitarians sometimes seem to suggest that this question can be answered by saying that happiness, in some abstract sense, 'has value' and therefore the more of it we create, the better. I must confess that I find this notion of happiness as some kind of free-floating 'value' quite unintelligible. Surely the reason why we are concerned to promote happiness is that we are concerned for the people who may be happy or unhappy. Many utilitarians talk as though what is logically prior is the requirement to maximise happiness, and as though we then need to make people happy because we need them to be the vehicles for this maximised happiness. The truth of the matter, however, is surely that happiness matters because people matter, not vice versa. And what I have been claiming about happiness goes also for all values, or at any rate for all human goods. If we value anything at all in people's lives, it must be because we respect those lives as such, and that is why our sense of the wrongness of destroying human lives is morally fundamental.

Can we go further and say that the wrongness of killing is an absolute principle—that is, that the taking of human life can never be justified? I do not think that this follows, but the preceding considerations do serve to establish how difficult it is to defend the idea of sacrificing a human life for the sake of some supposed greater good. I have alluded briefly to the idea of the *uniqueness* of each individual human life. That idea is important, but the connection between 'uniqueness' and 'value' needs clarifying. The point is not that, being qualitatively unique, each individual life has a kind of scarcity value, like a signed artistic masterpiece—as though the lives of identical twins thereby became less valuable because there were two of them. Rather, it is connected with my previous point about human lives as the bearer or the focus of value. Things have value because of the part they play in people's lives. Therefore, if one person's life is destroyed, this cannot be compensated for by the promotion of values in other people's lives. It cannot be compensated for, just because the values promoted for others will not compensate the person who has been killed. We could speak of the one person's loss being cancelled out by the other people's gains only if values could be computed in some impersonal way, apart from the context of separate human lives; but this is just what I am denying. There is no group consciousness, no supra-individual being which can experience both the losses and the gains and accept the former as an acceptable price to pay for the latter.

Nevertheless the fact also remains that people's lives do, inescapably, conflict. There just *are* cases where one person's life can be preserved only by sacrificing someone else's life. Consider the classic example where A is threatening B, and B's life can be saved only by killing A. If one kills A, the loss is, in the sense I have tried to indicate, a total loss. It is the extinction of one individual life, one consciousness for which things have value and within which goods are experienced. No preservation of values within B's life can cancel out that loss. On the other hand, exactly the same is true if one fails to save B's life. That loss, too, is total. A choice therefore has to be made, not because of some spurious computation of an overall impersonal good, but simply because, either way, someone will be killed. The only way to maintain an absolute prohibition against killing in such cases would be to invoke a distinction between 'killing' and 'failing to save someone's life', or to invoke the doctrine of 'double effect'. One could then say that it is always and absolutely wrong intentionally to kill any human being, and that therefore it would be wrong to kill A in this example; though B would then die, this would be describable as a failure to save his life rather than an act of killing him, or as a foreseen but unintended consequence of the refusal to kill A, and so would not be a violation of an absolute prohibition against intentional killing. Since however I do not want to say either of these things or invoke either of these distinctions, I have to say that in the light of such examples the principle of not taking human life cannot be maintained as an absolute principle.

I want to make two other points about the example. Given that a choice has to be made between two lives, how is it to be made? Again, not on utilitarian grounds. It would not be a matter of deciding which of the two is likely to have the happier life and/or to do more good in the world and, on those grounds, opting for the death of the other. (Similarly, to change the example, it would not be right to kill C in order to provide a liver transplant for D and thereby save D's life on the grounds that it could do more good than C's.) The relevant consideration is surely that A is threatening B's life, and that therefore if the choice has to be made it is A's life that must be taken, since it is he who is responsible for the fact that one or the other life must be sacrificed. The second point to be stressed is that all of this would remain true if it were B himself who had to make the choice. If B's life were threatened by A, and B could preserve himself only by killing A, he would be justified in doing so. Again, however, he would not be entitled to do so merely on utilitarian grounds. I stress these two points because between them they spell out the idea of justified killing in self-defence, to which we shall return in due course.

So far I have allowed that the principle of not taking human life cannot be an absolute principle because there are cases where a choice has to be made between two lives. Having made that concession, I think it also has to be conceded that the wrongness of killing could in principle be overridden by other considerations. I have argued that respect for human life is more fundamental than the value of freedom and than utilitarian values, and, as such, carries greater weight. That, however, is not enough to show that, in order to prevent oppression or suffering on a very great scale, it might not be necessary to take human lives. Once again the judgement cannot be a purely utilitarian one, nor can it be simply a matter of calculating alternative levels of freedom and oppression. The wrongness of killing carries an independent weight, and it weighs very heavily in the balance, but we cannot rule out the possibility that it might be outweighed by a sufficiently great prospect of the alleviation of oppression or suffering. Nor should we rule out the possibility that, in cases other than that of 'self-defence' in the narrow sense (as the defence of one's own life), it might be permissible to kill someone who has, through the wickedness of his own action, brought it upon himself. (An example might be killing in self-defence by a rape victim [4].) If anything is a candidate for being an absolute principle, then the principle of not taking human life is; but the trouble with any absolutism is that we simply cannot rule out, in advance, the possibility that considerations of one kind might come into conflict with considerations of any other kind and might, in some cases, be outweighed by them.

In summary, what I want to say about the principle of not taking human life is this. It is not an absolute principle, but it is a fundamental one and it carries very great weight. It can in principle be overridden, but only in special cases, and it cannot be overridden on the basis of a purely utilitarian calculation. This may look like a regrettably untidy and vague position. It is, however, a position of a recognisable kind in ethics. It is, for example, what many philosophers have wanted to say about the concept of basic moral rights. I am myself unenthusiastic about the concept of moral rights, finding it more confusing than helpful. Those who are more attached to the concept might nevertheless like to reformulate my discussion as a defence of a very strong right to life which, although it is not inviolable and although it can perhaps be forfeited in special cases, is more basic than any other moral right and more basic than utilitarian considerations.

To conclude this section I want to comment briefly on the relation between the *principle* of the wrongness of killing and the *attitude* of respect for human life. Pacifism, I have said, is a principled position, and the relevant principle to which it appeals is the principle of not taking human life. That, however, is not just an abstract principle whose validity is self-evident. The principle matters because it articulates the moral implications of the underlying basic response of a human being confronted with another human life. That is why the case for pacifism is made most powerfully not by rational arguments such as I am presenting in this paper, but by the portrayal of that basic response in works of imaginative literature. In war poems and novels and autobiographies one experience stands out: that of the soldier who kills an enemy and then confronts the fact that the person whom he has killed is not just an enemy but another human being like himself [5]. Through the direct personal encounter with the dying man—perhaps talking to him as he dies, perhaps looking through his personal documents—the killer comes face to face with the uniqueness of the individual human life which he has destroyed, with the enormity of what he has done, and with the fact that this is what war requires people to do. And this sense of the inviolability of another human life is what I refer to as the attitude of respect.

It may be said that a rational moral position cannot be founded on the emotional responses which people may or may not happen to feel on this or that occasion. I am not suggesting, however, that our moral commitments are the direct expression of felt emotional responses. The picture which I would offer is a more complex one. Our most fundamental, shared responses are embodied and expressed in the concepts of our shared moral vocabulary. It is in terms of this common vocabulary that we attempt to make sense of our moral world and to formulate the settled moral beliefs and principles with which we assess our actions. Ultimately, however, those beliefs and principles derive their force from the natural human responses on which they rest; and one example of this is the relation between the principle of the wrongness of killing and the underlying attitude of respect.

This, then, is the basis on which I shall build the case for pacifism. Respect for human life establishes a very strong presumption against killing, in war or in any other circumstances. What I now want to do is to show how difficult it is for this presumption to be overridden by the sorts of considerations which are normally thought to justify killing in war. I want to look at two kinds of justification which are standardly offered: first, those which feature in the tradition of 'just war' theory, and secondly, justifications couched in consequentialist terms.

'Just War' and Aggression

'Just war' theory is a complex body of doctrine, in an evolving tradition. I want to focus on the two points which have become central in recent discussions, and which are the twin pillars of the most recent extended defence of 'just war' theory, Michael Walzer's book *Just and Unjust Wars*. Walzer adopts the traditional distinction between *jus ad bellum* and *jus in bello*; the former provides the account of what justifies resort to war, the latter provides the account of what are just and unjust ways of fighting a war. According to Walzer the central principles of each are, respectively, that going to war is justified when it is the defence of a political community against aggression, and that a war is fought justly only if the immunity of non-combatants is respected.

Consider first, then, the suggestion that war can be justified as a response to aggression. Walzer defends this idea by reference to a morality of *rights*. "Individual rights (to life and liberty)", he says, "underlie the most important judgements that we make about war .... States' rights are simply their collective form" [6]. The comparison between individual rights and states' rights is then spelled out as follows.

> Over a long period of time, shared experiences and cooperative activity of many different kinds shape a common life. "Contract" is a metaphor for a process of association and mutuality, the on-going character of which the state claims to protect against external encroachment. The protection extends not only to the lives and liberties of individuals, but also to their shared life and liberty, the independent community they have made, for which individuals are sometimes sacrificed .... Given a genuine "contract," it makes sense to say that territorial integrity and political sovereignty can be defended in exactly the same way as individual life and liberty [7].

Walzer's case depends, then, on this analogy between a state's rights to territorial integrity and political sovereignty on the one hand and an individual's right to life and liberty on the other. Certainly there is something in this analogy. One can see a resemblance between the death of an individual and the destruction of the life of a political community when it is invaded and conquered; and between the oppression of an individual and the oppression of a community when its sovereign independence is violated. I want to say, however, that this analogy cannot do what is required of it for the argument. It is at best an imperfect analogy. And it is no more than an analogy; it does not show that the territorial integrity of a community has the *same* fundamental ethical status as the lives of human beings.

First, then, it is an imperfect analogy. Foreign conquest and domination may, in a loose sense, be construed as 'the death of a nation', but it rarely amounts to the complete destruction of a community. The shared way of life usually continues, in an attenuated form. Overall political control may be in the hands of the conqueror, but many other institutions, cultural and economic and religious, are likely to continue, and to embody at least some of the 'shared experiences and cooperative activity' which, as Walzer says, 'shape a common life'. Even in the minority of cases where the conquering power does aim at eliminating entirely the indigenous culture, it may well find it difficult to do so. The communal life may go underground, traditions may be preserved in secret, or in exile. I do not say that this is a happy state of affairs, but it is not the death of a community in the full sense which would make it entirely analogous to the death of an individual human being.

Suppose, however, that the analogy is complete, and that a whole way of life really is wiped out for ever. Then indeed a great wrong has been done, but it is still not a wrong of the same order as the taking of human lives. It may be analogous, but it is *only* analogous, it is not ethically equivalent. Even if their community has completely disintegrated, individuals live on. They may perhaps eventually create a new identity for themselves within the conquering society, or as refugees they may find a place in the life of some other community. Where this is not so, where the individual lives do not continue, we are no longer talking about the crime of aggression, we are talking about genocide, and we have then gone beyond Walzer's analogy altogether.

It may be objected that my position undervalues the importance which shared experiences and a common life have for individuals. Indeed, that objection might be held to carry particular weight since it seems to be supported by other features of my argument. My account of respect for life invoked a richer notion of a human life as more than a mere biological existence; but the relevant capacity to make sense of and give significance to their lives is something which individuals can acquire only through their participation in shared traditions and ways of life. Subtract from a human life everything which derives from the community and one is indeed left with a purely biological existence. Doesn't it follow, then, that the common way of life will be as valuable as life itself, and won't the principle of self-defence then have to embrace the defence of the community as well as the defence of the individual lives?

The starting-point of this objection is one which I would certainly accept. The capacity to live a meaningful life is a capacity derived from one's participation in a human community. However, I also want to reiterate that that capacity, once acquired, can survive the destruction of a particular community. Why is this? First, because there are many kinds and levels of community. A war of defence against aggression is normally thought of as a war in defence of one kind of community, a nation-state, identified by its territorial boundaries. The destruction of the nation-state, however, can leave intact many other overlapping communities, smaller and larger. There remain families and localities and networks of friendship. There remain intellectual, moral, religious, political or artistic movements and traditions, and though some of these may have been defining features of a particular nation, they are not necessarily destroyed when the nation loses its independence.

The second reason is the simple fact that the human capacities derived from participation in a community can be realised only in individual lives. This takes us, I think, to the element of truth in individualism. The philosophical conflict between individualism and communitarianism cannot be resolved by the simple vindication of one side. The truth of communitarianism is that distinctively human activities are made possible by participation in a community. The truth of individualism is the uniqueness and irreplaceability of each individual consciousness. If a community is destroyed, individuals retain the ability to speak the language and engage in the practices which they learned in that community, and they may be able, even under conditions of extreme hardship and persecution, to exercise that ability. When a human being dies, the value of that individual life is gone for good; in the sense I have tried to indicate, the life is irreplaceable and the loss is total. Tragic though the destruction of a community may be, the destruction of individual human lives is of a different order again.

I submit, then, that the analogy between individuals' rights and states' rights fails to establish that the need to resist aggression is a sufficient justification for resort to war. Given that there is a very strong presumption against the wholesale taking of life which war involves, the analogy is too weak to show that military resistance to aggression has sufficient ethical weight to override the presumption. There remains the possibility that resistance to genocide might be sufficient to justify waging war, and we shall have to return to that.

'Just War' and Non-combatant Immunity

The second principle of 'just war' theory which I want to consider is the principle of non-combatant immunity. This principle might at first be thought irrelevant to our present concerns, since its purpose is not to identify a possible justification for waging war, but to impose a further moral constraint which must limit the actions even of those who are justified in waging war. Nevertheless the principle does constitute an important point of disagreement with pacifism, and we can see this if we remind ourselves that the 'just war' theorist says about the killing of non-combatants what the pacifist says about all killing in war: that it must not be done, even as a means of resistance against aggression. This implies that, for the 'just war' theorist, there is something about the status of combatants which makes it permissible to kill them in resistance to aggression; and that is what the pacifist denies [8].

What are we to make of this suggestion? Why should there be an ethically significant distinction between combatants and non-combatants which makes it permissible to kill the one but not the other? The standard explanation is that the killing of non-combatants is wrong even in a justified war because it would be a case of killing the innocent. What contrast is implied here? If non-combatants are innocent, what are combatants? 'Guilty' is the contrast one would expect, but this immediately takes us to the heart of the problem, for it is difficult to find any convincing sense in which the ordinary combatant in war is guilty. In what sense, then, can non-combatants be called 'innocent', and what is the nature of the contrast with combatants?

One of the best discussions of this problem is Jeffrie Murphy's paper 'The Killing of the Innocent', and I shall consider that paper as an example of the attempt to make ethical sense of the 'combatant'/'non-combatant' distinction [9]. Murphy first points out that the 'innocence' of non-combatants can hardly be taken to mean moral innocence in a general sense. Military action against civilians, such as the bombing of a city, may kill all sorts of disreputable characters. Nor can 'innocence' mean moral innocence *of the war*. "Consider", says Murphy, "the octogenarian civilian in Dresden who is an avid supporter of Hitler's war effort ... and contrast his case with that of the poor, frightened, pacifist frontline soldier who is only where he is because of duress ...." [10]. The former is uncontroversially more responsible for the war than the latter. The relevant distinction, according to Murphy, is this: combatants are "all those of whom it is reasonable to believe that they are engaged in an attempt at your destruction" [11]. This includes not only soldiers but their military and political leaders, and others who contribute directly to the war effort such as, perhaps, workers in munitions factories. Because they are engaged in an attempt to destroy you, it is permissible to kill them. Non-combatants are not directly engaged in such an attempt, and in that sense they are 'innocent'.

The problem now shifts. Such a contrast can indeed be drawn, but why should it carry this ethical significance? If 'innocence' does not mean 'moral innocence', why should it determine who may be killed and who may not? There are two main elements in Murphy's answer. In general terms he appeals to a theory of rights. Normally, he says, to kill someone is to violate his right against interference. However, "when a person uses his freedom to invade the rights of others, he forfeits certain of his own rights and renders interference by others legitimate" [12]. This is why, when combatants are engaged in an attempt to destroy you, they forfeit their right not to be killed by you. However, if Murphy is going to talk about 'forfeiting one's rights', he surely needs to employ precisely those notions of moral guilt and innocence which he has shown to be unavailable in this context. One does not forfeit one's rights merely because one is, objectively, a danger to others. It must be the case that one is *morally guilty* of attempting to destroy others. We are then back with the fact that vast numbers of combatants, even if they are fighting an aggressive war, are not themselves morally responsible for the aggression, or at any rate are much less responsible than their leaders. Therefore they have not forfeited their rights, and killing them cannot be justified by claiming that they have done so.

Murphy also appeals more specifically to the idea of 'self-defence' to fill out his theory of rights. He says: "If one believes (as I do) that the only even remotely plausible justification for war is self-defence, then one must in waging war confine one's hostility to those against whom one is defending oneself...." [13]. And those against whom one is defending oneself are, he says, the combatants who are engaged in an attempt to destroy you and have thereby forfeited their rights.

Here we need to recall the problems with the idea of 'resistance to aggression'. A war of 'self-defence' is typically taken to mean a war to defend a nation's territorial integrity against an aggressive invader. I have argued that this justification for war is unconvincing. Murphy has his own doubts about it. He says:

> ... with respect to nations, the whole idea of self-defence is strongly in need of analysis. What, for example, is it for a state to die or be threatened with death?
>
> ... I am sceptical that the "self" to be legitimately defended must always be the nation or state. It is at least worth considering the possibility that the only moral problems arising in war are the oldest and most common and most important—namely, are human beings being hurt and killed, who are they, and why are they? [14]

And when he goes on to link the idea of self-defence with that of rights, he takes as his example the case of individual self-defence [15].

There are, of course, plenty of situations in war where the question of individual self-defence does arise. The combatant who is actually engaged in fighting is likely to find himself in situations where, unless he kills the person who is about to fire on him, he will himself be killed. But if that is the only killing which the 'combatant'/'non-combatant' distinction can justify, it is a great deal less than the theory is intended to justify. The theory is supposed to justify combatants killing enemy combatants in order to win; in fact it will only justify killing combatants in order to survive.

At this point we are, I think, forced back to the conclusion that the most that 'just war' theory can justify is a war against genocide. I suggested earlier that the first component of the theory, the principle of resistance to aggression, is plausible only if it goes beyond a mere analogy between 'territorial integrity' and 'the right to life'; it will justify resistance to aggression only if the aggression is *literally* an attempt to destroy the lives of the members of the community. Similarly the 'combatant'/'non-combatant' distinction, if it amounts to no more than a principle of self-defence, will justify a community only in fighting to defend the lives of its members. And note that even a principle of self-defence will still have to employ notions of moral responsibility, of moral guilt and innocence. I may not kill just anyone whose death would help to preserve my life or the life of another, but only someone who is morally responsible for the threat to that life. (Recall my earlier example of killing someone because you need a liver transplant.) So even if a community is justified in killing to defend itself against genocide, its resistance must be directed against those who are responsible for the threat of genocide. And if, as is likely, that means not the enemy combatants but their political leaders, then what will be justifed will be something rather different from war—a campaign of assassination, perhaps.

Consequentialist Justifications

I turn now from 'just war' theory to consequentialist considerations, that is, to the suggestion that wars can be justified by what they achieve. As I have said, something more is needed here than simply a utilitarian calculation. The fact that a war involves the taking of vast numbers of human lives must itself carry a very great independent weight, quite apart from the obvious disutilities of war such as the human grief and suffering, the massive destruction of resources and the dislocation of civil life. A consequentialist justification of war would have to show, in any particular case, that all of this can be outweighed by the good that waging war can achieve, or rather, by the even greater evils which it can prevent or eliminate. Can this be done?

There are strong reasons for doubting it. We might first look at the historical record. What is striking here is the way in which each war, in its outcome, sows the seeds of a future military conflict. Take the case of the Second World War. If ever any war has been justified by its aims and its results, then surely this war was. Of course it achieved its results at an immense cost, involving millions of deaths and appalling suffering, but by such means it brought about the overthrow of Nazism. At this point, however, we should remember that the purpose for which Britain declared war on Germany was not the defeat of Nazism as a political system, and that most of those who fought against it did so in complete ignorance of the concentration camps and the other distinctive features of Nazism. The occasion for Britain's entry into the war was the commitment to the independence of Poland, and it is at least debatable whether in 1945 this had been fully achieved. This should remind us that what the war did produce, as its direct consequence, was the division of Europe into two military power blocs, posing the danger of an even more destructive war, a nuclear war which would destroy European civilisation and perhaps even eliminate the human race altogether. If we then consider the possibility that Nazism could have been overthrown in other ways, without war, as Spanish fascism was eventually overcome, we may seriously wonder whether the achievements of the Second World War were as positive as they are usually thought to have been. And just as our present perilous situation is the outcome of that war, so also the ground for that war was laid by the Treaty of Versailles at the end of the First

World War; the First World War was in turn a product, in part, of the settlement at the end of the Franco-Prussian War of 1870–1; and so on.

That then is an example of the historical record, and of the way in which the outcome of one war becomes the cause for the next war. Nor should this surprise us. The settlement reached at the end of any war is, almost by definition, imposed by the military force of the victors, and as such it is bound to breed resentment and a smouldering desire for revenge. Pacifists would say that this illustrates a basic truth of human psychology: that violence breeds violence. It may be somewhat hazardous to infer from the facts of interpersonal behaviour to a conclusion about the political behaviour of states, but the inference does seem to be backed by historical experience. Of course causal claims about historical events are themselves notoriously conjectural. We can but guess at what might have happened if Nazism had not been resisted by military means, and at whether it could eventually have been overthrown without recourse to war. But this scepticism about predicting the consequences of waging or not waging war can itself be turned to account by pacifism. It is very difficult to tell whether fighting a war will achieve anything positive, and what its long-term consequences will be. We do know however, with very much greater certainty, that it will involve immense suffering and great loss of life. Therefore, weighing the certainty of suffering and death against the mere possibility of long-term good consequences, we may well conclude that war is never worth the risk.

Now scepticism about the positive achievements of war does not by itself entail pacifism. Nor does scepticism about 'just war' theory. Nor does respect for human life. What I have been claiming is that respect for human life sets up a very strong presumption against the justifiability of killing in war. Doubts about 'just war' theory, and doubts about the positive achievements of war, make it very difficult to see how that presumption could be overridden. That is the case for pacifism, and it is a very strong case.

Having No Choice

'And yet . . .' Those words of hesitation are inevitable, I think. Though I recognise the strength of the case, I still hesitate to accept it, and many people feel the same. Why is this? How is it that, though pacifism seems to be ethically compelling, doubts arise as soon as we start to think about actually applying it?

Those doubts are typically articulated by saying that, however ethically appalling it may be to contemplate fighting a war, there are situations in which people have no choice. I suggest that if we can pin down the sense of the statement 'We have no choice', we may be in a position to understand why pacifism remains difficult to accept.

Now of course it will never be the case literally and without qualification that one has no choice. One can always refuse to fight. But when people say that one sometimes has no choice, what they mean, I think, is that by refusing to fight, say, against aggression, or indeed against internal oppression, one is acquiescing in a very great evil, and by acquiescing in it one is tacitly endorsing it. Morally speaking, faced with that evil, we have no choice but to resist it, and if the only way to resist it is to fight, then we have no choice but to fight.

Now this reading of the situation might be challenged. Suppose that this country had been overrun by a Nazi invasion in 1940, and suppose that one had refused to fight against it. One might say: "I have not acquiesced in Nazism. I refuse to engage in military resistance to it, because that too would be ethically indefensible, but that does not mean that I accept Nazism. I reject it wholeheartedly, I will give no support to it, and if the Nazis order me to cooperate with their crimes I shall disobey even though I may be shot." One might say all this, and one might act accordingly.

Nevertheless, even if many people had thought and acted thus, it could remain true that, in an important sense, Nazism had not been resisted. This is because resistance to a social phenomenon such as aggression or oppression must, if it is really to count as resistance, take a socially identifiable form. It is here that the communitarian perspective may properly come into play. 'Aggression' or 'oppression' are constituted as such by the overall social meaning of innumerable individual human actions. Therefore one cannot resist them simply in virtue of one's own interpretation of one's own action— not because one will not be effective but because action does not count as 'resistance' unless it is socially understood as such. What forms of resistance are available will therefore depend upon the institutions and traditions of the community; and if the only recognised and organisable form of resistance is military resistance, then not fighting will mean not resisting. This, I think, is the significant sense in which people could say 'We have no choice but to fight'.

What also follows, however, is that what forms of resistance are socially available is itself something that can be changed, over time, by social action. In particular, institutional procedures for settling disputes without recourse to war, and traditions of non-violent resistance to invasion and oppression, can be gradually built up. And if they *can* be, they *should* be; for the stronger such traditions become, the less likely it is that people will find themselves in a situation where they have to say 'We have no choice but to fight.'

At the theoretical level, I find insoluble the dilemma posed by pacifism: that fighting in war is ethically indefensible, but is also sometimes the only thing that people can do. The interplay between individualist and communitarian perspectives, which has been a thread running through this paper, may perhaps help us to explain why the dilemma seems irresolvable. I have said that the truth of individualism is the irreplaceability of individual human lives. When we think in those terms the overwhelming fact of war is the loss of vast numbers of individual lives, and it is difficult to see how anything else can have a countervailing moral weight. But when we think in communitarian terms, we see war as a conflict between different social institutions or movements, and if the only socially recognised form of resistance to evil social practices is military resistance, then war may seem morally inescapable. The best conclusion I can offer, therefore, is this possibility of a solution at the practical level: that by building up a tradition of non-violent resistance to aggression and oppression, we can bring it about that people do have a choice and are not faced with an impossible ethical dilemma. It might then be possible to be unhesitatingly a pacifist [16].

Richard Norman, Darwin College, The University, Canterbury, Kent CT2 7NY, United Kingdom.

NOTES

[1] A notable exception is JENNY TEICHMAN (1986) *Pacifism and the Just War* (Oxford, Blackwell) and her earlier article 'Pacifism' in *Philosophical Investigations,* 5 (1982).
[2] MARTIN CEADEL (1987) *Thinking About Peace and War* (Oxford, Oxford University Press). Ceadel's typology of positions in the war-and-peace debate follows the sequence from 'militarism', through

'crusading', 'defencism', and 'pacific-ism', to 'pacifism'. He derives from A. J. P. Taylor the distinction between 'pacific-ism' and 'pacifism'.

[3] JAMES RACHELS (1986) *The End of Life* (Oxford, Oxford University Press), especially Chapter 2.

[4] Note, however, that such cases are controversial and that, even if it is accepted that they involve a right to kill, it is severely limited. Consider the recent legal case where a woman was acquitted of murder after killing a man who had raped her. "Judge Hazan warned that his ruling was not to be regarded in any way as a charter for victims of serious crimes—even rape—to kill their attackers. 'Revenge killings are unlawful and, depending on the circumstances, amount to murder or manslaughter,' he said. 'It is only killing in lawful self-defence that is justified'." (*The Guardian*, 1.10.87.) Note also that the woman had told the police: "I didn't mean to kill him, I only meant to get him off me—I was so frightened".

[5] Classic examples are Wilfred Owen's poem 'Strange Meeting', and chapter IX of Erich Maria Remarque's *All Quiet on the Western Front*.

[6] MICHAEL WALZER (1980) *Just and Unjust Wars* (London, Penguin), p. 54.

[7] Ibid.

[8] This conflict between pacifism and 'just war' theory is exemplified in G. E. M. ANSCOMBE (1961) War and murder. Anscombe suggests that "pacifism teaches people to make no distinction between the shedding of innocent blood and the shedding of any human blood. And in this way pacifism has corrupted enormous numbers of people who will not act according to its tenets". The paper first appeared in: WALTER STEIN (Ed.) *Nuclear Weapons: a Catholic response* (London, Merlin Press), and has been reprinted in various places including Anscombe's (1981) *Collected Papers*, III (Oxford, Blackwell).

[9] JEFFRIE MURPHY (1973) The killing of the innocent, *The Monist*, 57.

[10] Ibid., p. 531.

[11] Ibid., p. 536.

[12] Ibid., pp. 546–7. Cf. Walzer's linking of non-combatant immunity and rights, op. cit., p. 135.

[13] Ibid., p. 538.

[14] Ibid., p. 539.

[15] Ibid., p. 547.

[16] Many thanks for helpful comments from Tony Skillen, Karen Jones, Anne Seller, the *Journal of Applied Philosophy* referee, and philosophers at the University of Bristol and the Open University.

Part IV

Justice and Equality

17

Equity as an Economic Objective

JULIAN LE GRAND

ABSTRACT *Following Rawls' seminal work, political philosophers and economists have recently shown great interest in different conceptions of equity or justice. Apart from Rawls' own principles, these have included utilitarianism, need and desert, horizontal and vertical equity and envy-free distributions. None of these conceptions, however, seem to command general consensus; and this paper is an attempt to find out why. The conclusion is reached that they all fail because they do not take account of an essential element of equity: its relationship to the existence or otherwise of choice. An alternative conception is offered, based explicitly on that relationship; it is argued that this conception comes closer to capturing the essence of what is generally meant by the term equity than any of the others considered.*

In all societies there are a set of basic objectives that guide policy-making. For Western societies, these might include the achievement of efficiency, the attainment of equity or justice, the promotion of individual security and the preservation of individual liberty. Any policy recommendation concerning the allocation of scarce resources should therefore take account of all these objectives. However, to do so in any useful manner requires that they be defined in as precise a fashion as possible. Hence economists, as part of their efforts to advise on resource allocation questions, have found themselves on the terrain of political philosophers in attempting to formulate precise definitions for these objectives that would be useful for policy-making purposes.

This task has been far from easy. It has proved extremely difficult to find definitions which were simultaneously sufficiently general to command a broad consensus and sufficiently specific so as to permit useful application. However some success has been achieved in one area: that of efficiency. For several decades, there has been a definition which has commanded general agreement: Pareto-efficiency. That a pattern of resource allocation is efficient if it is impossible to make one person better off without making one or more persons worse off is one that has widespread intuitive appeal. Although not without its critics, this formulation has been immensely fruitful, providing the entire basis for welfare economics as conventionally considered.

Unfortunately, no comparable consensus has yet been achieved of another objective: that of equity. Although many alternative conceptions have been put forward, none has yet achieved a status comparable to that of Pareto-efficiency. This raises a number of questions. Is it possible to find a definition of equity that is sufficiently general so as to command consensus, while at the same time being sufficiently specific to be operationally useful? Why is it that none of the definitions and principles already proposed seem to meet these requirements? Should economists dismiss the whole exercise as futile and simply concentrate upon their traditional concern for efficiency? These are the questions which—in reverse order—I propose to address in this paper.

In the first section the arguments against even attempting to define equity or justice are discussed. The second section examines the criteria by which different conceptions of equity can be assessed. In the third section the conceptions that have been proposed are reviewed and some explanations offered as to their failure to command general consensus. An alternative definition is proposed in the fourth section which it is hoped captures the essential elements of the concept as it is generally used. Moreover, it has the advantage, for economists at least, that it relates the issue of equity to that of individual choice, and hence can be relatively easily translated into familiar economic concepts. The final section summarises the arguments.

To avoid possible misunderstanding, one thing should be made clear at the outset. By concentrating on the problem of defining equity, it is not intended to imply that equity criteria should dominate all others in determining policy. It is one of the tenets of this paper that objectives such as equity or efficiency are not ordered lexicographically in any social objective function. That is, they are not ranked such that a move towards the achievement of one objective, however small, will always be superior to a move towards the achievement of any other objective, however large. Thus an allocation of resources with less equity and more efficiency or liberty may be ranked higher or lower than one of greater equity but reduced efficiency or liberty, depending on the extent to which each objective is achieved in both allocations. There is no attempt here to specify how these objectives are or should be traded-off against one another. What is attempted, rather, is part of a task that is logically prior to any such specification: that of defining the objectives themselves.

It should be noted that this is a rather different approach to questions of equity or justice from that pioneered in Rawls great work (1971) and current in much of the political philosophy literature (see, for instance, Pettit, 1980). Under that approach, 'justice' is described as the "first virtue of social institutions" (Rawls, 1971, p. 1); principles derived from certain hypothetical procedures (such as the social contract) are said to be 'just', whether they concern equity, liberty or any other aim; and these principles of 'justice' are supposed lexicographically to dominate any other possible objective. Although I do not think that the interests of clarity have always been well served by this conflation of different aims under the same umbrella, I shall not argue the point here. Instead, to avoid possible confusion I shall describe the objective with which this paper is concerned as 'equity' rather than 'justice', and consider any conception put forward under the 'justice' umbrella that has obvious connections with equity (such as the Rawls maximin principle) as simply one among the many possible interpretations of the term.

Equity as an Economic Concern

Many economists have argued that equity is not a legitimate economic concern. There are three distinct arguments. First, there is the view that it is quite simply impractical to attempt to define equity in any general fashion; that individuals' views on the matter are so diverse that no consensus could ever be achieved. Second, it is argued that, unlike, for instance, efficiency considerations, matters of equity involve value-judgements and hence are not amenable to positive analysis. The third argument is that judgements concerning equity are not appropriate in many of the situations to which they are commonly applied, such as the distribution of income that emerges from the operation of a free market.

Since the purpose of the fourth section of this paper is an attempt to refute the first argument, it will not be considered further here. The dichotomy between equity and efficiency implied by the second argument is misleading. The definition of efficiency most commonly used by economists (that of Pareto) is not value-free [1]; nor would it be possible to find one that was. More generally, positive analysis is not inapplicable in cases where value-judgements are concerned. If an agreed definition of equity can be found, then positive analysis can be employed to determine whether a given allocation of resources is or is not equitable according to the definition; just as, with an agreed definition of what constitutes efficiency, positive analysis can be employed to determine whether a given resource allocation is efficient. The problem lies in the lack of consensus on the definition of equity, not in an alleged inapplicability of positive analysis.

The third argument is best put by Hayek (1978). He argues that (a) resources in non-socialist societies are largely allocated by the market mechanism and (b) the concept of equity (which he terms social justice) is inapplicable to the results of a spontaneous process such as a free market. Since no-one is responsible for a market-determined allocation of resources it is impossible to describe it as just or unjust, equitable or inequitable; indeed; to do so "does not belong to the category of error but that of nonsense" (p. 78).

However, this is not an argument against applying equity judgements in contemporary societies. Even if we accept the basic proposition that the outcomes of spontaneous processes cannot be judged in equity terms [2], it seems quite implausible to suggest that the allocation of resources in mixed Western economies is a 'spontaneous process'. There is substantial government intervention in the distribution of income; and government production of certain commodities is widespread. Indeed the very fact that the market is not allowed to allocate resources in some areas suggests that the continued operation of unfettered markets in others (and the consequent distribution of resources in those areas) is itself the result of human decision. Since Hayek admits (p. 69) that the concept of equity does have meaning when applied to non-spontaneous processes, it would seem that the search for a definition applicable in most existing societies is not a 'nonsense'.

Assessment Criteria

Innumerable conceptions of equity have appeared in the literature. These include the concepts of horizontal and vertical equity, 'desert'-based conceptions of need or merit, egalitarian proposals such as equality of income or utility, recent formulations relating justice to the existence or otherwise of envy, and the grand schemes of the utilitarians and Rawls. All seem in some sense to have 'failed'; and the third section examines the reason for this failure in some detail. But before that what is meant by failure in this context should be explained.

A number of different criteria have been suggested as a basis for evaluating different conceptions of equity. Among other things, it has been suggested that an 'ideal' definition of an equitable allocation of resources should have relatively small information requirements (in particular, it should not require that utility be interpersonally comparable or cardinally measurable); that it should be easily comprehensible; and that it should be possible to find allocations of resources that were simultaneously equitable and Pareto-efficient (see Rawls, 1974 and Pazner & Schmeidler, 1978).

However, the most important criterion, and one besides which these others seem essentially secondary, is that of intuitive acceptability. The aim is to find a definition of equity that will command general agreement. An essential requirement of such a definition is that it should not lead most people to judge as equitable situations which their intuition would regard as inequitable and vice versa. Any definition which did result in such a conflict would, *ipso facto,* not command a consensus; for, to be acceptable, a proposed definition has to conform to the way in which the term is commonly applied. As Rawls (1971) argues:

> There is, however, another side to justifying a particular (set of principles). That is to see if the principles... chosen match our considered convictions of justice or extend them in an acceptable way. We can note whether applying these principles would lead us to make the same judgements about the basic structure of society which we would make intuitively, and in which we have the greatest confidence. (p. 19)

Rawls' authority should not be invoked without some explanation as to why we do not use his other method of assessing the acceptability of a criterion of justice: the social contract. This is because, despite appearance, the method does not obviate the use of intuition. Its role now becomes one of assessing what conditions are likely to obtain in the 'initial position' where the social contract is to be drawn up. As Rawls says: "there are many possible interpretations of the social situation".. (and it is necessary) "to choose the interpretation... which best expresses the conditions that are *widely thought reasonable* to impose as choices of principles" (1971, p. 121, emphasis added). Hence, for Rawls, intuition enters twice: once in assessing the reasonableness of the conditions for the original position and once in assessing the conceptions which arise from the deliberations therein. Since there seems little advantage in adopting such a circuitous route to arrive at the same place, the more direct approach is adopted here [3].

To argue for the importance of intuition is in apparent conflict with Hare's (1981) rejection of 'intuitionism' as a means of establishing moral principles (chapter 1). But the disagreement is more apparent than real. Hare objects to the use of intuition as a means of establishing the essential 'right-ness' of moral propositions; he also points out that it offers little help in cases where moral propositions conflict. However, he accepts (p. 13) that intuition has a role in determining what people actually mean when they use moral terminology. Since the aim of this paper is to find a definition of equity that will command a measure of consensus, it is precisely this role that intuition is playing here; for, to command consensus, it is necessary to establish a definition that accords with the way in which the term is generally used. In Hare's terminology, we are using linguistic intuitions rather than moral ones.

Widespread acceptability thus has to be the principal basis for the evaluation of different conceptions of equity. However, this acceptability must not be bought at the expense of specificity. A vague conception which commands a measure of agreement only because it lacks specifics will do little to inform the debate. What is needed is a conception of equity that is both intuitively acceptable and is clearly defined; not one which obtains consensus by relying upon vague concepts about whose interpretation in any given situation there is little agreement.

Conceptions of Equity

Having specified the criterion for evaluating different conceptions of equity, let us now turn to the conceptions themselves. First, the concepts of *horizontal equity* (equals should be treated equally) and *vertical equity* (unequals should be treated unequally). These may meet the first part of our criterion (intuitive acceptability), but manifestly fail to meet the second (clearly defined teminology). Precisely who are equal and who unequal? What form should the different treatment of unequals take? These principles cannot be applied in any meaningful way until these questions are answered; but, as soon as any attempt is made to do so, consensus is likely to disappear. In fact, all the concepts embody is "the formal principle of all moralities which are not actually anti-rational: don't act capriciously" [4].

Similar difficulties arise with those conceptions where the equity or otherwise of a situation is judged by the degree to which distribution is according to *need* or to *merit*. For again there is little agreement as to what is meant by the basic terminology. So far as 'need' is concerned, on different occasions it has been argued that the old need less than the young, the low-born less than the high-born (because the former have not been brought up with the latter's expensive tastes), the mentally ill less than the sane, the physically healthy less than the physically handicapped, the clerk less than the coalminer. On the 'merit' side, at various times it has been claimed that free men are more meritorious than slaves, aristocrats more than labourers, the hard worker more than the idler, the intelligent more than the unintelligent, men more than women, white more than black. In either case, the fact that nowadays few would agree with most of these judgements suggests that definitions of equity in terms of need or merit are unlikely to be fruitful.

Definitions of equity that require *equality of income* or *utility* do not suffer from lack of specificity (at least, not to the same extent). However, it is far from clear that either would command universal acceptability. Consider first equality of income. Suppose we observe three individuals A, B and C, of whom B and C have the same income but A has an income greater than both. Suppose further we know that A and B have identical opportunities to obtain income, and that the reason why B has a lower income than A is simply because s/he has chosen to work less hard; while C, on the other hand, has a lower income than A because A is white while C, with identical skills and preferences, is black and working for a prejudiced employer. In that case, it is likely that we would judge the gap in income between A and B as more equitable than the *same* gap in income between A and C. Hence unequal incomes cannot be identified with inequity; nor equal incomes, equity.

To overcome objections of this kind it might be argued that the focus of concern should be equality of utilities or satisfactions rather than incomes. In the example considered, B's level of utility may well be on a par with A's, and therefore the difference between their respective situations would not, on this interpretation, constitute inequity. That an allocation of resources is equitable in which utilities are equal has considerable intuitive appeal, and has, not surprisingly, formed the basis of many interesting contributions to the literature: most notably, the equity axioms of Sen (1973) and Hammond (1976, 1977) [5]. These axioms are rules for distributing income so as increase the value of what Hammond (1977, p. 52) terms 'equity-regarding' social welfare functions: functions which show an increase in welfare when, *ceteris paribus*, the difference between any two individuals' utilities is decreased.

But this conception also has its problems. For instance, its information requirements are considerable; in particular, utilities have to be observable, measurable and interpersonally comparable. Yet more seriously from our point of view, it is quite easy to construct examples where its implications for policy conflict with intuitive judgements. For instance, suppose an individual tried unsuccessfully to steal another's handbag, but got hurt in the ensuing fracas. Should resources be transferred from the victim to the would-be criminal, now miserably nursing his/her injury, in order to equalise their utilities? To take another example, should an individual leading a life of penury after dissipating a large inheritance be compensated so as to bring his utility in line with that of his more parsimonious brother who received a similar inheritance but invested it? It seems unlikely that, in either case, the proposed compensation would be regarded as fair. More generally, just as with income, we cannot simply observe inequality in utilities and thereby judge, *on the basis of that inequality alone,* whether or not an allocation is equitable or inequitable. Hence a conception of equity that requires equality of utilities under all circumstances would be unlikely to command universal agreement.

Another interpretation has also recently received considerable attention in the economics literature (Foley, 1967; Varian, 1974; Pazner & Schmeidler, 1974). This defines an allocation as equitable if it is *envy-free:* that is, if no individual prefers any other individual's situation to his own. Although Foley is credited by Varian as being the originator of the idea, it has its origins in the older conception of 'how to cut a cake fairly'. If a cake is to be divided between two people, then a method of doing so is for one to cut the cake and for the other to choose his portion. The resulting allocation should be acceptable to both, hence envy-free and therefore equitable [6].

Once again, this conception does not seem to conform to the way in which the term is generally used. It is quite possible to conceive of situations which we might consider to be equitable, but where envy persists, or, alternatively situations where there is no envy, but which nonetheless might be considered as inequitable. An example of the first might be the case already mentioned of the profligate individual who dissipated his inheritance but who now envies his more careful brother [7]. An example of the second might be a caste society with great inequality in power and privilege, but in which the privileged had ensured by careful propaganda that those at the bottom 'knew their place'. The definition would have us consider the first as unfair and the second as fair; judgements with which it is unlikely that everyone would agree.

Similar objections can be levied against the 'envy-free' method of allocating the cake. For example, suppose there was an imbalance of information between the cutter and the chooser: the latter, say, having baked the cake, knew that some parts of it were more nutritious than other parts, but concealed this from the former. If we were aware of this, would we describe the resultant allocation as fair? Again it seems unlikely.

Let us now turn to the more comprehensive systems of the utilitarians and Rawls. The belief that *utilitarianism* has implications for equity is widespread. Quite why is not easy to understand; but two possible reasons come to mind. First it may be that those who make this connection wish to *define* equity in utiliarian terms. That is, an allocation is defined as equitable if it is the outcome of a specific application of utilitarian principles. Alternatively, the belief may arise because, under certain specific circumstances, utilitarian allocations are egalitarian in outcome. Unfortunately, as several writers have shown, neither view is convincing.

It is relatively easy to construct simple examples where utilitarian allocations are unlikely to be either equal or equitable. Sen (1973), for instance, gives the example of two individuals, one healthy and one crippled. The cripple, because of his handicap, finds it more difficult to 'generate' utility from his income than does the healthy individual; that is, each pound's worth of income is worth less to him. A utilitarian redistribution of income from a starting position of equal incomes would require taking income away from the cripple and giving it to the healthy. Hence the distribution of income would become unequal—and, in many people's eyes, inequitable.

To take another example, consider a utilitarian distribution of education. This would require that education be allocated to those who derive most utility from it. Now it is well established that children from wealthy backgrounds derive more benefit from a given amount of educational input than do the children of equal ability but from less advantaged homes. Hence utilitarianism would imply that education should be concentrated on the former rather than the latter. Again an inegalitarian outcome; and again one that few would consider as equitable.

Thus utilitarianism does not necessarily generate outcomes that are either equal or fair. Nor is this surprising. The focus of utilitarianism is on maximising the sum of individual utilities; hence, as Sen (1973, p. 16) puts it "it is supremely unconcerned with the interpersonal distribution of the sum".

Unfortunately, similar difficulties arise with the other major conception of equity or 'justice' current in the literature: *the maximin principle* of John Rawls (1971). This principle holds that inequality is only justified to the extent that it improves the position of the least well off (defined in terms of primary goods, rather than, as commonly assumed by economists, in terms of utilities). For our purposes this can be taken as implying that an allocation of resources can be defined as equitable if it is the outcome of maximising the position of those with the smallest quantity of primary goods.

This principle, and its derivation, has been subject to considerable critical attention and no full-scale critique will be attempted here [8]. Our concern is simply to judge the acceptability of the definition of equity implicit in the principle.

It is useful to begin by noting that the method of derivation of the principle is not concerned directly with equity. Rather, it is the outcome of decisions made by individuals concerned to maximise their own self-interest in a specific hypothetical situation: that of the social contract. These individuals are not concerned with what would be equitable in the society whose prospective organisation they are considering, but only with their own interests in that society. Their concern for the least advantaged expressed in the maximin principle derives not from any basic notion that the least advantaged suffer from inequity or injustice, but from a fear that they themselves might turn out to be the least advantaged.

This being the case, it is not surprising that as Nozick says (1974, p. 204), "the difference principle is on the face of it unfair". A given distribution may be totally 'just' in a Rawlsian sense, but unjust or inequitable when judged by more conventional standards of justice or equity. For example, under the principle, individuals who are naturally endowed with skills useful for raising the levels of the least advantaged would be 'bribed' to exercise those skills; that is, they would receive rewards on the basis of their natural endowment. Yet is it fair that one individual should receive more than another simply because he was born stronger, taller or more intelligent? Rawls (1971) himself says at the beginnning of his book that intuition requires "a conception of justice that nullifies the accidents of natural endowment and of social circumstances" (p. 15). Yet this is manifestly not provided by the maximin principle. As with utilitarianism, therefore, Rawls does not provide us with a specific definition of equity which is generally consistent with the way in which the concept is commonly used.

The fact that it seems to be possible to find examples for each of the conceptions considered where their application would produce outcomes inconsistent with intuitive judgements of equity suggests that there is some fundamental element in the latter which is not being taken into account. Nozick has gone some way towards finding out what this is. All the conceptions considered are what he terms 'end-result' principles. That is, the equity or otherwise of a given situation is determined by the structure of that situation itself. However, he argues, our judgements concerning the equity of that situation will generally depend on its *history*, or, in other words, how it came about. Simple observation of the fact that, say, two individuals have different incomes, is not sufficient to determine the equity of that distribution. Rather, Nozick says, we would want to know why they had different incomes before we could make such a judgement. In other words, what we need are *historical* principles: principles which require an investigation of the history of a given allocation of resources before then can help us determine its intrinsic equity or inequity. In the next section an attempt is made to provide such a principle [9].

An Alternative Conception

Consider some of the counter-examples used in the previous section. There situations were considered inequitable if within them:
one individual had a lower income than another because of his colour;
an individual received less than another due to his being prevented from acquiring information;
a congenital cripple received less than a healthy individual;
an individual received a larger income than another simply by virtue of his natural endowment.

What is the essential feature of these situations? In each case it seems to be regarded as inequitable if an individual is in a worse situation than another because of factors *beyond his control*. Thus the cripple, the poorly endowed individual, and the poorly informed one, all had little choice in determining their situation. Hence any allocation which discriminates against these individuals seems unfair. On the other hand, if an individual's eventual situation was the outcome of his own choice (for example, the individual who chose to consume less, or who acquired an injury through assaulting another), then discrimination does not seem so inequitable. Situations that are the outcome of unavoidable circumstances are generally considered inequitable; situations that are the outcome of unconstrained (or equally constrained) choice are not.

The crucial element which was missing from all the previous attempts to define equity thus appears to be its relationship to the existence of choice. For the examples considered suggest that *our judgements as to the degree of inequity inherent in a given situation depends on the degree to which we see that situation as the outcome of individual choice.* If one individual receives less than another due to his own choice, then the disparity is not considered inequitable; if it arises for reasons beyond his control, then it is inequitable.

This idea can be expressed more formally as follows. Define the factors beyond an individual's control as his *constraints*. These constraints limit the range of possibilities over which an individual can make his choices. Define the set of possibilities bounded by the individual's constraints as his *choice set*. Then *a situation is equitable if it is the outcome of individuals choosing over equal choice sets* [10].

Now this conception has several advantages. Its principal merit is that which forms the basis of its derivation, viz. that it conforms to the way in which the term is generally used. More examples of this are easily found. For instance, it is implicit in the judgement that inequalities of opportunity are inequitable. But it is also implicit in the view of many of those who advocate equality of outcome rather than equality of opportunity; for the reason they do so is generally because they believe differences in situations usually arise not through individual choices, but because of factors beyond individual control.

Another example is the economist's concept of 'merit goods'. It is widely believed that some commodities, such as health care, should not be distributed in accordance with the distribution of income. Quite why these commodities should be singled out for particular concern has often puzzled economists. The conventional efficiency justifications for non-market allocation (such as the presence of externalities or imperfect information) never seemed quite adequate to explain the degree of popular aversion to market distribution; but, if the chief aim was to promote equity in some sense, then direct cash subsidies seemed more appropriate than the subsidised provision of particular commodities. However, if equity is interpreted in the manner suggested here, then the selection of those commodities becomes more comprehensible. For example, take health care. Most people's demand for health care arises from something widely considered (at least until recently) as beyond individual control: the onset of ill-health. Hence if health care has to be purchased directly out of individuals' incomes, those with ill-health have to suffer a greater reduction in private consumption of other commodities than those in good health. Hence the pattern of commodity consumption would differ between individuals due to factors perceived as beyond their control; and therefore such an allocation would be inequitable.

A further advantage of the definition is that it may be acceptable to those with quite disparate social and political views. For it is possible to accept the definition, but to disagree upon its application in different situations. For example, consider two opposing political views concerning those in poverty; a 'right wing' view that they should receive little help, since they have presumably chosen not to avail themselves of the opportunities for making money in our society; and a 'left wing' view that the poor are proper recipients of aid, since they are 'locked into' poverty through a variety of social and economic impediments to social mobility. Now both sides of the argument could accept our definition of equity: that, to the extent the poor's income is the result of the constraints they face, then inequity exists. The disagreement would arise over precisely what factors constitute constraints and what did not. The discussion between them would therefore have shifted from a 'value' plane to an empirical one: the extent to which individual decisions are or are not constrained. This is an important aspect of the definition: if it is accepted, then questions concerning distributional issues cease to be matters of value, becoming instead matters of fact.

It could be objected to this last point that the shift of the debate from 'values' to 'facts' does not constitute a great improvement. For there may be just as many arguments concerning the extent to which differences in individual allocations arise from differences in constraints, as there are value-judgements about equity. Indeed, there has been intense philosophical controversy for centuries as to whether individuals can be said to have *any* freedom of choice: a debate which is not within sight of resolution.

To this there are three possible responses. First, even if the discussion here does not resolve the debate as to what is an equitable allocation and what is not, it is important to clarify what the battle is about. A disagreement concerning values is different from one concerning the extent of individual choice, and it is necessary to be clear which is being discussed. Second, in so far as this is a problem for useful application of the definition, it is one which it shares with almost the entire body of economic analysis. For the latter generally analyses economic behaviour by formulating it as a constrained optimisation problem: a procedure which requires specifying those factors which operate as constraints and those which do not. If it is possible for this purpose to obtain a plausible categorisation, it should be possible for the application of equity judgements. Thirdly, even if it is accepted that it will be difficult to obtain consensus on *all* the factors which may constitute constraints, it is likely that agreement can be reached on *some* of them. For example, most people would agree that an individual's genetic inheritance and his inheritance of non-human capital is generally beyond his control. It should therefore be possible to obtain agreement that a given allocation is inequitable, even if it is impossible to decide what would constitute one that was fully equitable. An illustration of how such judgements can be made in a specific practical case (the problem of fiscal federalism) can be found in Le Grand (1975, 1977).

The definition also has the advantage of meeting most of the alternative criteria for acceptability mentioned at the beginning of the third section. These concerned its comprehensibility, its compatibility with efficiency and its information requirements. The definition is easily comprehensible; moreover, it can be formulated in terms of conventional economic terminology. There is no reason to suppose that the equitable allocations, as defined, are necessarily inefficient: allocations with equal choice sets could be both equitable and Pareto-efficient. So far as information requirements are concerned, there are no doubt difficulties in measuring choice sets; but the requirements do seem low in comparison to most of the other definitions considered. In particular no interpersonal utility comparisons or assumptions concerning cardinal utility functions are necessary.

So far we have discussed the advantages of the conception. A possible disadvantage is that it may not be complete. It is possible there may be some situations which arise from different choice sets but which nonetheless an observer may judge as equitable. For instance, it could be considered that an individual whose possible choices did not include certain items of consumption might be 'compensated' by the extension of his choices to include different items. For instance the ability of an intelligent but crippled individual to obtain professional training and thereby increase his income could be viewed as compensating him for his inability to participate in extensive physical activity.

However, it is difficult to include considerations such as this in any formal conception of equity. What seems to be happening in such judgements is that the observer making the judgement is imposing his own preferences upon the choices concerned, and inferring that, if he were confronted with either set, the items he would choose would yield him the same level of satisfaction. Since doubtless different observers have different views as to what items would adequately compensate individuals for the absence of other items, it seems unlikely that any general consensus would be found as to whether different choice sets were 'equivalent' or not. Accordingly, it seems preferable to use the earlier conception of equal choice sets as the basic definition of equity, but with the acknowledgement that there may be distributions of choices which do not meet the criterion of equality, but which some observers might nonetheless consider equitable.

Another possible objection is the following. Someone who believes with Hayek that the concept of equity of justice is inapplicable to the outcomes of spontaneous processes, might question the view that *all* differences in choices are inequitable. What of those which arise from factors unconnected with social decision, such as genetic inheritance? Surely the fact that, for instance, men cannot have babies or that not everybody has blue eyes, is not in itself inequitable? This is a difficult issue. The answer probably depends on whether or not the differences in choices that result are amenable to social decision. If there is discrimination in, say, job opportunities, that favour those who do not have babies or who have blue eyes then those differences are inequitable—because they could be rectified by appropriate changes in social behaviour or organisation. But if the differences concerned have outcomes that are simply uncorrectable (for instance, the differences between the pains and pleasures associated with actually giving birth and those with watching it happen), then these are not so obviously inequitable. Differences in choices arising from spontaneous processes which can be corrected by social decision we could therefore consider as 'equity-relevant'; those which could not as 'equity-irrelevant'.

Conclusion

Despite its normative flavour, this paper has been an exercise in positive analysis. It constitutes an attempt to discover the common element in judgements concerning the equity or otherwise of particular situations. To this end, a number of conceptions have been examined. They can be conveniently summarised as follows:

An allocation of resources is equitable if:

it meets the requirements of horizontal and vertical equity;

resources are distributed according to need or merit;

income or utility are distributed equally;

it is envy-free;

it is the outcome of maximising the sum of individual utilities;

it is the outcome of maximising the position of the least well off;

all individuals have equal choices.

Of those, it was argued that only the last captures the essential element of the concept as it appears in general usage: its relationship to the existence or otherwise of choice.

Finally, let me re-emphasise a point made in the introduction. By concentrating on the problem of defining equity, it is not intended to imply that this should dominate all others in determining policy. In practice, it may prove impossible to equalise choices without seriously impeding social objectives in other areas, such as the attainment of efficiency or the preservation of liberty. Thus, for instance, to reduce the inequality between the choices of bed-ridden cripples and Olympic athletes may require, if it were possible at all, the allocation of virtually the whole GNP to the former or an unacceptable restriction of the latter's freedom of action (hanging weights around their necks?). But this does not invalidate the arguments of this paper. No claim is made here that equity should be ordered lexicographically among social objectives. That allocation of resources which represents the 'optimum optimorum' will presumably be the result of trading-off the degree of equity achieved with the degree of achievement of other objectives, such as efficiency or liberty. But specifying the optimum optimorum cannot be done until the objectives to be traded-off are themselves specified and defined; and it is to that part of the task that this paper has been addressed.

Acknowledgements

Many colleagues at the London School of Economics and Political Science and elsewhere have helped me with the many earlier versions of this paper. I must thank particularly John Broome, Peter Hammond, Philip Pettit and Amartya Sen for helping me avoid some of the pitfalls that await those who venture on to this tricky terrain.

Julian Le Grand, London School of Economics, Houghton Street, Aldwych, London WC2, United Kingdom.

NOTES

[1] It is generally considered as involving two value judgements: (a) that social welfare is increased if one person is made better off and no-one worse off, and (b) that individuals are the best judge of whether they are or are not better off. It might be noted that (b), although conventionally associated with the definition, is not a necessary element of it.

[2] Which could be questioned. For example, the phrase 'life is unfair' is not, as Hayek's argument would seem to imply, devoid of meaning in general usage.

[3] Qn Rawls' use of intuition, see Hare's article in Daniels (1975); on the effects of adopting different (yet 'reasonable') interpretations of the initial position on the principles adopted therein, see Arrow (1973).

[4] Watkins, quoted in Rees (1971, p. 95).

[5] More recently, Sen (1980) has advanced several cogent arguments against the use of equality of utilities as a foundation for social justice.

[6] See Dubins & Spanier (1961). To avoid confusion, it should be noted that Varian adopts a terminology which, instead of treating 'fair' as synonymous with 'equitable' (as we do), defines a fair allocation as one which is *both* equitable *and* efficient.

[7] Another example might be the case where male whites 'envy' affirmative action programmes for blacks and women. Actually, this raises another problem for the definition; what if an individual envies one *element* of another's situation (such as privileged access to university), but does not want the totality (e.g. male whites do not want to become black or female)?

[8] See, for example, Barry (1973), Daniels (1975), and Wolff (1972).

[9] Nozick says explicitly that he himself is not providing a theory of justice (p. 153). He does, however, propose an allocative rule, which he summarises as: "From each as he chooses, to each as he is chosen" (p. 160). However, his justification for this seems to be that it conforms to the (for him, lexicographic) requirements of individual liberty, rather than to some notion of equity or justice. If it *were* based on the latter, then the concept implied would be open to the same objection that has been levied against the other concepts discussed: viz., it does not conform to conventional usage. For example, the rule would be consistent with some individuals receiving large inheritances while others starve: an allocation that is not likely to be generally regarded as equitable.

[10] Sen (1980) has recently put forward a conception of equity based on equality of 'capabilities' that has clear links with the conception proposed here. I hope to explore the nature of those links in future work.

BIBLIOGRAPHY

Arrow, K.J. (1973) Some ordinalist-utilitarian notes on Rawls' theory of justice, *Journal of Philosophy*, 70, pp. 245–263.

BARRY, B. (1973) *The Liberal Theory of Justice* (Oxford University Press).

DANIELS, N. (Ed.) (1975) *Reading Rawls* (Oxford, Blackwell).

DUBINS, L.E. & SPANIER, E.H. (1961) How to cut a cake fairly, *American Mathematical Monthly*, 68, pp. 1–17.

FOLEY, D. (1967) Resource allocation and the public sector, *Yale Economic Essays*, 7, pp. 45–98.

HAMMOND, P.J. (1976) Equity, Arrow's conditions and Rawls' difference principle, *Econometrica*, 44, pp. 793–804.

HAMMOND, P.J. (1977) Dual interpersonal comparisons of utility and the welfare economics of income distribution, *Journal of Public Economics*, 7, pp. 51–71.

HARE, R.M. (1981) *Moral Thinking* (Oxford, Clarendon Press).

HAYEK, F.A. (1978) *The Mirage of Social Justice, Law, Legislation and Liberty*, vol. 2 (London, Routledge & Kegan Paul).

LE GRAND, J. (1975) Fiscal equity and central government grants to local authorities, *Economic Journal*, 85, pp. 531–547.

LE GRAND, J. (1977) Reply, *Economic Journal*, 87, pp. 780–782.

NOZICK, R. (1974) *Anarchy, State and Utopia* (New York, Basic Books).

PAZNER, E. & SCHMEIDLER, D. (1974) A difficulty in the concept of fairness, *Review of Economic Studies*, 41, pp. 441–443.

PAZNER, E. & SCHMEIDLER, D. (1978) Egalitarian equivalent allocations: a new concept of economic equity, *Quarterly Journal of Economics*, 92, pp. 671–687.

PETTIT, J. (1980) *Judging Justice* (London, Routledge & Kegan Paul).

RAWLS, J. (1971) *A Theory of Justice* (Cambridge, Harvard University Press).

RAWLS, J. (1974) Some reasons for the maximin criterion, *American Economic Review*, (Proc.), 64, pp. 141–146.

REES, J. (1971), *Equality* (London, Pall Mall Press).

SEN, A.K. (1973) *On Economic Inequality* (Oxford University Press).

SEN, A.K. (1980) Equality of what?, in: MCMURRIN, S. (Ed.) *Tanner Lectures on Human Values*, vol. 1 (Salt Lake City, University of Utah Press). Reprinted in SEN, A.K. (1982), *Choice, Welfare and Measurement* (Oxford, Blackwell).

VARIAN, H. (1974) Equity, envy and efficiency, *Journal of Economic Theory*, 9, pp. 63–91.

WOLFF, R.P. (1972) *Understanding Rawls* (Princeton University Press).

18

The Concept, and Conceptions, of Justice

ANTONY FLEW

ABSTRACT   *Occasioned by but not pretending to constitute a critique of Julian Le Grand's 'Equity as an Economic Objective', reproduced in Chapter 17 of this volume, this paper argues that the concept of justice must be distinguished from conceptions thereof. Once this is done it emerges that many of what are both offered and accepted as conceptions of justice really are not. By proceeding next both to enquire what are the incentives to such misrepresentations and to reveal some of their unrecognized costs, this is shown to be by no means a merely trifling and purely verbal matter. In particular, by misrepresenting the imposition of their peculiar and characteristic ideal of equality of outcome as the enforcement of the mandate of justice, Procrusteans unwittingly imply that they are themselves involved in appallingly shabby and discreditable practices.*

Julian Le Grand, in 'Equity as an Economic Objective' [1], is concerned with "different conceptions of equity or justice" [2]. He goes on to remark that here, as with other objectives that guide policy-making, "It has proved extremely difficult to find definitions which were simultaneously sufficiently general to command a broad consensus and sufficiently specific so as to permit useful application" [3]. Unfortunately he makes no distinction: between, on the one hand, providing an explication of the concept of justice, or a definition of the word; and, on the other hand, developing a conception of what—substantively and particularly—justice actually requires. Yet it is entirely possible, and common, for people to disagree pretty profoundly in their conceptions of justice, or chastity, or whatever else, while nevertheless employing the same concept, and hence the same definition of the word. Indeed, unless they are in this most fundamental though tenuous form of agreement, their different conceptions cannot be different conceptions of justice, or of chastity, or of whatever else is supposed to be under discussion.

Hopes that Le Grand is going to take this point rise when he proceeds to distinguish his own approach "from that pioneered in Rawls' great work (1971) and current in much of the political philosophy literature"... [4]. For Le Grand is clearly uneasy about the way in which "principles derived from certain hypothetical procedures (such as the social contract) are said to be 'just', whether they concern equity, liberty or any other aim" [5]. Nevertheless he concludes: "Although I do not think that the interests of clarity have always been well served by this conflation of aims under the same umbrella, I shall not argue the point here" [5]. Le Grand thus follows Rawls, as well as so many of the other critics of Rawls, ignoring the warning issued by Plato's Socrates in the final sentence of Book I of *The Republic:* "For if I do not know what justice is I am scarcely likely to find out whether it is an excellence and whether its possessor is happy or not happy".

Towards a Definition of 'Justice'

It is a remarkable fact, albeit a fact remarked remarkably rarely, that "Rawls' great work (1971)" would appear to be the first substantial treatise purporting to deal with justice which can, nevertheless, find no room to quote any version of the traditional definition. Instead, towards the end of his enormous book, the author indicates that he was eager "to leave questions of meaning and definition aside and to get on with the task of developing a substantive theory of justice" [6].

This impatience with any preliminary, narrowly philosophical, Socratic questions exposes Rawls to the charge that—whatever its other merits or demerits—what he is offering is simply not a conception of justice at all [7]. At times he himself comes close to recognizing that this may indeed be so. For instance, he offers his "justice as fairness", as a rival: not, in particular, to a Utilitarian account of justice; but, generally, to classical Utilitarianism as a whole. He wants it, so to speak, to replace not just Chapter V of J. S. Mill's *Utilitarianism* but the entire book. Yet certainly Rawls never sees all the implications of this misrepresentation, if such it be.

One version of the ancient definition tells us that to be just is *Honeste vivere, neminen laedere, suum cuique tribuere* [To live honourably, to harm no one, to yield to each their own]. In the *Institutes* of Justinian the mark of the just person is *Constans et perpetua voluntas jus suum cuique tribuere* [A constant and perpetual will to yield to each their own]. The last crucial phrase—*suum cuique tribuere*—can be traced back through the earlier Roman jurists till it is discovered in the definition wrongly rejected by Plato's Socrates in *The Republic*. For there, after old Cephalus has been politely seen off, his son Polemarchus inherits the argument. Following the poet Simonides, and improving on his father, Polemarchus suggests that justice is "to render to each their due" [8].

To become fully adequate such a definition would no doubt need both polishing and supplementation. But for present purposes it is sufficient to establish that the essential element is some variation on the theme of yielding, or allotting, or assigning, or resigning, to each their own. Were this conclusion being challenged directly, it would become necessary to deploy supporting argument. But, until and unless it is so challenged, that has to be superfluous.

Some Consequences of any such Definition

Once it is conceded that that constitutes the essential element, then it begins to be possible to draw some fairly substantial and sometimes rather disturbing conclusions. For some of what have been presented as conceptions of justice are now shown up as being not correctly so described. Nor is this, as is sometimes suggested, a matter merely verbal and trifling. Those who, on this account, have been misemploying the word 'justice' have not been simply careless, or indifferent as between one alternative and another. They employed, or misemployed, that deliberately chosen word because they wanted thereby to license the drawing of various practically important and strongly desired conclusions; albeit without, it seems, ever allowing themselves to notice that it must also, and by the same token, license the drawing of other equally important yet altogether unwelcome conclusions—conclusions often bound to be to the last degree embarrassing.

(i) What is justly due to people are their several, and presumably often very different and very unequal, deserts and entitlements. Those two key words are by no means synonymous: deserts are, necessarily, merited or deserved whereas entitlements may not be; while it would be at least odd to speak of an entitlement to something disagreeable. There is, therefore, plenty of room for, and there in fact are, different and competing conceptions of justice—conceptions differing in their accounts, not only of what people do in truth deserve and to what they are in truth entitled, but also of what really are the proper grounds both of desert and of undeserved entitlement.

So it follows that a theory which finds room neither for deserts nor for undeserved entitlements, however powerful its other claims to our acceptance, cannot be admitted as a theory of justice. Therefore, too, for Nozick to try to distinguish his own account as 'The Entitlement Theory', and for hostile critics to want to condemn it as such, is as if someone were to labour to pick out one particular conception of chastity as being peculiarly concerned with sexual restraint, while opponents were proposing on the same count to dismiss it out of hand [9].

(ii) A second consequence of the fact that the heart of the matter is given in the tag *suum cuique tribuere* is that the notion of justice is necessarily backward-looking. That is why, for instance, the *Shane* figures in good, old-original, American Westerns, or *The Four Just Men* of England's Edgar Wallace, cannot begin to do the justice "which a man has to do" without some preparatory research into the conduct and background of all the various persons concerned, and into their several and consequent deserts and entitlements.

The newer ideal of equality of outcome, equality of welfare, is by contrast essentially forward-looking. It commits its proponents to disregarding the past as irrelevant: their ideal future is to be very different and much more, if never perhaps perfectly, equal. That is why anyone attempting systematically to justify the currently common identification of the imposition of this Procrustean ideal with the enforcement of a kind of justice would be facing a formidable and perhaps impossible task. It would be so much easier, if only they could bring themselves to resign the enormous propaganda advantages of that identification, to present their own fresh and future-oriented ideal neither as, nor as a part of, but rather as a rival to justice—the pursuit of which they should therefore see and condemn as reactionary, backward-looking, irrelevant, unsociological, antique, and even gothic.

This is, after all, exactly how the most scientifically-minded and future-oriented reformers do present parallel proposals for replacing criminal justice by ortho-psychiatry. Karl Menninger, for instance, who was for years the recognised doyen of that discipline, had no backward-looking scruples, and no inhibitions against projecting what to dissident diehards will appear an unlovely image. Thus, in a book aggressively entitled *The Crime of Punishment*, he wrote: "The very word 'justice' irritates scientists. No surgeon expects to be asked whether an operation for cancer is just or not. No doctor will be reproached on the grounds that the dose of penicillin he has prescribed is less or more than justice would stipulate. Behavioural scientists regard it as equally absurd to invoke the question of justice.... This (to the scientist) is a matter of public safety and amicable coexistence, not justice" [10].

What is in the present paper offered as the second consequence of a minimum definition of 'justice' Le Grand derives from a consideration of what he quotes Nozick as calling "end-result" principles of distribution: "what we need", Le Grand argues, "are *historical* principles" [11]. This is, as far as it goes, all very well. But, through not attending at the beginning to the concept of justice, Le Grand fails to make room for undeserved entitlements.

Someone with less respect for popular intuitions might at this point make so rash as to assert that there are none. To do this however, would be rash indeed. For all claims to universal human rights are and can only be grounded on what people are rather than on what they have done or not done. Also, the very possibility of desert seems to presuppose that of undeserved entitlement. Certainly it is awkward to speak of property rights where the putative owner cannot be substantially distinguished from what is said to be owned. Nevertheless very few of us could bring ourselves to accept all the implications of denying to individuals some sort of (necessarily undeserved) rights or entitlement, not only to their several bodily parts, but also to those very various native talents and dispositions which are both inherent in and consequent upon their several and equally various physical constitutions.

The most explosive challenge to any such denial demands to know whether, in a world in which half the children were born with two eyes and half with none, and in which eye transplants were possible, the two-eyed would have no right to their second eyes, but should, as a matter of social justice, be forced to surrender these unequal and hence illicit holdings to the transplant surgeons. It ought, by the way, to be noticed that to speak of the distribution either of bodily parts or of the talents and dispositions native to the human individual is to lay yourself open to the objection previously urged against talk of property rights here. To whom were those various bodily parts, talents and dispositions—all of which, uninstructedly, I should have been inclined to describe as mine—originally allocated; or by whom were they originally inherited? And who were all the others among whom God or Nature might have made a different and fairer allocation of all such things [12]?

(iii) The third practically important implication of this logical truth, that justice refers to deserts and entitlements, is that the claims of justice, unlike some other moral claims, may properly be enforced by the public power; though to say this is not, of course, to say that they always ought to be. This is a conclusion upon which there appears to be for once near universal agreement; although awareness of what it follows from is much less than unanimous. For instance, in his other masterpiece, the great Smith wrote: "Mere justice is, upon most occasions, but a negative virtue, and only hinders us from hurting our neighbour. The man who barely abstains from violating either the person, or the estate, or the reputation of his neighbours, has, surely, little positive merit. He fulfils, however, all the rules of what is peculiarly called justice, and does everything which his equals can with propriety force him to do, or which they can punish him for not doing" [13]. J. S. Mill concurs: "When we think a person is bound in justice to do a thing, it is an ordinary form of language to say that he ought to be compelled to do it" [14].

This is one of the implications which makes people value the word 'justice'; and often they insist on applying it without sufficient attention to the upsetting question whether their applications are justified. Suppose, for instance, that Rawls was challenged to justify his famous manifesto proclaiming the absolute indefeasibility of the demands of justice. He could support it only, if perhaps still not sufficiently, by maintaining that these are claims of desert and right, trumping all claims of other and necessarily weaker kinds.

Again, suppose that our Procrusteans were both inclined and able to make good on the contention that justice demands (a no doubt always to some extent qualified) equality of outcome. Then they would have equipped themselves with a knock-down decisive response to the protest of anyone daring to ask: "By what right are you proposing to impose your peculiar and personal idea of the Good Society upon those who do not share that ideal?"

For, on the present supposition, what they would be striving to impose is not merely a "peculiar and personal ideal of the Good Society". On the contrary: they would now be fully entitled to the splendid *Shane* image. For they would all be proven and paradigmatic exemplars of justice, devoted to ensuring that everyone should have and should hold their several deserts and entitlements, their own, their due; no less and no more.

A Sting in the Tail

Those who, with unfriendly fairness, I characterise as Procrusteans are always and only people who strive to ensure that their sort of egalitarianism is achieved by social engineering exercises of state power. It would be quite unfair to attach that same studiously unflattering label to those very few who are dedicated to pursuing the same ultimate end by non-coercive persuasion, and sometimes sacrificial personal example. Those very few entirely escape: not only that unfriendly labelling—hard words break no bones; but also another challenge too—one which is far more discomfiting.

It emerges that there is a price to be paid for making out that it is justice which demands equality of outcome. For once we have taken even a brief look at the concept of justice, it becomes clear that this conception carries a truly devastating implication. Inescapably it implies that equal shares are: not just something which it would be nice for everyone to have, and which in some ideal and future world they perhaps would and will enjoy; but instead something to which they have now, and always have had, a presumptively indefeasible right. So what is the corollary implication for those who are at present enjoying what is, by these bleakly bureaucratic standards, too much?

Certainly all the Procrusteans of my own acquaintance are, they should say, rather conspicuously underdeprived. If they were prepared to put their doctrine forward only as a remote ideal, then we might perhaps find some reasons to allow that they can in the meantime, consistently and with clear consciences, continue to enjoy their privileged excesses. But if, as is in fact usually the case, they choose to identify Procrusteanism with (social) justice, if they therefore also both arrogate to themselves a *Shane* image and denounce opponents as enemies of justice; then it becomes imperative to point out—and this is, remember, precisely and only on their own account of the matter—that everyone who is at this time holding anything above the ideally equal share is necessarily in possession of stolen property; and, most shameful of all, property stolen from others worse off than themselves [15].

Once the presence of this sting in the tail is more widely appreciated, we may expect to hear much less about equality of outcome as the supposedly obvious and imperative mandate of (social) justice, as well as far fewer preposterous denunciations of anti-Procrusteans as by their cloth committed enemies of (unqualified) justice.

Antony Flew, 26 Alexandra Road, Reading RG1 5PD, England.

NOTES

[1] Le Grand, Julian (1984) Equity as an Economic Objective, originally published in *Journal of Applied Philosophy*, 1, pp. 39–51.

[2] Ibid., p. 39.

[3] Ibid., p. 39.

[4] Ibid., p. 40.

[5] Ibid., p. 40: the hesitation quotes around the word 'just' are, surely, significant of Le Grand's own reservations?

[6] RAWLS, JOHN (1971) *A Theory of Justice*, p. 579 (Cambridge, Mass., Harvard University Press).

[7] See, for pressings of this charge, MATSON (1978) What Rawls calls justice, *The Occasional Review 8/9* (San Diego, World Research) and FLEW, ANTONY (1981) *The Politics of Procrustes* Chapter III (London, Temple Smith).

[8] 331E. For support for the claim that this definition is wrongly rejected by Plato's Socrates, and for a more comprehensive consideration of the relations and lack of relations between Rawls and Plato, as well as Rawls and Aristotle, see FLEW, ANTONY (1983) Justice: real or social?, *Social Philosophy and Policy*, 1, pp. 151–70.

[9] NOZICK, ROBERT (1976) *Anarchy, State and Utopia*, p. 150 (Oxford, Blackwell) I borrow this comparison from MATSON (1978), above.

[10] MENNINGER, KARL (1968) *The Crime of Punishment*, p. 17 (New York, Viking), For much more of the similar compare FLEW, ANTONY (1973) *Crime or Disease?* (Basingstoke, Macmillan).

[11] Op. cit., p. 46.

[12] Compare, again, FLEW, ANTONY (1981), Chapter IV.

[13] SMITH, ADAM (1759) *The Theory of Moral Sentiments*, II (ii) 1.

[14] MILL, J.S. (1910) *Utilitarianism*, p. 44 (London, Dent).

[15] For an abundance of examples of such identifications, arrogations and denunciations, compare FLEW (1981) and (1983).

19

Welfare State versus Welfare Society?

ANTHONY SKILLEN

ABSTRACT   *The welfare state is not just a system of personal insurance but an expression of community, of concern for our fellows. It places some things beyond the question of purchasing power. Yet its structures are often criticised as subverting personal and social cares and responsibilities. Arguably there is a 'dialectic of self-destruction' here, a tendency for the institution to undermine its own support. At the same time this problem is inherent in the capitalist state itself, as is brought out by a study of the philosophers of 'civil society' from Mandeville to Green. It is schematically argued that the welfare state needs reconstructing as an articulation rather than a substitute for 'community'. Implications for the class, gender and age structures of society are sketched.*

The Beveridge Report

In 1942 Beveridge wrote: "A revolutionary moment in the world's history is a time for revolutions". His report insisted that the new order would have, on its first principle, to serve all, and not only 'sectional interests'. Its 'second principle' was that the British National Insurance Scheme was "part only of a comprehensive policy of social progress. Social insurance . . . is an attack on Want. But Want is one only of the five giants on the road to reconstruction . . . The others are Disease, Ignorance, Squalor and Idleness". Its third, linking social service with 'service and contribution', was that "the state in organizing security should not stifle incentive, opportunity, or responsibility; in establishing a national minimum, it should leave room and encouragement for voluntary action for each individual to provide more than a minimum for himself and his family" [1]. Many have noted this principle's acceptance of the private enterprise system and its consecration of the domestic status of women. But I would like to emphasise as well its ideas of a 'co-operative' relation between state and citizenry, and its conception of private enterprise as justified only by its role in generating goods from which *all* could benefit. In other words, as was implied in Archbishop Temple's talk at the time of a transition from a 'Warfare' to a 'Welfare' state, the idea of 'the Welfare State' should be considered as a whole order of welfare in which the state is seen as playing the central role, guaranteeing the conditions of universal welfare, of faring well.

It can be said then, that whatever else might be implied in the word 'paternalism' (or 'the Nanny State', as Mrs Thatcher calls it) Beveridge and the ensuing 'Butskellite' consensus accepted the 'family' model in at least this sense: independently of one's capacity to make effective market demands, membership, citizenship, was a sufficient condition of societal provision for one's fundamental needs [2].

For such reasons we need to be wary of our tendency to talk of the Welfare State, as I shall to some extent myself, in terms of a notion of 'residuum': of especially needy and dependent people, or of especially needy and dependent times in our lives. This tendency it seems to me distorts the focus, both of its uncritical supporters and its hostile demolitionists, by generating a picture of the Welfare State as the Great Provider and individual people as dependent and disgustingly grateful or disgustingly ungrateful receivers. This drip-feed model draws us into conceptualising as central to the Welfare State what is not central in Beveridge's three principles: a division of society into burdened contributors, professional officials and nursed beneficiaries. To ignore the latter aspect, to play down the necessity in any community for recognition that there are more or less dependent and needy members whose capacity for active contribution is severely limited would, as the Eugenic tendencies of the early Fabians show, be most dangerous [3]. But Beveridge, for all his mandarin limits, foresaw a world in which the class of contributors, as far as possible, is the class of beneficiaries, so that the state's role is one of orchestrating among the community's members a flow of the goods and services essential to human welfare. At least in the sense of Anthony Crosland's *The Future of Socialism* [4], it is an egalitarian vision and a vision of a common good.

Current Controversies

Now, of course, the context of this article is one in which this whole outlook is being attacked and its constructions dismantled. I have talked of the Welfare State ideal as one in which there is social responsibility, democratically endorsed, for each other's needs; of the Welfare State as the expression of reciprocity, moral community and altruism. But here is what Rhodes Boyson had to say in an article called 'Farewell to Paternalism':

> The moral fibre of our people has been weakened. A state which does for its citizens what they can do for themselves is an evil state; and a state which removes all choice and responsibility from its people and makes them like broiler hens will create the irresponsible society. In such an irresponsible society, no one cares, no one saves, no one bothers—why should they when the state spends all its energies taking money from the energetic, successful and thrifty to give it to the idle, the failures and the feckless [5].

Now Boyson is no doubt living partly in a fairyland where there is good land enough for a good family man to make 'independent provision' for his dependents and to "grow in moral stature by his free gift" to those few whose physical handicaps incapacitate them from emulating *him*—a corollary of this of course is that where men lack such benevolence the poor, however deserving, will be left to suffer. But, despite the constraint that many to Boyson's left might feel, in fighting the cuts, to treat what Mr Cyril Smith called "our great National Health Service" as the quintessence of humanity and justice, the kind of thing Boyson, and now Thatcher, are saying needs to be accorded some sort of respect. After all, it is not as if some of what these advocates of the Blue Revolution are saying does not coincide with what many socialists were arguing when the Welfare State was unquestioned by the establishment.

Consider the following situation; you may recall it.

Early in 1984, a BBC radio presenter was questioning a Liverpool Social Services official over the fact that a mentally handicapped child had been sexually assaulted by her foster-father, a man already known to be under police suspicion of a similar offence. In response to the interviewer's attack, which echoed the trumpetings of those sections of the press for whom sex and social-worker bungling is a lucrative concoction, the squirming official finally made the point, not only that this man was 'in other respects' an excellent foster-parent but that it is in any case exceedingly difficult to find families who will take on fostering of handicapped people. These remarks were pounced on by the spokesman of the community as a feeble excuse. But the truth is that a high proportion of mentally handicapped people in this country presently live, out of our sight and out of our mind, in conditions which make life in such a family home, with its perversion, a relative blessing.

I would argue that the official's riposte is deeply pertinent, especially now, when the government of cost-cutting and individual 'go-getting' is actually talking about returning the residents of state homes and hospitals—people in need of many times as much devoted attention as most of us—to something which they call 'the community'. How, I want to ask, can we, through the BBC interviewer identify ourselves with communal moral indignation against officials whose predicament is that they are operating in circumstances where the caring and moral capacities of 'the community' are so cruelly feeble? On the other hand, how can public official-dom bemoan this lack of community involvement when it has taken over 'care' as its private business, so that, as Boyson hyperbolically says, "no one cares"? Does this mutual buck-passing, which is historically represented by cycles of state advance and withdrawal, not reflect the problematic status of 'the moral community' in modern industrial society? The Welfare State seems on the one hand an expression of moral community, a rejection of the amoral baby-farming society, of the banana republicanism that is capitalism's tendency. On the other hand, it seems at least to suck up into itself institutions, networks and 'Friendly Society' values that nourish and protect human welfare in a harsh modern world. The State, by taking on the mantle of that which does good, consecrates egoistic indifference among its subjects [6]. What do you expect them to do as voting citizens?

Here is another anecdote which I think illustrates this point. In some seminars on John Stuart Mill's ethics, recently I introduced the following example, whose chlorinated waters might have a familiar odour.

> You have just finished twenty brisk laps of the hotel swimming pool when you see your little sister on a poolside seat looking miserable and in need of attention. You are going to her side when suddenly two boys, before rushing off, throw another child into the deep end, where he splashes about helplessly. A large man turns to you: "you can swim; I can't; save my son!" You tell him that you are attending to your sister and turn away. He grabs you violently: "Get in there and don't come out until you bring my child to safety". You obey him. Do you think the man was entitled to force you to rescue his child?

Now despite his rather dim view of children, Mill would certainly have said yes. His ground of legitimate coercion was "the prevention of harm to others" and he thought that 'positive acts of benefit" such as labour on public work and military service could legitimately be required. He specifically mentions "acts of personal beneficence" such as "saving a fellow creature's life" as legitimately forced on one if such force is necessary [7]. I asked each of my seminar members. Nearly all responded that although the selfish swimmer had acted badly, the drowning child's father, though understandably desperate, had no real right to use force. One line among these 'anti-wets' was that the selfish swimmer had undertaken no lifeguard duties. A minority view (for which non-swimming children might on occasion be grateful) was that the father's duties to his son gave him an overriding right to take the action he did despite this being at the expense of your right to go about your business. When asked whether a stranger would therefore not be so entitled this student thought on reflection that a stranger would have this right. Here are people who seem to exhibit Dr Boyson's stereotype of the Welfare State's products, combining personal indifference to human priorities with what strikes me as a pathological obsession with officially constituted obligations. At the same time, paradoxically, their argument, on the face of it, would undermine a central principle, the 'rescue principle' of the Welfare State itself. And what would Dr Boyson think?

A Dialectic of Self-destruction?

The Welfare State is analogous in some ways to the helpless father, who can do nothing unless he obtains and redirects capacities to where they are needed. He has to use force because people can't be trusted or expected to offer the needed help voluntarily or for any material reward. What is different is the face-to-face and one-off nature of the swimming pool situation, which is precisely what makes the selfish swimmer's attitude so outrageous. The Welfare State operates through compulsory taxation whereby resources to meet need are extracted and transferred. (One would like to say 'redistributed' but that term might suggest what is contrary to fact: that the Welfare State soaks the rich to help the poor) [8]. Through this process, then, we are forced to render benefit to be spread among indeterminate recipients, (who include ourselves in sickness, study, unemployment or old age) as well as the chronic equivalents of the drowning child. This indirectness, indeterminacy and dilution contrasts with diving into a pool or with the Good Samaritan's actions. The 'abstractness' of this situation, where beneficience is expressed as compulsory subtraction from income, is further seen in the absurdity of my asking how much of my tax goes to this or that state 'department'. Yet I think Robert Nozick was right to connect being taxed with being forced to do things, with forced labour [9] (something both Rousseau and Mill were prepared to countenance). He was right to note, if not to exaggerate, the common character of the two sorts of case. Does the legitimacy of this sort of compulsion reside in its being democratically endorsed at the polls, in its being consented to by a majority? I do not think so. But if my students are typical, many are of a cast of mind opposed to it. They are potential tax rebels, objecting to being made to support others, let alone themselves, and insisting on the right to carry on their lives undisturbed as long as they do not harm others. Why should they have to give up what they legitimately hold to people to whom they owe nothing? The dialectic of self-destruction in the Welfare State seems to be simply this: it depends for its support precisely on the communal attitudes and values which it undermines.

Hume and the Precariousness of Justice in Civil Society

Now Nozick did not invent or claim to invent these ideas and attitudes. And it would be wrong to suggest, in line with current trends of thought, that they are essentially *reactive* attitudes to the Welfare State whose structure as compulsory charity-monger is responsible for them. The Welfare State developed after generations of rampant capitalism and despite the entrenched and conscious hostility of Political Economy and Liberal Philosophy at its threatening to interfere with the law of value and natural rights [10]. I want, then, to survey briefly some of this outlook of the Old Right.

Hume wrote in the *Treatise* in the chapter 'On Justice',

A man naturally loves his children better than his nephews, his nephews better than his cousins, his cousins better than strangers, where everything else is equal. Hence arises our common measure of duty in preferring the one to the other. Our sense of duty always follows the common and natural course of our passions [11].

Yet Hume recognised that civil society was, in contrast with earlier social formations, essentially a collection of *strangers*. Moreover, to that sort of collection, the partialities of love presented a problem:

But tho' this generosity must be acknowledged to the honour of human nature, we may at the same time remark that so noble an affection, instead of fitting man for large societies, is almost as contrary to them as narrow selfishness. For, while each person loves himself better than any other single person and in his love for others bears the greatest affection to his relations and acquaintance, this must necessarily produce an opposition of passions which cannot but be dangerous to the newly established union [12].

Hence 'justice', that 'artificial', 'abstract' and 'indirectly' utilitarian virtue, often apparently cruel in its dictates, is needed as a remedy. But this virtue must, on Hume's account, be most precarious. For it is kept in our hearts by a reflective and *ex hypothesi* feeble sympathy for 'humanity'. No wonder justice is so closely tied to the coercive role of the state and its laws. No wonder either, we might note, since for Hume nine tenths of law is possession, that it is in the hands of the section of society most obviously interested in upholding it.

The need for justice in Civil Society then, connects with the mutual indifference, anonymity, isolation, mistrust and competitiveness of its members. Justice, to the extent that it exists, countervails our tendency to tread on and exploit those to whom we are indifferent or opposed. There is little left of the 'natural' community of families and pre-commercial societies. As Adam Ferguson put it, their "bands (sic.) of affection" have broken and civil man tends to "deal with his fellows as he does with his cattle or his soil; for the sake of the profits they bring" [13]. Mandeville, more brutal, had 'proved' that private vices, especially pride and greed are, (at least among the propertied) public virtues [14]. Adam Smith, 'showed' that the state should largely keep its clumsy fist out of the national economy and leave the invisible hand to generate public benefit from private interest [15]. But all recognised the necessity for a state to maintain by force the public order within which private transactions took place. Markets, after all, entail private property and this institution entails compulsory exclusion. But though it was said to be in the interests of most that this overall order was maintained, both Hume and Kant sought to root this organizing force in principles of a different order from interests. Bentham who is perhaps the spiritual grandfather, along with Kant, of modern bureaucracy (General Good; Universal Principles) sought to foster personal, especially monetary, interests in promoting general utility; but he had a problem in postulating agencies of general utility in a world of individual hedonism. In all these systems of State, as of Morals, the universal principle and agency are fragile. This is signalled by the perpetual quest, mocked in advance by Mandeville, to show that even if you have to die to find out, duty coincides with interest. But since the rich could evade its net and the poor fell through it, some avoided the burdens and others missed the benefits, leaving an order exposed on one side of the highway to free riders, on the other to the resentful street mobs threatening to seize what they felt under no obligation to respect. So civil society had a problem: its motivating principle was private interest, but not only were there those whose interests were *not* served by this order, even those whose interests were so served had reason to break the order's rules when that was in their interest. Justice is not only blind, she could hardly hold the scales up.

But political Economy showed that direct charity, or any other enthusiasm, was on the whole a menace to its putative beneficiaries—why induce poor parents to disable their children so as to render them eligible for relief? asked Mandeville. Hence, at the same time as non-private sentiments were seen to play little role in civil society, their absence was a good thing. Kant, for example, not only thought that compassion lacked '*moral* worth'; he endorsed Political Economy's view of the social play of inclination:

> Nature should be thanked for fostering social incompatibility, enviously competitive vanity and insatiable desire for possession and even power. Without these desires, all men's excellent natural capacities would never be roused to develop . . . [16]

Yet as these remarks imply, and as Mandeville, Smith, Ricardo, Bentham and Mill accepted, civil society does have its casualties, its helplessly destroyed victims, as well as its normal mass of workers whose dreadful lot was excusable only by the idea that any other system would be worse. And so, as well as having free rider problems among its obvious beneficiaries, civil society, requiring a mass of stupefied labourers and a reserve army of unemployed, offered little to maintain the constant allegiance of its losers. It is small consolation to a starving rioter to be told that under a different order he would not have been born.

Bentham, Green and 'Scientific Charity'

With hindsight we can see, I think, that Bentham and T. H. Green, for all their commitment to the market and contract principles, were among what we would, until recently, have called gravediggers of *laissez-faire*. Bentham, that author of 'Pauper Management' that designer, almost inventor, of factory and prison, that choreographer of executions, sought with mad sensibleness to develop a vertical scale of sanctions, from the gallows through to the country mansion, such that government could put its finger on the social scales to correct disutilities in the spontaneous order. He even worked out the relative comfort of bedding between prison and workhouse. He sought to minimise the pain of the least eligible, compatible with overall utility. After all, the lowest were motivated by the same "sovereign masters, pleasure and pain" as their betters, and were no more ultimately to blame than their superiors were to be credited. To this end Bentham proposed official, though 'private', agents who would profit from the output of workhouse or prison. He endorsed, like Beveridge, and like old Mandeville, full employment; even for prisoners. We know of course that the Poor Law Act of 1834 with its principle of 'less eligibility' and the system of factory legislation to render honest labour more 'eligible' than idleness or crime, were Benthamite developments that are still around us today in the talk of the 'disincentive to work' that a semi-decent unemployment allowance constitutes.

Green was a High Victorian, a liberal philanthropist and a Philosophical Idealist. He was a father of modern English professional philosophy and the grandfather of modern English social work [17]. His influence extended through Bernard and

Helen Bosanquet and other disciples. Through the 'Charity Organization Society' (1869–1909), they at once developed Benthamite social investigation techniques for separating the deserving poor from the undeserving residuum ('scientific charity' as it was called) that are with us still, and opposed state 'provision' for reasons which I find it difficult wholly to understand. Green was a liberal and regarded the direct state enforcement of morality and responsibility as a contradiction in terms. But he was an advocate, on grounds of 'positive liberty', of state intervention to prevent contracts not genuinely free because compelled by poverty and because destructive of 'autonomy', of "the positive power ... of doing or enjoying something worth doing or enjoying" [18]. Not only in his great 'Lecture on Liberal Legislation and Freedom of Contract' (1880) but in the more abstract *Prolegonema to Ethics,* Green attacked the vulgar model according to which the hungry freely contract with their powerful exploiters:

> ... left to sink or swim in the stream of unrelenting competition ... so far as negative rights go—rights to be left alone—they are admitted to membership of civil society, but the good things to which the pursuits of society are in fact directed turn out to be no good things for them [19].

So Green, though a supporter of the principle of free and equal contract, saw the *laissez-faire* system tending to divide society into exploiters and unfree exploited, as unjust and wantonly destructive of individuals. Yet his advocacy of state intervention was sharply limited, not as much by a sense of its economic as of its moral danger. Private charity might be as misdirected and corrupting as statutory provision. But State charity is a contradiction in terms while the impersonality and indiscriminateness of State provision must transform morally elevating and productive charity into a debilitating mechanism. As the Christian Socialist, Canon Samuel Barnett wrote:

> Men at the University, especially those who directly or indirectly felt the influence of T. H. Green, were asking for some other way than that of institutions by which to reach their neighbours ... Thus it came about that a group of men and women at the University distrusted machinery for doing good ... Their desire was, as human beings, to help human beings, and their human feelings protested against forms of help which put the interest of a class or of a party before that of individuals [20].

So here we have the phenomenon of a major, highly organised, volunteer social work movement of dedicated philanthropists, sincerely if arrogantly committed to good works among the poor but resisting statutory provision. This can be seen in their conservative Royal Commission Report on the Poor Law Act (1909), opposed by the famous Minority Report of the Webbs, with its advocacy of wholesale state management. It is interesting to note here that, whereas the Utilitarians had been as deterministic as Robert Owen in their recognition of the role of social environment in shaping individual character, Helen Bonsanquet expressed the individualist voluntarism that is to be found in so much right-wing thinking today:

> But what if the social conditions will not permit them (the poor) to meet the responsibility (to family)? It is a vain hypothesis. The social conditions *will* permit them; for their very efforts to do so will make them steady and efficient workers, whose service will be valued by the community (*that word again*) and will be supplemented by the help of the young people who will grow up into such a family as their's will be [21].

How easy then to see poverty as a just punishment, and wealth as a deserved reward. In this voluntarist spirit, they insist that if enough men and women of compassionate good will and scientific outlook would come forward, the poor could be helped, through their agency, to accept their responsibilities to work (in an order in which, alas, compassionate good will had little place). Meanwhile, Green's advocacy of state intervention in area after area left anomalous his support for the Charity Organization Society and his resistance to state welfare institutions. I admire Green, but it must be through a deep sickness that so many, like him, think that spontaneous charity requires desperate and spectacular misery before it can exercise itself. If, as Green saw, the state's role was one of maintaining the conditions of free citizenship and if he was an advocate of state provision for education, he could hardly in all consistency leave 'charity', Boyson-style, to the earthly grace of 'free men'.

Alienations

The space at my disposal combines with the withdrawal of twentieth century British philosophers to their institutions, to stop this tour of ancestral homes. Therefore I leave Green, reluctantly and implicitly pointing towards Beveridge's position and beyond. An interlocking story would point from the growing role of the state in the capital accumulation process itself, towards Keynes and beyond. I can think of no major British philosopher until this century, certainly not that very political animal Berkeley, who was not deeply immersed in social and political and economic issues, none who were not 'applied philosophers'. What has interested me is the way in which problems about the relation of 'the State' to 'civil society', problems we have all studied in terms of the 'social contract' and so on, have very real significance in terms of problems of allegiance and material support for an overall public order whose motivating principle at the personal level was private interest and whose dominant institution was capitalism, accepted as a given frame of reference. How, in the absence of supernatural intervention, could there be an institution which did have the will *and* the way to promote the general good? No wonder Welfare legislation has typically had a sectional motivation; mainly fear of revolt. No wonder Hegel thought war, with the intoxicated consciousness of unity it brings, the 'health of the state'; and no wonder that Beveridge's vision of Britain as a fair and caring community triumphed in wartime. No wonder, either, that it needed Keynesian economics, with its rejection of the Ricardian doctrine of the poor as eternally with us, to provide an economic rationale in terms of rescuing capitalism from its own defects.

The moral culture of the welfare state, as we are familiar with it, is deeply ambiguous. Openly divisive appeals to 'burdened taxpayers' (healthy, insured to the eyeballs, affluent, secure in employment, go-getting) that accompany the present cuts, invertedly testify to the Welfare State's status as an expression of moral community, of a form of collective mutality and altruism. The very existence of a welfare state, even in a capitalist society, testifies to the sense among a society's members that membership is sufficient grounds for a 'decent' start and decent support in life. The denial of this, as Disraeli's 'two-nations' phrase brings out, is the denial of citizenship's rights and hence its obligations. This sense of belonging, of fellowship, is not I think fully captured in the phrase 'as of right', though it entails it insofar as state guarantees and administration are necessary to protect it. If I perceive my welfare solely in terms of an 'entitlement', as something I claim from the State 'as of right', I express the relative absence of that sense of common belonging or fellowship. I see myself as existing through coerced sufferance, albeit that I, *qua* contributor, suffer you too.

The fact that the Welfare State in liberal capitalist society is sustained through compulsory deductions from personal incomes of people who are thereby left to mind their own business with what remains (paid life-guards, supported by my money, will see to small children in the pool, as I pursue my own pleasures), generates a sense of utter separateness between my interests and interests which I compulsorily and indirectly support, even when these interests are my own. The welfare state is staffed and administered, by a combination of Benthamites and Greenians: professionals, who do what they do, not necessarily as a vocation with a 'sacramental' dimension, but as a job or career for the living and associated status it brings. They necessarily form a particular interest group as *employees*—with more or less power and with jobs to protect, often against non-professional involvement. As *officials*, these same individuals many of them with class identifications way above the station of their 'clients', have rights to intrude in, interfere with, categorise and control the lives of the cohorts with which they deal. Hence their practices are frequently seen as those of alien authority by those at the receiving end, whose dignity and even identity are subject to wholesale undermining. And where the goods they are 'delivering' include spiritual values such as 'care', 'attention', 'concern', the strain reaches a conceptual pitch emotionally reflected in 'burn-out'. This all looks like an unstable solution, a divisive and crumbly form of social cementation. The Welfare State's mode of operation in civil society seems deeply characterised by the horizontal and vertical divisions in society that make it necessary.

Rights, Care and Moral Culture

Returning to Hume, we can see that on his reasonable account 'justice' (that necessary benevolence-surrogate) must be a fragile force. If civil society is the arena of mutual indifference and egoistic competition, then even though I benefit I will be constantly prone to free-ride the system and to escape its burdens. Yet if all followed this path the system would collapse. The problem is bad enough for its bourgeois beneficiaries; how much more precarious is the situation of one forced to 'free-ride' because he or she cannot get a job, cannot *be* an active contributor, whatever consolations he may derive from his passive role in helping to hold down wages. Here we seem to have an injustice that excludes people from the very sphere of reciprocal justice.

My focus, however, is not so much on *whether* there is a right in justice to work, the conditions of health, knowledge, material sufficiency, or care in childhood and old age, though I would want to argue so. I am not centrally concerned with the Rawls, Hare, Nozick, Dworkin and others' debate about the *criteria* of justice. What I would here draw attention to in their writings is the intellectualist individualism that these positions tend to share and which I have been tracing in my historical survey. All devise variations of the 'how-would-you-like-it-if-you-were-in-that-position?' model. And a powerful model it is too, by which we are encouraged to function as impartial spectators 'of our own and others' competing interests. But suppose the impartial spectator is an idle voyeur. Suppose he isn't disposed to 'take rights seriously'. The sort of point I am making is suggested by a remark of Philippa Foot in response to a lecture of the rationalist altruist, Thomas Nagel: "Surely you could be perfectly aware of the unfairness of your position. But if you are not nice, you won't care". Leaving aside problems about their hypothetical status, Rawls' initially 'ignorant' contractors, in a state of mutual indifference, are as likely to behave as the mutually mistrusting prisoners of recent philosophical fable as they are to produce an outcome equivalent to the dictates of humane benevolence. Why should they not gamble on not being handicapped?

A moral community may require but is not constituted by agreements in judgement alone; it must arguably have a sufficiency of common mutual and overlapping concerns and consequently identifications beyond that of private subject. The free rider knows that he is unjustly exploiting his fellows. The sense of justice requires not only the imagination and the intellect but the capacity to care about, to respect, the more or less conflicting needs, interests and claims that are at stake. It is this sort of thought, I suspect, which prompted Aristotle to stress the friendship of the Polis, for friendship is the paradigm—of justice and community—of the ideal of a common good in which individuality flourishes.

On the other hand, to a degree that confused Marx into subverting concern for it, justice is a reluctant virtue. It implies rights, obligations and rules and, further back, conflict and separateness of interests. Mill says, for example, that if something is a requirement of justice you can be compelled to do it. The negative and formal virtue of justice seems equipped to be the cardinal virtue of liberalism. Any political morality which gives it the central place, or in Rawl's case, virtually the whole stage, will tend to play down community values as individual motives. Justice is the 'umpiring' virtue. Yet, as I say, and the same goes for tolerance and mutual respect, justice itself cannot exist, save as an internalised policeman, without the capacity for humane care and appreciation. But as earlier social philosophers were aware, such qualities are not the ultimate springs of individual conduct but are themselves formed and modified by forms of social life. Bourgeois liberalism affirms justice, but it fails to account for the social basis of justice.

In his 'The Public Use of Private Interest', Charles Schultze wrote in 1977:

> Market-like arrangements not only minimise the need for coercion as a means of organizing society; they also reduce the need for compassion, patriotism, brotherly love and cultural solidarity as motivating forces behind social improvements. Harnessing the 'base' motive of material self-interest to promote the common good is perhaps the most important social incentive mankind has yet achieved [22]?

On this account, whose direct claims I leave aside, who does the harnessing and why? Where does the support come from? Micro materialism seems to entail macro idealism. Saints would have to run the nightwatchman state—or be into all sorts of corruption. We are back with the problem with which I burdened Hume. Schultze's utopia would, I suggest, rapidly slip on the skin of banana republicanism.

What I am stressing, then, is that justice, with fragile support from the political infrastructure, needs to be imposed against the grain and principle of market society. To the extent that it is not necessary to the operations of that principle or hinders them it will meet resistances from taxpayers and capitalists. Rawlsian counterfactuals, about what rational individuals abstracted from their social position and interests would choose, will not stabilise the Welfare State.

Now you will rightly infer that I am stressing the Welfare State's attachment to capitalism. And I would be inclined to do so. But I am not, as some socialists would be, and as the Webbs were, for setting up the Welfare State as if it were distorted in its potentially benign operations solely by this precarious attachment. The state gets its form in large measure from its task of 'controlling' civil society—"keeping the show on the road" in Joan Robinson's phrase. But the authoritarian form of the state hardly softens automatically when the State no longer has capital to push it about. The Soviet State drains what I am calling the moral and self-organising capacity of the society to the degree that, in the name of community, it pursues its tasks. The Welfare State in its very statist' form consecrates society's selfish swimmers even as it counters the consequences of the sink-or-swim outlook. However, at least on my view, were the sink-or-swim principle of the market to be directly extended into areas that citizens have in the past seen as needing to be placed beyond the market, then this would be disastrous. Powerful private firms with, *ex hypothesi*, no vocational interest and no status as *our* public servants vie with each other to exploit the vulnerable *and* the taxpayer (always himself prone to demand further reductions and bet on his own security), while the shrunken public authority, with an unimpressive record of control over capital, announces toothless controls over the welfare entrepreneurs. Other right-wing proposals for means tests and negative income taxes regenerate the nineteenth century's 'residuum'; widen the poverty trap, while simultaneously exacerbating the sense among the fortunate that they are being milked to keep the idle alive. At the same time, assuming they are not privatised —and why not?—the police, whose authoritarianism is praised almost in the same breath as the same trait in 'welfare' state practices is condemned, would have its work cut out to maintain order (with appropriate tax-burdens).

Moreover, any thought about human welfare today and tomorrow needs to recognise that continuing industrial revolution, having slashed industrial employment, is rapidly automating the service sector and poses the prospect of spontaneous technological unemployment for a major part of the population over a major part of their lives while others' employment is dependent on the decisions of globe-trotting firms not committed or subject to any particular 'commonwealth'. Can the welfare state be discarded in those circumstances? Short of platonic devices to exterminate the dysfunctional or modest infanticidal proposals of a Swiftian kind, an *expanded* welfare state' will be required. But I have given reasons, I hope, for doubting the stability of such an order if we think of it as more of what we now have.

Conditions of Community

It might reflect pessimism as much as timidity that positive remarks will take up comparatively little space. I have so far, while using words like 'community' in a gestural sort of way, tended to confine myself to writing in terms of the received categories of State, Market, Family, Individual; good for a circulating tag-wrestle. But I think that we ought to emulate the boldness of the 'applied philosophers' we have surveyed, people who consecrated and almost invented the school and the prison, 'Utopian' institutions, we nowadays foolishly take for granted. I have been emphasising the precariousness of modern societies with their 'dialectic of dissolution' and even 'self-destruction'. There has been hyperbole and idealisation (of a base kind) in this picture in so far as it has played down the cultural meanings of 'bourgeois' practices that are not adequately represented by terms like 'self-interest': even status-seeking, after all, presupposes some shared honourings and admirings that transcend mere consumer appetite. Nonetheless, I would contend, our kind of society is radically deficient in social institutions and practices that foster the integration of free individuals into forms of life characterised by justice.

No society, it seems to me, can be just or humane when its forms fail to generate a well-founded common sense of contributing and gaining, of pride and indebtedness, of benefits and burdens, of give and take, of power and dependency; of community, justice and freedom. This cannot be a matter of strict equality; some people, for example, must be less able than others to contribute, some less capable of receiving. But divisions and inequalities in power, knowledge, wealth and status which are false to humans' capacities, needs and contributions mark an unjust, inhumane and mutually irresponsible society; one which lacks, in Rawls' terms, the 'bases' of mutuality and self-respect [23].

What I have been suggesting is that the official paternalist forms of welfare, funded through taxation, insurance payments and nothing else, atrophy and block a society's capacities for generating more direct mutual and common values and responsibilities. The alternative to statism is not capitalism (which any way secures its own welfare-handouts from the state) but a form which, though it does not do without states as authoritative central institutions, or for that matter without markets as communicators of demand, opens up spaces for, institutionalises and supports, community networks and facilities with appropriate territorial and functional definitions. In the absence of such reproducible and reproducing networks of co-operation it is cant to speak as the government does, of 'deinstitutionalising', for example, mentally ill and mentally handicapped people, whose need is for more, not less, intensive care and support, and 'returning' them from hospitals to 'the community'. For in our society, for all its voluntary agencies, that generally means either private entrepreneurs or private families: institutions in some ways more antithetical to 'community' than is a public hospital.

At this stage one of the premises implicit in many of the writings mentioned should be made explicit: Hume, Beveridge and Boyson think, as they talk about economic *man*, of *domestic* woman. The categorisation is taken for granted as reflecting the nature of things. So the moral burden of altruistic care which capitalist ideology lifts from the egoistic male 'go-getter' is in the same motion transferred to his wife, his children's mother and his parents' daughter-in-law (not to mention her job as a nurse). Indeed, we could almost speak of this 'private' realm of femininity, this circumscribed and downgraded sphere of micro-community, as constituted by its complementary exclusion from the 'public' masculine realm of rational self-interest [24]. But if the capitalist *order* requires this sexist structure, this realm where services are rendered not as commodities (just as it requires an established 'bourgeois morality'), the market itself is as genderblind (and as age-blind) as it is amoral; hence it subverts the conditions of its own continuance. Firms, in the absence of special legal constraints, will employ women if they are cheaper, more patient, dexterous, docile or easily dismissed than men. So what can the capitalist *state* do (except pontificate)? We ought to be sceptical, on the other hand, of expectations that men be both breadwinners and domestic authorities and examples. These points, even when added to the familiar left-platonic list of 'the family's' anti-social tendencies in virtue of its architecturally reinforced enclosing of passions and interests, do not amount to the call to 'smash the family'. Despite the fact that family institutions, bolstered by inheritance laws, have evolved in ways that promote a stupid narrowness and amplify injustice, the 'domestic principle' of intimate love and unconditional support is a precious good, needing social support and compatible with wider identifications and networks. Indeed without these networks domestic life suffocates while those outside the range of the family hearth are left out in the cold as wards of charity or state. To place 'family responsibility' at the centre of a modern society's welfare system is to over-burden it and to sentence countless individuals to virtual orphanhood [25].

To discuss the moral economy of the family is at once to speak of a structure of care (and of the conflicts it entails), and also of a sphere where children acquire their moral outlook and habits. Any ongoing moral order reproduces itself; any social form gives its members a moral education, builds or jerrybuilds their character. Hence we should look at the sort of moral education the capitalist-statist order promotes and consider whether there are alternative forms of education to those dominated by 'family' and 'school', whose connection with capitalist-statist values are clear enough, if not quite transparent. But what we find is that the argument between 'left' and 'right' over 'education' is restricted to issues of discipline, curriculum and finance within the established framework. But schools are bizarre institutions in which to spend such a large part of one's life, 'institutionalising' their charges at the same time as they isolate them. If responsible, just, generous, skilled, enterprising, democratic, inquiring and critical people, male and female, are to be brought up to populate a just and humane society, they have to be provided with the conditions which foster these qualities through their graduated exercise. Yet, although compulsory schooling was commonly responded to in its earliest days as state abduction, it has become accepted as a natural, almost a conceptual, context of childhood. And so people find nothing odd in effervescent young people's brains going flat week by week, year by year, in the ever-decaying containers of classroom and school. Now that there is no excuse for *any one* being forced to crawl up chimneys and down mines there is no excuse for the absolute gulf that 'protects' children from the responsibilities and rights, necessities and freedoms appropriate to growing citizens. It is time that university teachers, who are and who get the stale cream of this process, reflected on the implications of a system that hands over its finest in a mental state blocked to further education. Youth needs enfranchisement.

I have focused, in looking towards alternative social forms, on two social 'categories' at present essential to but locked out of the dominant chambers of 'public' life: women and children. This focus, in part recognition of the inadequacy of a purely 'class analysis' of what is wrong with our society, makes us seek to grasp the conditions under which women's equality in and children's membership of community would be a reality. The focus, I suggest, highlights not just the need for a radically altered organization of 'working life' so that all *can* contribute and be recognised as contributing ('the right to work') but a radically altered vision of 'public' and 'private' life so that the contrast is not an imprisoning dichotomy [26].

Any modern society is a huge community of people who are mostly strangers to one another. But it is through active and co-operative contact, through direct initially local experience that they discover and are able to generalise from their own and others' talents, needs and limits. Martin Buber was wrong to think of the ideal society as a community of face-to-face communities, as a tribe of tribes; so many of our central links are 'activity' not 'territory' based. But unless we can develop institutional forms which foster rather than atrophy 'bands of affection' among strangers, unless we go beyond alternating welfare mixed of mothers, markets and ministries, we shall travel further down the path now strewn with increased domestic chaos, increased poverty and increased cynicism about citizenship. At present we have undeniable if twisted evidence of the 'need for community' in racism, localist hooliganism, militarism and consumer-conformism. These are illusory forms of community; at the same time they make the question as to the truer meanings of that term more urgent. Anarchists as much as state apologists have assumed that state forms must destroy community and have failed to speculate on diverse ways in which the 'mutual aid' so central to their vision might be feasible. As there is no alternative to it in some form, we need to develop models of 'the state' in which community resources and initiatives are seen to be represented and fostered, in which the state is a vehicle for circulating resources that come 'from below'. 'Welfare state' would then be a way of talking about rather than a way of burying questions about 'welfare society'.

Acknowledgement

I was helped in working on this paper which was presented as the Conference Address to the Society for Applied Philosophy in May 1984 by Rod Edmond, Brian Munday, Peter Taylor-Gooby, Janet Thomas, Chris Arthur and Brenda Cohen. I should like to thank the Society for Applied Philosophy for a stimulating discussion which should issue in developments and changes in my thinking on these issues.

Anthony Skillen, Keynes College, University of Kent, Canterbury, United Kingdom.

NOTES

[1] *Report on Social Insurance and Allied Services*, H.M.S.O., 1942, page 6.
[2] T.H. Marshall (see his *Citizenship and Social Class*, Cambridge University Press, 1950) developed this citizenship model. Its 'activist' implication sits uneasily with the problematic status of 'citizenship' (contrast 'subjecthood') in British society. The theme is brilliantly revived in Michael Walzer's *Spheres of Justice*, Martin Robertson, 1983.
[3] Any socialism which allows the functional categories of producers' or 'contributors' as central place needs to beware of marginalising or even conceptually 'liquidating' those who are *unable* to be anything but 'parasites'.
[4] Crosland's book was reprinted by Jonathan Cape in 1981.
[5] In *Down With The Poor*, 1971, R. BOYSON (Ed.) Churchill Press, page 5.
[6] MARX, in a famous passage of his *Civil War in France* wrote of the French state:

> Every common interest was straightway severed from society, counterposed to it as a higher *general* interest, snatched from the activity of society's members themselves and made an object of government activity; from a bridge, a schoolhouse ... to the railways ... (*Selected Works of Marx and Engels*, Moscow 1962, Vol. 1, page 333).

[7] MILL, J.S. *On Liberty* Introduction. See M. Warnock (Ed.) *Utilitarianism*, Fontana 1962, pages 136–7.
[8] See, among many, Julian Le Grand; *The Strategy of Equality*, Allen & Unwin, 1982. RAMESH MISHRA, *Society and Social Policy*, Macmillan, 1978; IAN GOUGH, *The Political Economy of the Welfare State*, Macmillan, 1979.
[9] *Anarchy, State and Utopia*, 1974 (Oxford, Blackwell) page 169.
[10] As Locke is often held up as *the* ancestral sanctifier of right-wing callousness, it would be well to read section 42 of the *First Treatise of Civil Government* which asserts that "it would always be a sin in any man of estate to let his brother perish for want of affording him relief out of his plenty". (*Everyman*, 1924, page 30). The 'Lockean Proviso "provides" quite a bit!
[11] HUME, D. *Treatise* Book 111, Part 11, Section 1, *Oxford*, 1888, page 483.
[12] Ibid., page 487.
[13] FERGUSON, ADAM (1767) *An Essay on the History of Civil Society* page 19, page 34.
[14] MANDEVILLE, *The Fable of the Bees*.
[15] SMITH, ADAM *The Wealth of Nations*.
[16] 'Ideas for a universal history with a cosmopolitan purpose' in *Kant's Political Writings* edited H. Reiss; Cambridge University Press, 1970, page 45.
[17] See the excellent discussion in Melvin Richter's *The Politics of Conscience*, WEIDENFIELD &

NICOLSON, 1964, and the introduction by C.S. YEO to HELEN BOSANQUET, *Social Work in London,* 1869–1912, Harvester, 1973.

[18] 'Liberal Legislation and Freedom of Contract', *Works of T.H. Green,* Vol. 111, Longmans Green & Co, 1890, page 371.

[19] GREEN, T.H. *Prolegomena,* Oxford, page 245.

[20] Quoted by RICHTER, op. cit. page 323.

[21] Quoted by RICHTER, op. cit. pages 331–332.

[22] CHARLES SCHULTZ (1977) *The Public Use of Private Interest,* Brookings Institute pages 17–18.

[23] RAWLS, J. (1971) *A Theory of Justice,* Harvard, especially page 440.

[24] See CLARE UNGERSON 'Women and Caring' in *The Public and the Private* edited by E. GAMARNIKOW *et. al.,* Hinemann, 1983. My thinking on this and all the issues discussed was deepened by William Connolly; *Appearance and Reality in Politics,* Cambridge University Press, 1981, Chapter 5.

[25] See ALAN WALKER, 'A Caring Community', in *The Future of the Welfare State* edited by H. Glennester, Hennemann, 1983.

[26] A most suggestive discussion linking the need to break from the State/Market/School framework is *Not For Sale,* The Swedish National Youth Council Report of 1981, summarised by Benny Henriksson Aberdeen University Press translation, 1983. My *Ruling Illusions,* Harvester 1978, attempts without adequate grasp of the potential for change in the state's 'ways of working' to outline dimensions of such 'grass roots' politics.

20

Market Equality and Social Freedom

MARTIN HOLLIS

ABSTRACT *Conflicts between the good of each and the good of all are often presented in terms of freedom versus equality, with liberals pulled one way by libertarians and the other by social democrats. When we distinguish between negative and positive notions not only of freedom but also of equality, the liberal freedom 'to pursue our own good in our own way' is a positive freedom involving a negative idea of equality (or 'equity'). Yet 'equity' is not strong enough to deal with the problem of public goods. Trust is a public good, essential if markets are to work and dependable only where there is a moral commitment to a positive basic equality among citizens.*

Headfield School, in the town of Dewsbury in the north of England, added a footnote to political theory in 1988. At the time it was one of several local state schools admitting children at the age of eight. It differed from others in that 85% of its pupils were of Asian origin, a proportion which the local Council thought far too high and which it was trying to lower in the name of a policy of 'social mix'. So, although parents in Dewsbury were asked to list their preferences among schools for their eight-year-olds, these wishes were not altogether respected. In particular some white parents found their children assigned to Headfield School against their will. Twenty-two of them took the Council to court in 1988, arguing that their statutory freedom of choice had been denied them. There were other schools which could take more children, they pointed out, and children of many other parents with the same preferences had not been assigned to Headfield. They asked the court to overrule the Council's decisions and have their children allocated to schools more acceptable to them.

The Council maintained that it had done its legal duty by providing school places. It defended its policy of 'social mix' as a legitimate way to ensure a balanced intake of backgrounds and abilities in all its schools. The policy had been in its election manifesto and was aimed at equal education for all and hence equality of opportunity in later life. (It could not declare openly that ethnic mix was involved because the Race Relations Act forbids discrimination on grounds of race.) Moreover, the Council had indeed consulted all the parents in its area and accepted their preferences in most cases. It could not follow all parents' wishes without abandoning its policy of social mix but it had not singled out the 22 complainants in particular when it came to adjusting the intake for Headfield.

The court ruled in favour of the parents, who were hailed in Conservative circles as winners of a great victory for the freedom of the individual. To be precise the ruling was given on the technical ground that the Council had failed to publicise its policy properly, and side-stepped the deeper questions of freedom and equality. But public interest was caught by the ideological argument, construed as one between the individual rights of parents, congenial to the militant individualism of a Thatcherite central government, and the social concern for the public good expressed in the 'social mix' policy of a local Labour council. The rhetoric is, of course, misleading. It is not obvious that the freedom of an articulate few instances a freedom which all could share. Nor is it obvious that champions of equality are enemies of individual freedom. Indeed my purpose is to argue for equality in the name of freedom. But the strong passions aroused by schooling in Dewsbury are an instructive sign that the age of ideology is not dead in Mrs Thatcher's third term of office.

That perhaps strikes too overtly political a note. The Dewsbury parents also exemplify a cool question about the relation of the good of each to the good of all. For instance, no one wants the new by-pass through *his* garden, the new flight path over *his* rooftop or the new community home for alcoholics sited next door to *him*. But, if one looks to the general good, then cars, planes and alcoholics are pieces in a public jig-saw and they have to go somewhere. Much effort by government, especially by local government, is spent in fiddling the pieces so as to minimise discontent and to persuade or compensate the aggrieved. This is cool, largely non-party work, pragmatic in its detail, even if ideological in some of its priorities and its choices of which pieces to include. It takes a very fervent ideologue to maintain either that individual freedom gives each citizen an invariable right of veto or that the common good admits no losers. But the cool work of negotiation is not purely pragmatic. There is also a cool, philosophical question about the nature of both freedom and equality, which needs addressing before one dons a political rosette even of pastel hue.

The New Right contends that freedom conflicts with equality and should be preferred. In so far as the model of freedom here is market freedom, the Old Left agrees that there is a conflict and contends that equality should be preferred. Abstractly, if my freedom consists in my being able to do what I want, then it will sometimes clash with your freedom to do what you want. All societies have ways of intervening. They range from providing a market-style arena, policed by the rule of law to ensure fair play, to radical arbitration which may involve redealing the hands or even reconstituting the wants which produced the conflict. If equality consists in uniformity imposed in the name of social planning, then the tension between freedom and equality is palpable. By this test the Dewsbury parents were indeed claiming a freedom of choice the Council's aim of equality flatly denied.

But neither concept is clear or simple. Both can be given what I shall call 'negative' and 'positive' definitions (at some risk of confusion, as these terms have various usages in social philosophy). By 'negative freedom' I mean freedom defined as an absence of obstacles to desire, so that an agent is negatively free if nothing prevents his doing what he wants to do. One might bear in mind J. S. Mill's remark that "freedom consists in doing what one desires" (*On Liberty*, Ch. 5) and Thomas Hobbes's that "the liberty of subjects depends on the silence of the law" (*Leviathan*, Ch. XXI). My notion of 'positive freedom' starts from the idea that there is a kind of life proper for a free agent and that freedom is to be defined as the ability to live it. One might bear in mind Rousseau's dictum that "freedom is obedience to a law which we prescribe to ourselves" (*Le Contrat Social*, Book I, Ch. 8), coupled with his case for thinking that it flourishes in its moral form only where a General Will prevails.

That reference serves also for 'positive equality' or what I shall term 'egality', the idea that you and I are equal only if we have the same full, participating share in the costs and benefits of the social enterprise. That is to contemplate a more radical egalitarianism that Rousseau's but one which sets up a limiting, social, ideal-type to contrast with 'negative equality' or what I shall term 'equity'. This is an idea of basic, minimal rights, typified or even constituted by equality before the law. You and I are negatively equal, if your penny is as good as mine and your vote and mine both count for exactly one in the election. But there is no suggestion in equity that we must both have the same number of pennies or that your political influence cannot be greater than mine. We might recall Aristotle's saying that justice consists in treating unequal people unequally.

The negative concepts go with an individualism which begins, or perhaps even ends, by considering society from the standpoint of individual rights. They embody the libertarian pull on liberalism, as witnessed currently by the tendency to think of social freedom by analogy with the standard idea of market freedom. Negatively, a market is free, if anyone may offer to buy or sell whatever he wants and if all resulting transactions are by mutual consent. Equality is a matter of an equal right to engage in the process, not of an equal power to get what one wants. Although even libertarians usually grant some case for restricting a free market in, for instance, sex, drugs or guns, or for limiting those who may take part, for example, by excluding children or foreigners, these clauses are to be seen as limitations and restrictions, not as enhancements of a more genuine freedom. There is no more genuine freedom than that of consent.

There is much in a negative approach to attract a liberal. J. S. Mill declared early in *On Liberty* that "the only freedom which deserves the name is that of pursuing our own good in own way". This catches the central theme of liberalism that society must leave each of us a choice of ends, even if it may prescribe the means of pursuing them in order to prevent harm to others. The libertarian pull is towards silence about ends and towards only such interferences in the choice of means as will increase the scope for capitalist acts between consenting adults (in Robert Nozick's pleasing phrase). Law and government offer an impersonal, even-handed arbitration which is neutral about the content of the good life.

An obvious doubt arises about the sum of the consequences of leaving people free to transact as they will within the limits of equity. A free and equal society, negatively defined, might be a thoroughly nasty one. The libertarian has two kinds of reply. The more austere is that it is irrelevant whether the results are nasty in sum, because no greater collective activity can be justified. If there is a price for freedom and equity, so be it. The more ambitious is that the results will not be nasty, or, at any rate, that the results of central planning are nastier. These replies raise different sorts of questions and we need to keep them apart. I begin with the more austere.

In Chapter 7 of *Anarchy, State and Utopia* Nozick presents a sweeping argument to show that the claims of freedom conflict with those of egality and, indeed, of almost any other policy of redistribution. It is an objection to all attempts at imposing a 'pattern' on a society for the sake of general welfare, social justice or some other aspect of the common good. In essence it goes like this. Suppose there is a revolution one Monday morning and a new government installs a distribution of resources intended to embody what is good, right or just. Suppose, for instance, that it decrees equality of wealth and income. Then think what will happen if people are left free to act as they see fit in this new situation. They will, of course, upset the pattern, not necessarily because they dislike it but because they make individual choices which will sum to defeat it. Those whose talents are in demand will get richer, while others with less to offer will get poorer. Entrepreneurs will wax fat, alcoholics and their families thin. By the following Monday the society will no longer be a good, right or just one as judged by whatever the test was. The pattern will have to be reimposed constantly. No patterned society can be a free society.

The Dewsbury case is a nice illustration. Parents have their individual aims for their own children. These aims, if allowed free rein in the choice of school, have no tendency to sum to a social mix. On the contrary, they will sum to differentiate schools into white and coloured, middle class and working class and so forth. The Council cannot hope to prevent it merely by an initial imposing of its social mix. It must constantly correct departures and constantly restrict choices. Equality is the enemy of freedom in education, exactly as Thatcherites maintain.

But the Council's supporters need not take Nozick lying down. Even liberals should find his libertarian argument too sweeping, since even equity falls victim to it. It is possible to sell one's birthright for a mess of potage, as Esau did (*Genesis*, Chapter 25) and so to dispossess one's descendants. One can do so not only because one is lazy, careless or stupid but because cumulative inequalities of power can erode the bargaining position of the losers and then their rights. Left to itself, an uneven distribution of power will presently erode the ability of many to pursue their own good in their own way, which is the cornerstone of a liberal society. Here is one pattern which freedom seems to demand.

Nozick thinks of basic rights as a 'side-condition' on what can be left to market-style activity rather than as a pattern, as a base-line rather than an end-state. But, in any case, a corrective mechanism is called for on the instructive ground that free choices can sum to defeat the conditions of free choice. This is slippery terrain for libertarians, because it invites further thought about the conditions for even negative freedom and introduces the other pull on liberalism. So libertarians may be inclined to retort that the only correction needed is the removal of defects in the working of free markets. If the inequalities which destroy freedom arise only where there are obstacles to market-style activity, then removing the obstacles is not to limit freedom. This retort introduces the more ambitious line that a free and equitable society is one where life goes better than with central planning, including redistribution.

I have space here only to gesture to what I take to be the crux for the more ambitious line, which is market failure in the case of public goods. A public good is of benefit to all and cannot be confined to persons who have contributed to it. Street lighting, clean air and civil defence are standard examples. Given the stock definition of a rational agent and assuming that no agent or small group gets enough benefit to make it worth paying the whole cost, there is a simple demonstration that indivisible public goods will not be provided by voluntary action. The nub of it is that it is better for each not to contribute, both if others will contribute and if others will not. Hence it is better not to contribute whatever others do. Hence no rational agent contributes and the good is not provided. For a lucid analysis I know of no better source than J. S. Mill's *Principles of Political Economy* (Book V, Ch. XI), nor of any more recent ways of avoiding his conclusion that only government can provide public goods.

Mill argues that, although the great business of society goes best if it is left to individuals, in these cases intervention is needed not to frustrate individual interests but to give expression to them. In the modern language of game theory, there are cases where individually rational choices sum to Pareto-inferior outcomes, not because of failure to solve a co-ordination problem but because the game is of the Prisoner's Dilemma type. If the Pareto-superior outcome is wanted, it must be imposed. Furthermore, since it remains vulnerable to the free-riding, which would have prevented it, it must be constantly reimposed. The crux for the more ambitious libertarian line is what to do about this diagnosis of generic market failure.

The usual libertarian reply is, I think, to concede the case for imposing some public goods but to deny the threat to individual freedom. Since *everyone* prefers that everyone contributes, over what happens if no one contributes, *everyone* has had his preferences better satisfied. Since these are 'goods' in the sense merely that everyone would rather have them than not, and there is no suggestion of imposing a moral or objective good, no damage is done to the negative concept of freedom. All the same, however, this is where libertarians and liberals begin to part company. Mill himself discusses the case in terms not of preferences but of interests. That this is no slip of the pen is clear from *On Liberty*, where his plea for individuality, and for a form of society where it can flourish, rests on the true interests of human beings. There is no ultimate conflict between wants and interests, because interests are treated as the wants which one would have in the absence of false consciousness. But such deeper, reflective wants are distinct from wants-of-the-moment and so from the given preferences of market economics.

I take *On Liberty* to be evidence that, even within a negative theory of freedom, liberals are at odds with libertarians. The liberal's idea of freedom as the ability to pursue 'our own good in our own way' involves social preconditions stronger than the libertarian's, namely conditions in which the desires of a mature and developed individual truly indicate where his own good lies. This, however, creates a gap between consumer sovereignty, where the customer is always right, and individual autonomy, which the customer often fails to achieve. Once introduced, the gap widens swiftly.

Public goods, which are public in the strict economist's sense that *everyone* wants them, *no one* can be excluded and contributions *cannot* be enforced, are pretty rare. Even the famous examples, street lighting, civil defence and clean air, are not strictly public goods by this test. Burglars like the dark, the deployment of defence brings differing costs and benefits to different areas, the bill for clean air can be levied differentially. In general, norms which resolve Prisoner's Dilemmas and prevent free-riding, do *not* in fact bring about a Pareto-superior outcome, if one is strict about benefit to *everyone*. For instance, laws against dealing in drugs are very reasonably held to be in the general interest and are an important example of the state's providing a good which individuals cannot provide for themselves. But they are not a 'public good'. There are plenty of customers for drugs, ready to exercise consumer sovereignty, if allowed, and plenty of suppliers, ready to persuade, beguile and induct new customers. Addiction changes preferences and its encouragement is an exercise in power. There is, indeed, a libertarian view that there should be a free market in drugs; but liberals usually resist on the ground that the wants of addicts are not the true wants and consent to buy is not genuine consent.

To defend the reasonable idea that laws against drug dealing are a public good, one must therefore go behind existing wants to some prior baseline. The point applies in general whenever the liberal invokes the idea that law is often needed not to frustrate the interests of individuals but to give expression to them. As a proposition about *wants* it is rarely true and so can be stated in terms of wants only by idealising to what individuals would want in baseline conditions. Indeed the very theory of the social contract is a theory of what all individuals would want in conditions schematised as a state of nature. The social contract is not a Pareto-improvement on any existing state of society, since it deals the cards more equally than would suit everyone as things are.

This is familiar enough liberal ground. Preconditions are set and enforced for pursuing our own good in our own way but all is well, the liberal hopes, because preconditions are not conceptions of the good. Yet are they not? The line between negative and positive notions of freedom is by now very thin. The mark of a positive notion is to identify the sort of life proper for a truly free agent and to insist on social arrangements which make it possible. It will not take much to show that there are enough social commitments in arranging for the pursuit of our own good in our own way to overstep the line. I shall offer two arguments, one concerned with power in relation to market freedom and the other with the thought that a shared conception of the good is itself a public good.

One difference between equity and egality is that egalitarians argue for equality of power, if there is to be equal freedom of choice. Equity does not involve equality of power: each of my pennies is worth the same as each of yours, even if you have millions more than me. Neither position is attractive undiluted. An equity which lets the widow starve, provided that her one mite matches one mite from the rich man's hoard, is surely too abstract. The rich man can afford to be careless with one mite. He can afford to wait or to gamble. He is cushioned against bad luck or inflation. There are plenty more where it came from. The widow, whose one mite is her whole income, lives in fear, at the mercy of her poverty and with horizons narrowed to a desperate subsistence. Perhaps it is easier for a camel to pass through the eye of a needle than for a rich man to enter the kingdom of heaven. But on earth even spiritual happiness is not free. For the very poor even the spirit is harrassed and confined in ways which do not threaten the rich. Equity does not involve equal power but it needs to set a limit to the inequality.

On the other hand egality is too dogmatic. The freedom to be exactly equal to everyone else is no freedom. Even Rousseau, in invoking the General Will in order to force citizens to be free, does not first force them to be exactly equal in material things. A rough equality of wealth and income seemed to him enough. An extreme egality, which removes all advantages, also flattens all differences. So why favour it? I find no answer to that simple question. Egality is not an end-in-itself. It is a means to ends like individuality or self-realisation which, however communitarian in their conception, require variety of possessions. Egalitarian limits to unequal power must not make it impossible to pursue our own good in our own way.

There is plenty of scope for compromise by insisting on an equal, sufficient minimum for all and thereafter leaving people to their own pursuits. Naturally there is also plenty of scope for argument about what this minimum should include. The current disputes about the proper function of the state in matters of welfare and taxation rage fiercely. That is partly because conviction politics have been weakening consensus politics. But consensus politics can agree on, for instance, the need for a welfare state without agreeing how far it shall extend, how high to set the guaranteed minimum or how much of its processes should be left to the market. I cannot enter the dispute now but I mention it in answer to Nozick's argument about patterns being incompatible with freedom. I see no threat to freedom in a taxation policy which takes 50% of income above a certain level and redistributes it to those below the level. Indeed, as a very rich great-uncle of mine remarked in the days of the post-war Labour government when British income tax rose to nineteen shillings and sixpence in every pound, "you should see how the sixpences mount up".

Believers in equity can thus recognise that there are welfare preconditions for equity without becoming egalitarians. For instance, this is as far as a local Council needs to go, when insisting on a social mix in its schools. The recognition, however, involves a related thought about market freedom. Enoch Powell, in the days when he was a leading Conservative spokesman, once described a cash register as "an unseen ballot box". Whenever I buy something in a shop, he declared, I am as if voting for that product against others and so exercising a democratic freedom of choice which influences what is produced by signalling my preferences to would-be producers. The market economy is the counterpart of political democracy, he added. In a sense he is plainly right—free markets allocate goods responsively to individual preferences. But, at the same time, the analogy is outrageous. If a purchase is a vote, then a huge purchase is a huge vote and a million pennies purchase a million votes. From a democratic point of view, the widow is effectively disenfranchised.

Applying the thought more moderately, we still find the converse, that democratic freedom implies a market equality connected with purchasing power. Again, whereas egality might insist on complete equality of power in the market, equity need only recognise that the widow and the rich man, the individual worker and the multinational, the small supplier and the conglomerate buyer are too unequal to have equal freedom. The Brandt Commission, for instance, reflecting on disparities between North and South, is not egalitarian but was very clear that, viewed through Southern eyes, the market in primary products is not free. A free market is one where consent to a transaction is a sign that both parties have made a free choice. The mere fact of consent does not signal freedom of choice. The idea of a fair price is involved and that is far more complicated.

That is as much as I can say about the 'market equality' of my title, if I am to take the idea of 'social freedom' further. When Mill speaks of the only freedom which deserves the name as that of "pursuing our own good in our own way", he creates an ambiguity. Is the phrase to be taken as saying that you shall pursue your good in your way, while I pursue mine in my own way? Or are *we* to pursue *our* good in *our* own way? Even the first, wholly individualist, reading makes the point that for each person there is a 'good' which governs the freedoms which should be allowed—the developed life of a mature individual with individuality. But the second goes further by suggesting some notion of a common good. I shall argue that a free society needs a shared moral bond between its members and that this public morality is a public good involving a positive notion of freedom.

Even the most fervent defenders of free markets see the need for a framework of law and enforced social order to prevent the breaking of contracts. A free market will not work to mutual advantage unless you can trust me to keep our bargain even when it would pay me not to. Yet why should you, if we are rational, self-interested individuals? Hobbes's famous answer in *Leviathan* is that, human nature being what it is, "covenants without the sword are but vain breath" and hence we cannot trust one another, unless we are subject to a "common power to keep all in awe". But, it seems to me, if free-riding is checked only by fear of sanctions, then the common power will be either ineffective in detail or appallingly intrusive. Hence the usual view is that we need a public morality with enough grip to ensure that each of us acts as he promised.

To put flesh on this abstract line of thought, think in terms of an Enterprise Culture spreading the word that, as Mrs Thatcher has famously put it, "there is no such thing as society; there are only individual men and women" and that each is to reap whatever he has sown. The encouragement to individual enterprise is a threat to social harmony and, witness trends in crime and hooliganism, one which penalties alone cannot confine. Yet the shared morality which might confine it is eroded by rampant individualism. If it is a good, then it is a public good in the technical sense which implies that it is individually rational not to contribute. It must be imposed, on the ground that even those like Yuppies, who will erode it if they can, are better off by not being given the chance.

It is not obvious that such a shared morality amounts to a shared conception of the good which restricts the choice of ends. Indeed a crucial claim in liberal works like John Rawls's *A Theory of Justice* has been that it does not—an instructive point of reference, seeing that Rawls himself has changed his mind lately and declared for a shared conception, or at least overlapping conceptions of the good. I agree. If the public good in question is *merely* trust that bargains will be kept, then it can be imposed by inculcating some very illiberal values. For instance, a strongly hierarchical system which preaches the subjection of the lower orders and of women can do it. But neither liberals nor, for different reasons, Yuppies will buy trust at this price. They insist that the moral bond be between equal persons with equal opportunities; and hence, I submit, pass from a thin to a thick theory of the good.

Thus, broadly, what starts as a precondition of freedom becomes a rough but committal view of the proper way for free agents to conduct their business in the pursuit of proper ends. The view gains precision, however, when we reflect on its implication for the nature of free markets. Market freedom is often thought of as a rational anarchy of unfettered choice within parameters: law, government and social convention set a framework but one which leaves all choices *à la carte* rather than *table d'hôte*. Relatedly, orthodox neo-classical economics separates the economy from society at large, and cordons off political and social matters by putting them in *ceteris paribus* clauses. I do not find this artificial approach consistent with the terms on which it wants to solve the problem of public goods.

To see why the approach is artificial, reflect that an economy comprises all production, exchange and distribution of goods and services in a society. These are all rule-governed activities, not merely in that they are constrained and regulated by rules but also in that they are enabled, constituted and permeated by rules. For instance religion, in a society which takes religion seriously, penetrates the work undertaken and the ways of doing it. It affects social and hence economic relationships. It constitutes at least some economic activities, like the funeral business, where there is no external goal to which a funeral is an efficient means and no test of the efficient conduct of funerals independent of the meaning of the burial of the dead. What is plainly true of religion is no less true of any activity whose meaning is expressive before it is instrumental.

Someone might retort that, although there is a case for defining freedom internally to the meaning of activities in a traditional society, the case does not apply to modern societies with rational-legal systems framing a world without magic (to echo Weber on *die Entzauberung der Welt*). But the point stands, I think. What counts as a good or service depends on what exactly is valued. Cars, for example, do not sell just on their ability to get people about fast or cheaply. They are vehicles of self-expression, witness the famous campaign which Mercedes ran in Sweden on the slogan 'You are what you drive'. Similarly production of goods and services is a complex activity mainly conducted in organisations, where people enact roles and embody norms. Here the slogan might be 'You are what you do'—not an ultimate truth, I dare say, but one which captures part of the relation between self and role in modern societies as much as in traditional ones.

I am putting in a plea against thinking of men and women as social atoms connected only by the instrumental rationality of a cash nexus. This would indeed imply that, to repeat Mrs Thatcher, "there is no such thing as society"; but it would also imply that the attempt to create a shared morality as a public good will fail. Whatever the ultimate truth about human nature, a shared morality will bind only if it permeates relationships and so transforms atoms into citizens. Hence the only freedom which deserves the name is that of citizens to pursue the common good in their own way.

That will sound too like Rousseau for liberal comfort. But there have always been two ways to take *Le Contrat Social*. One makes the General Will central and works back to the individual citizen, whose freedom consists in humble obedience on pain of being forced to be free. The other is content to regard as the General Will *whatever* emerges from the free association of independent-minded citizens, who, be it noted, retain an individual will, enjoy private property and are not forced to be equal in an egalitarian sense. The liberal can, I hope, accept the pull of a positive notion of freedom which can be described as social freedom and yet combined with individuality.

Dewsbury parents, like others, want the best for their own children. If asked whether they care about other people's children, they can make the ambitious reply that it sums to the best for all children if the parents of each make a free choice for the good of their own. The Council wants the best for all children. If asked how this can be best for the children of the disaffected parents, it can make the ambitious reply that those parents are mistaken. Neither reply is compelling as it stands. The parents are content with a social order whose notion of equality of opportunity means a flying start for their own children. But this cannot mean a flying start for *all* children without changing the rules of competition. The Council is trying to change these rules and cannot easily maintain that *all* children will thereby have better chances. Conducted on this level, therefore, the dispute is so far unresolved.

I have not tried to resolve it directly. But I do hope to have complicated it. The parents are not the obvious champions of freedom because the only freedom which deserves the name is a positive one, which involves a common morality and shared conception of the good. The council, however, is not entitled to insist on an egalitarian conception of the good. The argument allows only something more nuanced, that even market freedom implies a measure of market equality and that human relationships in a free society start from a baseline of moral equity. Yet it follows that there is no inherent objection in the name of freedom to a policy of 'social mix'. Indeed it also follows, I submit, that some such policy is implicit in the very idea of a free society.

The crux is whether there is a public good involved which takes the form of a shared morality beyond the scope of a market theory of the social contract. If there is, and if it can flourish only by transforming market relations between social atoms into social relations between citizens, then the Dewsbury parents must look to their defences. My final word on freedom and equality is that all turns on the relation of rights to duties. The message of current individualism too often sounds as if rights come before duties, thus leaving it unclear why a rational agent should not shirk the duties whenever possible. But there is an older view of individuals, which says firmly that duties come before rights. In that case there *is* such a thing as society, and it should not be beyond the wit of individualists to recognise that individuals are social actors at heart. There is more to autonomy than consumer sovereignty.

Martin Hollis, School of Economic and Social Studies, University of East Anglia, Norwich NR4 7TJ, United Kingdom.

21

Paternalism and the Criminal Law

RICHARD TUR

ABSTRACT   *If it could be shown that law is, in some sense, a moral system the apparent contradiction between (moral) autonomy and (legal) heteronomy might be challenged. In order to prepare for such a challenge this paper questions the prevailing view that law is not in the business of enforcing morals. That is done primarily by using decisions of the criminal courts to show that the law does not always criminalise conduct merely to prevent harm to others. Paternalism is distinguished from the harm principle in order to show that the law (rightly or wrongly) sometimes seeks to secure that which is (thought to be) morally good, irrespective of the prevention of harm, at least overall harm.*

If such an insight is well founded there are consequences for legal theory in that neither of the ruling paradigms (naturalism and positivism) seems able adequately to accommodate the view of law which emerges. Consequently, an attempt is made in the essay to develop a middle theory of law, between naturalism and positivism, which is referred to as 'normative positivism'. The theory presented has, in turn, consequences for political practice. If law can be seen as community morality rather than as merely the morality of officials, then everyone has a stake in the moral content of law and there may be good moral reasons for disobeying official laws. Civil disobedience is the citizen's ultimate resort against the official morality that has appropriated to itself the eulogistic name of 'law'. That law may be seen as community morality also calls into question some ruling paradigms as to the nature of morality but, if the claim can be sustained, then the legal system may be seen as applied moral philosophy in action.

The general question which I seek to answer is whether law should be used for the enforcement of moral values. That, I take it, is itself a moral question. A well-known and powerfully advocated answer is that law should *not* be used solely for the purpose of enforcing moral values. Neil MacCormick has helpfully christened this answer as "the principle of moral disestablishment" [1]. The principle has been supported by John Stuart Mill and H. L. A. Hart primarily on the ground of individual liberty and the autonomy of the moral agent [2]. If moral values were enforced by law, heteronomy rather than autonomy would prevail. Liberalism thus draws upon the nature of the moral agent in order to limit the extent to which the state may pursue 'welfare' objectives. Anything beyond the minimalist encroachment (however defined) upon liberty leads inevitably, so it is thought, down the "road to serfdom" [3]. The acceptability of the principle of moral disestablishment therefore bears upon central issues not only in ethics and jurisprudence but also in political philosophy and practice especially given current tendencies to dismantle the welfare state.

MacCormick offers a list of examples against which we might test the principle of moral disestablishment:

(1) murder;
(2) assault;
(3) theft;
(4) abortion;
(5) obscenity;
(6) sodomy;
(7) adultery and fornication;
(8) cruelty to animals.

Now I take it that most people would regard some, if not all, of these as immoral and I hazard the guess that most people would regard most of the examples as involving greater or lesser degrees of immorality. Most of the examples, (4), (6) and (7) apart, are crimes according to English law. Can the existence of such crimes be justified *solely* by the fact (if fact it is) that the majority of people regard the conduct as morally wrong? Is positive morality the justification of criminal law? Moral disestablishmentarians must answer these questions negatively.

The principle is, of course, wholly negative; it states not what law-makers may do but merely what they may *not* do. As MacCormick observes, disestablishmentarians have usually offered the harm principle as the positive corollary. Different proponents have, of course, interpreted 'harm' differently. Not all have agreed with Mill that harm to others is the *only* ground for legislation. Feinberg usefully lists a range of possible justifications for encroaching upon liberty:

(1)(a) the private harm principle—prevent harm to others;
(1)(b) the public harm principle—prevent harm to essential institutions;
(2) the offence principle—prevent offence to others;
(3) legal paternalism—prevent harm to self;
(4) legal moralism—prevent sin or enforce morality;
(5) extreme paternalism—benefit self;
(6) the welfare principle—benefit others [4].

Unrepentant minimalists, advocating the night-watchman state, draw the line above (1)(b). Feinberg, himself, interprets Mill to include (1)(a) and (1)(b). Others go still further down the list. Hart, for example, includes both the offence principle and paternalism and thus draws a line between (3) and (4) though he still claims to be adopting the harm principle. This has appeared to some to proceed "far beyond the permissible limits of exegesis or even amendment" [5].

Notoriously, the powerful advocacy of Lord Devlin has been marshalled against all such principles. His profound point is that no *a priori* principles can be established to limit the legitimate scope of the criminal law. Thus there are no theoretical limitations upon law. In balancing conflicting values of law makers "... cannot be constrained by rule ... [or] suffer a definite limitation upon their powers" [6]. Lord Devlin is widely interpreted as an advocate of legal moralism, that is the view that there exists, independently of law, a coherent and identifiable common morality which it is the business of the law to enforce. It is not absurd to hold that a large and complex society requires common standards of conduct. *Ibi societas, ubi jus*—wherever there is society there is a right way and therefore a wrong way of doing things. If, however, it is Lord Devlin's case that there is some pre-existing, independent moral code or consensus, then I respectfully disagree. It is the *absence* of any such moral consensus in the modern national or multinational state which necessitates law. Law, it might be thought, would be redundant in the presence of complete moral consensus. In the absence of such consensus the law determines the conduct that ought to be in the face of particular and concrete problems. Such determination is tentative in the sense that it is hostage to acceptance but in many cases what the law determines becomes the current standard of conduct. Thus the law in general and the criminal law in particular can be represented as constitutive of a common morality. As MacCormick observes, the law does not *reflect* but it tends to *generate* a common morality. One might then regard law as the most comprehensive, extensive, articulated and detailed positive moral order of a community. Furthermore, it is the *dominant* positive morality although this dominance may be that of incorporation of societal values rather then exclusion. The law at various times has respected the autonomy of the church, of trade unions, of the family, of civil society and of individuals thereby, in a sense delegating crucial decision-making and thus incorporating values not of its own creation.

Whereas I part company from Lord Devlin in so far as he proposes an independent, fully-formed morality, I rejoin him in asserting that law is in some sense necessarily in the business of enforcing moral values. The consent of the victim is not universally treated as a defence in English criminal law. Murder is one obvious example. Consequently, euthanasia is regarded as a crime. Consider, next, this ancient case reported by Coke in 1604:

> a young and lustie rogue, to make himself impotent, thereby to have the more colour to begge or to be relieved without putting himself to any labour, caused his companion to strike off his left hand [7].

Both were convicted of mayhem. More recently, in *Bravery* v. *Bravery* (1954) Lord Denning M.R. (as he then was) observed of a sterilisation operation:

> when it is done for a just cause, it is quite lawful, as, for instance...to prevent an hereditary disease; but when it is done without just cause it is unlawful, even though the man consents to it. Take a case where a sterilisation operation is done so as to enable a man to have the pleasure of sexual intercourse without shouldering the responsibilities attaching to it. The operation is then plainly injurious to the public interest [8].

Another example is *Donovan* (1934) [9]. Here the defendant, for his own sexual gratification, beat a 17-year-old girl with a cane in circumstances of indecency. The evidence suggested that the girl had gone willingly with the defendant to his garage in full knowledge of his perversion and ready to submit to it. Nonetheless, Donovan was convicted of both common assault and indecent assault. The Court of Appeal acquitted on a misdirection but upheld the legal proposition that if the blows were likely or intended to cause bodily harm then the defendant is guilty even though the victim fully consented. In *Attorney-General's Reference (No. 6 of 1980)* [10] the Court of Appeal held that where two men agree to settle their dispute by a 'square go' both are guilty of assault. Thus most fights are unlawful regardless of consent.

Finally, I turn to the very recent decision of the Court of Appeal in *R.* v. *Tan* [11]. Miss Tan had advertised in 'contact magazines' as follows:

> Humiliation enthusiast, my favourite pastime is humiliating and disciplining mature male submissives, in strict bondage, lovely tan coloured mistress

invites humble applicants, T.V., C.P., B., D. and rubber wear. 12 noon to 7. p.m., Mon. to Fri. Basement Flat 89 Warwick Way, Victoria SW1.

The law report records:

> The services provided at ... [the] premises were of a particularly revolting and perverted kind. Straightforward sexual intercourse was not provided at all. With the aid of a mass of equipment, some manual (such as whips and chains), some mechanical and some electrical, clients were subjected, at their own wish and with their full consent, to a variety of forms of humiliation, flagellation, bondage and torture, accompanied often by masturbation.

Miss Tan could not be charged with running a brothel because she worked alone in her basement flat. She was charged with and convicted of running a disorderly house, sentenced to 18 months imprisonment and subjected to a property confiscation order in respect of the apparatus. In order to secure this conviction the trial court itself had to massage the current legal definition of a 'disorderly house' which hitherto has always involved some element of concurrent multiplicity of parties. The jury were directed:

> a single prostitute who provides services in private premises to one client at a time without spectators is guilty of the common law offence of keeping a disorderly house if it is proved that the services provided are of such a character and are conducted in such a manner ... that their provision amounts to an outrage of public decency or is otherwise calculated to harm the public interest to such an extent as to call for condemnation and punishment.

On appeal, the Court of Appeal upheld the new definition of a disorderly house, upheld the direction to the jury, upheld the property confiscation order but reduced the custodial sentence to six months which is, as it happens, the statutory maximum for running a brothel, a consideration which influenced the same court in *R. v. Payne* [12]. Then, in open recognition of the novelty of the charge and the conviction, and the circumstance that Tan genuinely believed herself to be operating within current criminal law, the Court of Appeal suspended the custodial sentence for two years with, however, a stern warning that others offending in like manner would receive immediate and substantial custodial sentences [13].

Lord Devlin's response to cases which override the victim's consent is that the law is thereby enforcing moral values, rather than adopting the harm principle. He writes, "there is only one explanation—there are certain standards of behaviour or moral principles which society requires to be observed", for example sanctity of life and the physical integrity of the person. He therefore argues that the function of the criminal law is clearly revealed in such cases; it is "to enforce a moral principle and nothing else" [14].

Hart's response is to deny what Lord Devlin asserts. All such cases are examples of legal paternalism and "paternalism is a perfectly coherent policy" [15]. And, of course, it is. But like the harm principle itself, paternalism needs some notion of 'harm' in order to bite. Most people would, I suppose, regard killing and maiming other human beings as 'harmful'. Surely only philosophers, professionally disposed to doubt, could question a proposition so self-evident. Yet a moment's reflection reveals that there is no one-to-one relationship between 'harm' and death or between physical injury and 'harm'. Legal systems of my acquaintance allow for cases of justifiable homicide as, for example, in self-defence [16]. The euthanasia lobby clearly does not regard death as necessarily a 'harm' and death with dignity might justifiably be regarded as a good worth striving for. Coke's "lustie rogue" clearly did not regard maim as an unqualified harm nor can surgical operations which remove organs or limbs necessarily be regarded as 'harms'. It is at least doubtful whether any significant 'harm' is present in the case of a 'square go' and in *Donovan* the evidence suggested only that there were seven or eight red marks on the girl's buttocks. Clearly not all reasonable men would regard a vasectomy as 'harmful' and I suppose that it would be a feat of unparalleled perspicacity to detect 'harm' in the *Tan* case. And even if there is some 'harm' in such cases it is far from clear that there is 'harm' overall. If there is not, then either these cases are wrongly decided or, if right, some justification other than 'harm' must be sought.

Devotees of paternalism who seek to maintain that paternalism is consistent with the harm principle could argue that cases which exhibit no significant harm do not fall within the paternalist principle and have therefore been wrongly decided in the courts. This may appear rather like an *ad hoc* immunisation of a suspect thesis. The paternalist principle *is* suspect because it offers no explanation of why some values, including the prevention of freely chosen harms to self, are to be preferred to the value of freedom. Labelling the policy of the law 'paternalism' does not explain why it is sometimes right to override individual choices. Nor does it explain why, in the face of identical harms, for example, death or physical injury, it is sometimes appropriate for the law to adopt a dual posture, criminalising some deaths and physical injuries and legitimating others. Only with some reason for overriding freedom and only with some explanation of the different reaction to identical harms can paternalism be "a perfectly coherent policy". Since (at least in my scheme of things) freedom is a moral value, reasons for overriding it must be moral reasons. Further, the decision whether there are *any* circumstances in which deliberately killing or injuring other human beings is justified is irreducibly a moral decision. Consequently the paternalist covertly presupposes moral principles and his policy cannot be applied independently of these. It is the suppressed moral presuppositions which determine the issues and not the presence or absence of harm. Therefore paternalism is "a perfectly coherent policy" only by virtue of moral presuppositions. Thus paternalism is itself a moral principle and its admission into the justification of the criminal law is inconsistent with the principle of moral disestablishment.

The argument that paternalism is based not upon 'harm' but upon morality would be more strongly made out if it could be shown that 'harm' itself is irreducibly a morally loaded concept. MacCormick offers such an argument. Surveying his examples, he concludes that murder, assault and theft obviously ought to be punished under the harm principle and are so regarded by the majority of its devotees. Abortion ought to be punished only if the fetus is regarded as a person. I pause to remark that *that* is, of course, contested, which reveals that it is not the 'harm' but a prior moral commitment which informs the law. Returning to MacCormick's survey, cruelty to animals ought to be punished if "harm" is extended to all sentient beings. Obscenity ought to be punished only if it causes offence and thus, so long as sex-shops come in plain brown wrappers, no sanction is appropriate. Adultery would only be punishable if it were regarded as a harm to the cuckold. Sodomy and fornication would not call for punishment at all on the harm principle.

Presumably MacCormick would treat prostitution, lesbianism and sexual perversion in a similar manner. He observes that the criminal law tends to follow this analysis pretty closely and that crimes not fitting the principle have been seen as objects of law reform. Thus Wolfenden and Williams. Clearly the harm principle has been influential.

Looking only at murder, MacCormick observes that few would argue that the deliberate killing of another human being is not morally wrong. Consequently, in this case at least, the harm principle justifies punishing conduct which is (also) immoral. The same argument could be put as forcibly regarding assault with intent to do grievous bodily harm. In such cases the criminal law is enforcing moral values and it therefore contradicts the principle of moral disestablishment. Obviously one response for disestablishmentarians is that this is merely a coincidence. *The* reason, they might re-affirm, for punishment is the harm, not the immorality. It is an accidental not a necessary property of the conduct that it is immoral. I am not persuaded. Nor is MacCormick.

He argues, first, that harm itself is a morally loaded and essentially contested concept. He observes that the harm principle necessarily presupposes a prior determination of legitimate private interests and a conception of the public good. In passing, it can be added that if one, with Feinberg, interprets Mill as embracing 1(a) *and* 1(b) then the harm principle is internally indeterminate because it provides for no resolution of conflicts between private interests and the public good. In any event the principle can only bite if such interests and goods are, as it were, given. But such interests and goods are not given. They must be determined. Such determination of private interests and the public good and their relative merits irreducibly involves making moral choices. MacCormick instances theft. Most advocates of the harm principle hold it, together with murder and assault, as falling foursquare within the sphere of legitimate legal prohibition. Theft is, however, rather obviously parasitic upon the concept of property. The question whether an individual's interest in property is legitimate is a moral question. Furthermore the definition of theft in English law includes a requirement of dishonesty which, as things stand, is a question of fact for the jury. Thus theft is defined by reference to a moral criterion [17].

My comment on these three examples (murder, assault and theft) is that it does appear that the criminal law is dependent upon moral values such as the sanctity of life, physical integrity and inviolability of property. Such values are legitimated or ratified by the moral-and-legal order. Indeed, as Hart suggests, given some fairly obvious truisms abut the human predicament, it is difficult to imagine a moral-and-legal order enduring if it does not uphold such values to some extent [18]. Different moral-and-legal orders concretise these values in particular and practical applications rather differently. Circumstances constituting murder in Scotland do not constitute murder in England [19]. What is theft in Victoria may not be theft in England [20]. Even so, the point remains that without *some* conception of legitimate interests or values the harm principle simply cannot be applied. The harm principle therefore presupposes and is parasitic upon some conceptions of a just ordering of persons, actions and things. Consequently such criminal laws as are justified by the harm principle do not merely *coincide* with positive morality; these laws are *necessarily* related to the protection of interests and values which are legitimated by current positive morality. Some interests and values, such as the sanctity of life and physical integrity, are so embedded in positive morality as to require an earthquake to shake them. Others are more fragile and susceptible of alteration by a moral pioneer winning the hearts and minds of the people.

MacCormick's second argument against the harm principle rests upon his conception of the nature of punishment. The harm principle is, after all, a principle justifying punishment. MacCormick adopts a widely canvassed but currently dormant account, namely, the expressive theory of punishment [21]. On such a view, punishment can be regarded as an expressive and symbolic act, evincing an attitude of very serious disapprobation. Theorists of punishment frequently ignore parental punishment of children. MacCormick does not. He suggests that when a parent punishes a child this does not merely invest conduct with harmful consequences; it also evinces the parent's serious *disapproval.* MacCormick acknowledges that punishment by the law is altogether more complex. The law is the millenary labour of many heads, hearts and hands. Yet the law is also in some sense an organised and purposive system. In deciding to stigmatise conduct as criminal, the law maker bespeaks *his* judgment that the conduct in question is somehow reprehensible and worthy of disapprobation. When a judge imposes sentence he can be seen as expressing public disapprobation. Judges certainly do claim to be imposing *society's* values but it bears repeating that society has no coherent and systematic values, independent of the system of values institutionalised in the law. Consequently, judges, whatever they may say, may be interpreted as evincing the law's disapprobation of the conduct in question. Punishment, therefore, can be interpreted as the expression of moral attitudes.

MacCormick can therefore draw the conclusion that the harm principle directly contemplates the immoral quality of immoral acts. Consequently the harm principle is incompatible with the principle of moral disestablishment. His conclusion is, I think, fortified by the considerations raised in the treatment of paternalism and the law's reaction to the victim's consent. The matter can be put even more strongly. Those who jointly espouse moral disestablishment and the harm principle (even broadly interpreted to include offence and paternalism) presuppose a false moral ontology. They appear to believe that there exist, independently of legal rule or moral principle, identifiable harms, finite in number and fixed in form. They then suppose that the law maker may take in his left hand a list of such pre-legal, extra-moral harms and produce in his right hand the equivalent list of criminal laws. But such harms do not exist independently of and prior to law and morals. Harm is not only a morally loaded and essentially contested concept; it is also a rule-dependent concept. Far from harm existing independently of and prior to legal and moral rules as a condition, identifiable and determinate harm is a consequence of moral and legal rules. Only if the moral and legal rules are known can one determine whether or not a particular event constitutes harm. Thus the harm principle, like the social contract, is viciously circular. One can extract from it only what one has tacitly projected into it. Therefore the harm principle is incapable of determining a line between legitimate and illegitimate uses of coercion.

If, then, the law is necessarily in the business of enforcing moral values the question is not whether but what values it should enforce. That, too, is a moral question. MacCormick's answer is that law should enforce other-regarding moral values but not self-regarding moral values. I remain to be persuaded that this classification is any sharper than the notoriously opaque distinction between 'public' and 'private' activities canvassed by many disestablishmentarians. However it is clear that the demolition of the harm principle and the principle of moral disestablishment opens the way for laws which, upon threat of punishment, seek not to prevent harm but to benefit self and others. The welfare principle explains what the harm principle excludes, for example, compulsory schooling, compulsory national insurance contributions and compulsory taxation to provide health, education, housing and employment for members of a civilised and caring community.

The view of law canvassed in this essay, namely that law is the dominant positive morality of a community, calls for some explanation and defence because it does not seem to fit readily into any of the established paradigms. Legal theory has long been bedevilled by a sterile debate between positivists and natural lawyers. The debate has been sterile because each side has begged the question by assuming itself to be correct. But of course natural law theory is false judged by positivist assumptions just as positivism is false judged by natural law assumptions. Since no further theory is available whereby the competitors might be assessed legal theory appears to have reached an impasse. Here I can merely indicate how an alternative theory might be constructed. I shall attempt to demonstrate that a synthesis of positivism and natural law is possible and that what I shall call 'normative positivism' is consistent with the account of law canvassed in this essay. Ideal-typically, positivism may be characterised by its use of such notions as 'fact', 'will', 'power', 'instrumentalism', 'discretion', '*mala prohibita*', etc. The dialetical contraries to these notions are 'value', 'reason', 'authority', 'legitimacy', 'deduction', '*mala in se*', etc. These characterise natural law thinking. If positivism and natural law, ideally conceived, represent the end points on a spectrum, 'normative positivism' might occupy a middle position. Various authors can be placed notionally at different points on the spectrum depending on how closely they approach the ideal model of positivism or natural law. The idea can be illustrated schematically:

POSITIVISM	'NORMATIVE POSITIVISM'	NATURAL LAW
◄──►
no ought	formal ought	material ought
fact		value
will		reason
power		authority
instrumentalism		legitimacy
discretion		deduction
mala prohibita		*mala in se*
Bentham	Hart Kelsen	Blackstone
Austin	Aquinas [Finnis]	Fuller
Scandinavian Realism		Dworkin
American Realism		

Of course actual authors are dialectically difficult to classify and my examples are fairly arbitrarily drawn, the diagram being illustrative rather than an exercise in exegesis. For present purposes it suffices to concentrate on two important aspects of the diagram, the discretion-deduction spectrum and the nature of the 'ought'. Natural law thinking is characterised by two major problems: first, the identification of its fundamental principle or principles and, secondly, the correct application of such principles to fact situations. I shall allow my hypothetical ideal natural lawyer his fundamental prinicple or principles and enter no objections as to the difficulties of conflicts between, and priorities amongst, fundamental principles where more than one is in question. *All* such principles are general and abstract and even if there were complete agreement as to *the* principle the problem of application to particular and concrete facts would remain.

John Finnis criticises positivists for attributing to natural law thinking a wholly deductive methodology such that given the fundamental principle as major premise and a statement of fact as minor premise the one right answer pops out automatically. Finnis remarks that the relationship between principles and decisions is too complex to be characterised as pure deduction and nothing else [22]. This is no new thought and many theorists, although moving from quite different assumptions, could readily give assent. Holmes, for example, held that "General propositions do not decide particular cases" [23]. Hart exhorts us that "we should not cherish even as an ideal a rule so detailed that no new choices arise at the point of application" [24]. Unger remarks that "language is no longer credited with the fixidity of categories and the transparent representation of the world that would make formalism plausible in legal reasoning or in ideas about justice" [25]. Kelsen insists that "every law-applying act is only partly determined by law" [26] and presents actual legal systems as a synthesis of formal, static deduction and informal, dynamic determination. It is, therefore, difficult to find and exhibit in captivity a pure deductivist.

Finnis explains that Aquinas regarded law as consisting in part of rules which are "derived from natural law like conclusions deduced from principles" and for the rest of "rules which are derived from natural laws like implementations [*determinationes*] of general directives" [27]. Finnis observes in a footnote that there is no happy English equivalent of "*determinatio*" but suggests that "implementation" is more elegant then Kelsen's "concretisation" [28]. What Finnis does not comment upon is the remarkable similarity between this doctrine and the Kelsenian account of the legal norm or rule as a 'frame' within which a range of determinations is possible [29]. Thus it would appear that Kelsen and Aquinas agree that law sometimes involves applications of general rules by way of subsumption of the particular under the general, that is a deductive process, and sometimes concretisation by way of delegation and determination. Kelsen distinguishes, as ideal types, 'static' and 'dynamic' systems. A static system is one in which the content of all individual applications of the rules is at least tacitly contained within the general rules and principles and is discoverable therefore by a purely intellectual process. By contrast, a dynamic system involves delegation to the law maker of the determination of the content of the decision. For Kelsen, the dynamic principle is characteristic of legal positivism which understands law to be in some sense a product of human acts and decisions rather than a deduction from timeless and immutable principles. However, he also acknowledges that any actual legal system synthesises the static and the dynamic principles. Kelsen further holds, in one of his most mysterious doctrines, that the primacy of the principle of delegation means that even a determination *outside* the frame is valid and binding unless and until set aside by a higher decision. Thus for Kelsen as for legal positivism in general, law can have any content [30].

Clearly these Kelsenian doctrines go well beyond what Finnis would concede on behalf of Aquinas. However it is difficult to see how, having once admitted determinations into his system, Aquinas can hold the line against such Kelsenian conclusions. Finnis illustrates the notion of a determination by the example of an architect's instructions to an artificer to put a 'doorway' in a wall of a building [31]. Clearly there are minimum and maximum dimensions without which no opening in a human habitation can count as a 'doorway'. Equally clearly the doorway when installed must have precise dimensions. Since these dimensions cannot be read off intellectually from the concept of doorway, the artificer, by decision, determines the general and abstract instruction in its particular and concrete application. The important thing to note about this example is just how favourable it is to the general natural law case which Finnis, I take it, is at pains to defend. All that has been conceded so far is that law, consistent with natural law methodology, can have, within limits, a variable content. It does not follow that law can have *any* content. However, 'doorway' is a concept exhibiting what I shall call 'middle order generality', that is a concept the descriptive content of which is relatively clearly defined. Clearly not all determinations of the artificer could reasonably be regarded as doorways and even more clearly should be step outside the "frame" and instal a window no one could reasonably regard that as a determination of the architect's concept.

However, another example given by Finnis is somewhat more problematical. He correctly observes that "if material goods are to be used efficiently for human well-being there must be a regime of private property" [32]. He acknowledges that precisely what rules of property there should be is undetermined by this "general requirement of justice" and he also concedes that the choice of rules will be to some extent arbitrary. Even so, Finnis remains committed to the proposition that in determining the concept of property the legislator's choice cannot be regarded as wholly unfettered or arbitrary. With respect, this is altogether less plausible with 'property' than with 'doorway'. Even allowing Finnis his large claim that *private* property is a general requirement of justice it must be evident that a remarkably wide range of possible determinations presents itself to the legislator. Once the legislator's choice is admitted as a source of content it is entirely possible that two positive legislators will not only determine a concept differently but will determine a concept in a contradictory fashion. It is one thing to concede, as Finnis does, that the determination of the general requirements of justice leaves open a variable content but it is quite another if the concession is held to entail that, given determination, *any* content is possible. Indeed, if it could be shown that any content is possible consistent with the general requirements of justice then 'justice' or 'natural law' would be stripped of its crucial function whereby that which does not exhibit conformity of content with 'justice' or with 'natural law' is disqualified as law or, at least, is in some way a law less compelling upon conscience.

It seems to me possible to demonstrate that some of the general requirements of justice are compatible with any determination including mutually contradictory determinations. The quintessential formulation of justice is "live honestly, harm no one and render to each his due". This is not the doctrine adopted by Finnis and I would have to show that the arguments canvassed here could be applied equally effectively to the very much more sophisticated account presented in *Natural Law and Natural Rights*. However, the classical formulation serves as an initial and simplified target. Presumably, the law maker must determine the content of these general requirements of justice. Suppose, as I have already indicated, the law makers in England and Victoria have determined the concept of 'honesty' not only differently but in such a manner that on identical facts an individual would be 'dishonest' and therefore liable to conviction for theft in Victoria but 'honest' and therefore fall to be acquitted in England. I believe something like this to be the case [33]. Can one accept that both decisions are determinations of the concept of 'honesty'? If so, then the whole edifice so carefully reconstructed by Finnis is in danger of collapse. Once logical contradiction is admitted to a system of proposition any other proposition and its negation can be proved to be true by virtue of the rules of formal logic [34]. Consequently, Finnis must either deny that one or other of the mutually contradictory determinations is a genuine determination or accept that his account of natural law is, ultimately, consistent with any positive law whatever. If he admits that his account of natural law is consistent with any positive law whatever he has, in my submission, conceded that natural law, like positive law, can have any content. Then, of course, any critical function which natural law might be supposed to have in constraining the content of positive law is dissolved and Finnis's natural law with a variable and changing content is revealed as serving the purely ideological function of justification and not an epistemological function in relation to the moral-and-legal system.

Similar considerations present themselves as regards "rendering to each his due". Suppose the law makers in England and in Scotland have determined differently the question whether a man is entitled to whatever another has gratuitously promised. Again, I believe something like this to be the case [35]. Are both genuine determinations of a man's due? If so, natural law is again exposed as consistent with any possible content of positive law and it thereby loses its critical function. If not, as with 'honesty', the onus remains on Finnis to explain what, consistent with his methodology, distinguishes genuine or legitimate determinations from false or illegitimate determinations. If this burden is not discharged one may conclude that there is very little difference indeed between some versions of positivism and Finnis's account of natural law. This suspicion is reinforced by another concession whereby Finnis allows that an unjust law may be a *law* for all that [36]. Of course if determination is as open-ended as I have argued it is, in the absence of any criterion to distinguish the genuine from the false determination, no positive law could be unjust because every positive law, whatever its content, being a determination of the natural law, will necessarily be consistent with the natural law and therefore valid. It follows that it is at least possible in principle to regard some versions of positivism and some versions of natural law as tending towards a middle position on my spectrum. Both Kelsen and Aquinas acknowledge the role of determination and subsumption and both regard positive law as normative in the sense that it consists of precepts intimating how men ought to behave under particular circumstances. Doubtless Finnis would be disposed to argue that Kelsen (unlike Aquinas) allows that law may have *any* content whatever but if the general requirements of justice are indeed so indeterminate as to allow even of mutually contradictory determinations then this objection falls. Further, the quaint Kelsenian point that the law maker can determine outside the frame cannot offer Finnis much of a target because if the frame is as indeterminate as to admit of mutually contradictory determinations then the distinction between a determination within and a determination without the frame is meaningless.

As to "harming no one", arguments have already been presented to the effect that 'harm', being a rule-dependent concept, is indeterminate unless and until moral principles or legal rules are brought into play to define with greater or lesser precision the legitimate interests and the general good. It appeared that even death does not necessarily constitute a 'harm'. Whether the physical fact of death is a 'harm' depends upon circumstances. Thus to those who favour euthanasia death is not a 'harm'. There is therefore no direct inference ticket from physical harm to harm normatively defined. Thus the general requirement of justice, "harm no one" is utterly indeterminate and can accommodate the content of any positive law whatever in so far as 'harm' is not a precondition of a legal rule or moral principle but a consequence of the definitions of legitimate interests and the common good established by such rules and principles.

So far, I have attempted in limited compass to render plausible the claim that an account of law which synthesises salient features of natural law and positivism is possible. A detailed exposition and defence would require considerably more ingenuity and effort. The argument thus far can be fortified by a consideration of the nature of the 'ought'. The schematic account suggested that legal positivism first presented law as reducible to fact without remainder. Such (fact-based) theorists sought to reduce law to one or other favoured fact. Austin thus reduced law to the psychological fact of command and American Realism is associated with the predictive account of law. Hart's most significant criticism of both is that they leave no or little room for a normative conception of law. One cannot, he says, arrive at the normative concept of a rule from the factual elements of commands and habits of obedience. Thus, crude or naive positivism might well be characterised as including no 'ought' whatever. Natural law thinking, however, is overtly normative and therefore includes an 'ought'. The 'ought' of natural law thinking is, in my view, irreducibly a material 'ought', that is to say that somehow the 'ought' of natural law predetermines to some extent what can be the content of an 'ought' statement.

Consider the related concept of 'good' as an illustration. The notion of a 'good thumbscrew' is troublesome if the meaning of 'good' is not exhausted by 'efficient' and if, but only if, 'good' necessarily imports some generalised conception of human welfare. If one operates with such a material concept of 'good' then the idea of a 'good thumbscrew' is a contradiction in terms. A formal concept of 'good' would be wholly indeterminate as to content such that anything, irrespective of its impact upon human welfare, could be characterised as 'good'. 'Good' on such a formal account is wholly indefinable *a priori* because, to adopt Moore's reasoning, moral propositions would otherwise be tautologies or self-contradictions [37]. The argument as to 'ought' is similar. Natural law thinking adopts an 'ought' which somehow incorporates some material content such that, for example, the statement "You ought to kill" is not merely immoral but incoherent. I seek to contrast that material 'ought' with a formal 'ought' whichis a necessary element in the theory of law which I shall refer to as 'normative positivism'. Such an utterly formal and indefinable concept of 'ought' is necessary if law is to be regarded as normative and if the positivist proposition that law may have any content is to be sustained.

One could then regard law conceptually as, initially, a wholly empty series of 'ought'—formulae, to which content is added not by any logical deductions from some fundamental principles or from any material content lurking within the 'ought' itself but from the act and decisions of the law makers in a society. What content the law has would then be entirely a contingent and empirical matter dependent upon the values, beliefs, intuitions, ideals, interests and emotions of whosoever has the law making function in hand. But even the most detailed body of laws will still themselves require concretisation in particular applications and the final stage of law creation is the actual human conduct that occurs. In a sense, therefore one may adopt Hare's significant point that what people *do* is a matter of some importance [38]. Not only may law influence human conduct but human conduct may influence the content of the law. It follows, too, for anyone who refuses to believe that universalizability is a necessary element in the meaning of 'ought' as it is in that of 'all', that such a normative system, replete with content flowing from the 'millenary labour' of many heads, hearts and hands, constantly in flux, but also sufficiently determinate to guide conduct, may be regarded as a socially valid, positive system of morality [39]. If so, 'normative positivism' legitimates the view that law is *necessarily* in the business of upholding moral values. With a formal 'ought' it seems possible to move from the anormativity of crude, fact-based positivism to a position short of the material 'ought' of natural law and thus, as we saw in regard to determination so with the 'ought', a theory occupying a middle position between classical positivism and classical natural law appears possible.

The formal 'ought' may look rather too like an artificial construct brought in to make the theory work and some might well wonder how the special functional legal 'ought' could simultaneously be regarded, as I purport to regard it, as a *moral* 'ought'. On this point I pray Kelsen in aid, "... in this relative sense, every law is moral; every law constitutes a—relative—moral value. And this means; the question about the relationship between law and morals is not a question about the content of the law but one about its form" [40]. Hart's account of law may be interpreted in similar fashion. Others have observed that, for a 'positivist', he makes significant concessions to natural law thought [41]. But it is not merely the minimal content of natural law which supports such a view. Consider Hart's account of what it is for a social rule to exist and his distinction between the internal and the external points of view [42]. The crucial point about rules, as opposed to habits, is the critical reflective attitude which *justifies* hostile reactions and, ultimately, sanctions. In a 'healthy' legal system the citizens and the officials alike exhibit such an internal attitude. Even in a healthy society, however, it is enough that the officials accept the secondary rules of recognition, adjudication and change and that the citizens acquiesce [43]. Since 'acceptance', for Hart, involves a critical, hostile attitude, his concept of law comes very close to being the morality of the legal officials of the society or even the morality of the 'ruling class'.

Such a vision of law, as the morality of the ruling officials, must strike many as unattractive in that it distances the citizens from the law and thereby leads to feelings of impotence and alienation. Although there is no relationship of entailment between legal positivism and liberalism the two are mutually supportive and as long as law is perceived as a non-moral datum the principle of moral disestablishment is the more secure. Normative positivism challenges the principle of moral disestablishment by asserting what legal positivists deny, namely that there is a *necessary* connection between law and positive morality. At the same time, by refusing to adopt a material 'ought', normative positivism radically separates itself from any suggestion that there is a necessary connection between law and any critical morality. Unless they commit the naturalistic fallacy, all critical moralities, utilitarianism just as much as natural law, rest upon an unproved and unprovable axiom. Mill's famous 'proof' is unpersuasive as all such proofs must be, given either the infinite regress of supposed justification higher than the ultimate justification or the viciously circular proposition that the ultimate justification is, illogically, its own justification [44].

All the foregoing has consequences for political practice. Ultimately there is a dialectic between the current content of the positive moral-and-legal order and the actual 'intuitions', common sense beliefs, gut feelings, emotions, ideals or interests of *individuals* who are, in my view of things, the sole bearers of moral commitments. From a democratic point of view, these 'intuitions' ought to be brought to bear upon the content of the law. The good legal system would provide mechanisms for informing the content of the law of the current standards of ordinary decent people. Thus the theory of law canvassed in this essay leads on to a series of political and constitutional reforms. In any case, from a pragmatic point of view, these 'intuitions' must necessarily influence the content of the law. Ultimately, the law can endure only if it attracts sufficient support from enough individuals. Such support is measured less by what people say and more by what people do. Consequently, law breaking in order to alter the law is a legitimate option. Consider the posture struck first by students and subsequently by lecturers at the Polytechnic of North London that (a) the National Front is an organisation undeserving of the freedoms and rights normally secured in a liberal democratic society and (b) that a tutor's loyalty to his students is such that imprisonment might be morally preferable to its breach. Consider also the behaviour of Mr Arthur Scargill and the miners widely reported at the time of writing. It is not difficult to understand that the miners are unhappy because the labour laws were framed by a sectional interest with a particular axe to grind against them. Where laws diverge significantly from the ideals, interests or intuitions of their addresses there will be pressure to change the law and such pressure will manifest itself in behaviour, all the more so where the beliefs are deeply held. Lord Devlin catches the point perfectly:

> there is a natural respect for opinions which are sincerely held. When such opinions accumulate enough weight, the law must either yield or it is broken. In a democratic society there is a strong tendency for it to yield—not to abandon all defences so as to let in the horde, but to give ground to those who are prepared to fight for something they prize. To fight may be to suffer. A willingness to suffer is the most convincing proof of sincerity. Without the law there would be no proof. The law is the anvil upon which the hammer strikes [45].

There is, however, another side to law breaking in order to change the law and Lord Devlin is wholly alert to it. First, he observes that "Society must be the judge of what is necessary to its own integrity if only because there is no other tribunal to which the question can be submitted" [46]. Secondly, there is "the understanding in the heart of every man that he must not condemn what another does unless he honestly considers it to be a threat to the integrity or good government of . . . [his] society" [47]. Of course, thirdly, "there may be times in the future, as there have been in the past, when a man has to set himself up against society. But if he does so, he must expect to find the law on the side of society. If in his struggle he is armed with a good conscience, he must put his trust, firstly, in the rightness of his conviction, secondly, in the knowledge that nothing that law-makers and lawyers can do can fetter the mind of man, only his body; and last but not least, in the certainty that law can be made effective only through human agents and that a law that is truly tyrannical will not for long command the services of free men" [49]. Consequently he who would break the law in order to change it must recognise that if the value he pursues is less than the value he challenges in his attempt to change the law he is more than likely to fail. It follows that violence is almost always a fruitless mode of civil disobedience, simply because personal integrity is so deeply entrenched a value in our society, and that the more directly the law addresses an individual's conduct the better is he placed to thwart it by his policy of non-co-operation, precisely because the disobedience will necessarily be directly associated with the law in question.

In this paper I have tried to show that law, especially criminal law, may be understood as the positive morality of a community. As such, law is necessarily in the business of enforcing moral values, and principles that counsel otherwise, such as the principle of moral disestablishment and the harm principle, fall to be rejected. In so far as legal positivism involves either (i) a wholly fact-based approach to law or (ii) a radical separation of law and morals, then it, too, falls to be rejected, or at least qualified in order to bring out that law is indeed a system of moral values. The most significant argument awaiting response is that law cannot be 'moral' because law is jurisdictionally limited in its sphere of validity whereas morality is universally applicable in time and space. Indeed, powerful arguments have been advanced to the effect that universalizability is the distinctive feature of the moral 'ought' and therefore that law consists not of moral norms but merely of imperatives [49]. One response is to argue that legal rules and decisions are no less universalizable than moral rules and decisions [50]. This I reject as descriptively false of legal systems or, at best, trivially true [51]. Rather, I ask *why* must one accept that the moral 'ought' is necessarily universalizable? Surely particular moral judgments are possible; e.g. "Richard Tur ought to tell Dick Hare the truth on Sunday, 27 May 1984, between 12 noon and 3.30 p.m. at the White House, Isle of Thorns". Given that this is a moral judgment or norm, then the argument would be whether it is validated by some universalizable 'ought' such as that everyone, always and in all circumstances ought to tell the truth. That is a moral judgment which I do not share, but the example reveals that the allegedly formal criterion of universalizability may incorporate a substantive or material element rather as natural law thinking, as explained in this essay, may be said to do. Nor is the universalizable 'ought' saved by a parenthetical interpolation after 'everyone' to the effect of his being like Richard Tur in the relevant respects save the position. First, because what the *relevant* respects are calls for further moral judgment and, secondly, because there may be a morally significant sense in which individuals are unique. Introducing criteria such as universalizability or rationality into the *definition* of morality [52] relegates positive morality to *mores*, merely, and positive law to fact, alone. Simultaneously, it elevates critical morality to the exclusive status of morality, properly so-called. I reject the definitionalist claim so to stipulate a meaning for 'morality' such as to exclude sociologically valid systems of positive morality and positive law and to include only a sociologically invalid critical morality such as, say, natural law thinking or utilitarianism. Thus the concept of law that I am at pains to defend may involve challenging ruling paradigms as to the nature of morality [53]. I am fortified in my prejudice that law may be understood as the positive morality of a community by the following observation, recently come to hand: "The law itself, binding on everyone in society, whatever their beliefs, is the embodiment of a common moral position. It sets out a broad framework for what is morally acceptable within society" [54].

Richard Tur, Oriel College, Oxford OX1 4EN, United Kingdom.

NOTES

[1] MacCormick, Neil (1982) Against moral disestablishment, in: MacCormick, Neil (1982) *Legal Right and Social Democracy*, Ch. 2, pp. 18–38 (Oxford, Clarendon Press).

[2] MILL, JOHN STUART (1859) On liberty, in: McCALLUM, R.B. (Ed.) (1946) *On Liberty and Considerations on Representative Government* (Oxford, Blackwell); HART, H.L.A. (1962) *Law, Liberty and Morality* (Oxford, Oxford University Press). This work is referred to subsequently as 'LLM'.

[3] HAYEK, F.A. (1944) *The Road to Serfdom* (London, Routledge & Kegan Paul).

[4] FEINBERG, JOEL (1973) *Social Philosophy*, Ch. 2 (Englewood Cliffs, N.J., Prentice-Hall).

[5] DEVLIN, PATRICK (1965) *The Enforcement of Morals*, p. 138 (Oxford, Oxford University Press). This work is referred to subsequently as 'EM'.

[6] EM, 117.

[7] Co. Inst. 127a & b.

[8] [1954] 3 All E.R. 59, 67–68.

[9] [1934] KB 498.

[10] [1981] 2 All E.R. 1059.

[11] [1983] 2 All E.R. 12.

[12] (1980) 2 Cr App Rep (S) 161.

[13] TUR, RICHARD (1978) Varieties of overruling and judicial law-making; prospective overruling in a comparative perspective, *Juridicial Review*, pp. 33–64.

[14] EM, 8.

[15] LLM, 31–32.

[16] cf. *Cousins* [1982] 2 All E.R. 115.

[17] See TUR, RICHARD (1985) Dishonesty and the jury, in: Phillips Griffiths, A. (Ed.) 1985, *Philosophy and Practice*, pp. 75–96 (Cambridge, Cambridge University Press).

[18] HART, H.L.A. (1961) *The Concept of Law*, pp. 189–195 (Oxford, Clarendon Press); this work is referred to subsequently as 'CL'.

[19] See *Hyam* [1975] AC 55, *Majewski* [1976] 2 All E.R. 142, *Caldwell* [1982] AC 341; cf *Brennan* 1977 S.L.T. 151.

[20] *Salvo* [1980] V.R. 401; see ELLIOT, D.W. (1982) Dishonesty in theft; a dispensable concept, *Criminal Law Review*, pp. 395–410; cf TUR, RICHARD (1983) Dishonesty and the jury [note 17 refers].

[21] FEINBERG, JOEL (1970) *Doing and Deserving*, ch. 5 (Princeton, Princeton University Press).

[22] FINNIS, JOHN (1980) *Natural Law and Natural Rights*, ch. X.7 (Oxford, Clarendon Press); this work is referred to subsequently as 'NLNR'.

[23] *Lochner* v. *New York* (1905) 198 U.S. 76.

[24] CL, 125.

[25] UNGER, R.M. (1976) *Law in Modern Society* (New York, The Free Press), p. 196.

[26] KELSEN, HANS (1967) *Pure Theory of Law* (Berkeley and Los Angeles, University of California Press), p. 349; this work is referred to subsequently as 'PTL'.

[27] NLNR, 284.

[28] NLNR, 284, n. 16.

[29] PTL, 245.

[30] PTL, 198.

[31] NLNR, 284–285.

[32] NLNR, 285.

[33] *Salvo* [1980] V.R. 401; TUR, RICHARD (1983) Dishonesty and the jury [note 17 refers].

[34] POPPER, KARL R. (1974) *Conjectures and Refutations*, p. 317, 5th edn. (London, Routledge & Kegan Paul).

[35] WALKER, D.M. (1979) *The Law of Contracts and Related Obligations in Scotland* (London, Butterworth), p. 34, "... valuable consideration ... is not a requisite of a Scottish contract". TREITEL, G.H. (1983) *The Law of Contract*, 6th ed, p. 51 (London, Stevens) "In English law, a promise is not, as a general rule, binding as a contract unless ... supported by some 'consideration' ". It follows that the content of a gratuitous promise is man's due in Scotland but not in England and that the two legal systems have determined the concept in different, indeed mutually contradictory, fashion.

[36] NLNR, 351.

[37] MOORE, G.E. (1903) *Principia Ethica* (London, Cambridge University Press), p. 15, "... whatever definition be offered, it may be always asked, with significance, of the complex so defined, whether it is itself good".

[38] HARE, R.M. (1952) *The Language of Morals* (Oxford, Oxford University Press), p. 1.

[39] cf. HARE, R.M. (1963) *Freedom and Reason* (Oxford, Oxford University Press), p. 35, "... the word

'ought' cannot be used in making legal judgments; if a person has a certain legal obligation, we cannot express this by saying that he *ought* to do such and such a thing, for the reason that 'ought'—judgments have to be universalizable, which in a strict sense, legal judgments are not. The reason why they are not is that a statement of law always contains an implicit reference to a particular jurisdiction".

[40] PTL, 65.

[41] D'ENTREVES, A.P. (1951) *Natural Law: an introduction to legal philosophy* (London, Hutchinson's University Library), p. 185; "... represents a remarkable effort on the part of an avowed positivist to recognise the merits of that ancient and venerable notion"; pp. 185–186, "... to recognise a core of good sense ... is to show an understanding that goes beyond tolerance".

[42] CL, 54–59.

[43] CL, 113.

[44] See GLOVER, J. (1977) *Causing Death and Saving Lives*, pp. 23–26 (Harmondsworth, Penguin).

[45] EM, 116.

[46] EM, 118.

[47] EM, 118.

[48] EM, 119; and see PTL, 43, "Even under the most totalitarian legal order there exists something like inalienable freedom; not as a right innate and natural, but as a consequence of the technically limited possibility of positively regulating human behaviour".

[49] HARE, R.M. (1963) *Freedom and Reason*, p. 35 (Oxford, Oxford University Press).

[50] MacCORMICK, NEIL (1978) *Legal Reasoning and Legal Theory* (Oxford, Clarendon Press), p. 99, "... the notion of formal justice requires that the justification of decisions in individual cases be always on the basis of universal propositions to which the judge is prepared to adhere as a basis for determining other like cases...".

[51] TUR, RICHARD (1978) Varieties of Overruling ... [note 13 refers].

[52] CL, 176–177.

[53] COOPER, NEIL (1966) Two concepts of morality, *Philosophy*, pp. 19–33; STRAWSON, P.F. (1961) Social morality and individual ideal, *Philosophy*, pp. 1–17; cf HARE, R.M. (1963) *Freedom and Reason*, pp. 151 ff. (Oxford, Oxford University Press).

[54] Report of the Committee of Inquiry into Human Fertilisation and Embryology, Cmnd 9314 (1984), Foreword, para. 6.

Part V

Ethics and Medicine

22

Thinking Critically in Medicine and its Ethics: relating applied science and applied ethics

DANIEL A. MOROS, ROSAMOND RHODES, BERNARD BAUMRIN &
JAMES J. STRAIN

ABSTRACT   *While interest in philosophy and medicine has burgeoned in the past two decades, there remains a need for an analysis of the intellectual activity embodied in good medical practice. In this setting, ethical and scientific decision-making are complexly interrelated. The following paper, collaboratively written by physicians and philosophers, presents a view of applied (clinical) science and applied ethics. Making extensive use of illustrations drawn from routine case material, we seek to indicate a variety of philosophic issues to be found in daily practice, elucidate various levels of critical reasoning within the medical setting, and demonstrate a remarkable similarity between medical and ethical decision-making.*

The purpose of this paper is to provide an analysis of the role of ethics within the framework of medical practice and medical education. In these settings scientific and ethical decision-making have immense and immediate consequences and cannot be considered in isolation from each other.

In recent years medical practice and education have come under increasing scrutiny. Two frequent criticisms have been: (1) the emphasis placed on the mastery of techniques and memorization of facts with a concomitant neglect of the skills of critical reasoning, and (2) inattention to ethical and humanistic concerns [1]. Though often regarded as distinct issues, these two failures are more closely related than is usually appreciated. Almost every action within the medical setting either explicitly or implicitly contains two judgements, one ethical and one scientific, and there is a constant interplay between what is technically possible and what is morally desirable. Consequently, issues within the philosophy of science need to be considered so that questions of medical ethics can be adequately examined. Furthermore, as will be demonstrated in what follows, the process of careful critical thought is similar both in evaluating claims to scientific knowledge and in evaluating moral issues and applying moral principles. With this perspective in mind, the elaboration of a concept of critical thinking and an examination of the nature of clinical science and applied ethics should contribute to the teaching and practice of medicine and is an important prelude to curriculum reform [2].

In what follows we will present parallel schema that we consider to be the elements of critical reasoning in medicine. The first is devoted to the evaluation of factual claims. The focus here is not on the issue of scientific proof but rather on the application of science to practice. The second is concerned with the analysis of moral decisions. These schema are organized in a hierarchical fashion from more basic to more sophisticated abilities. They are not intended to mirror the actual developmental process of increasing sophistication within individuals, or to be taken as rigid directions for how to think. Rather they are a framework for the critical evaluation of factual claims and moral decisions in medicine. In addition, the parallelism of these two outlines underscores the similarity between technical and moral reasoning within the setting of an applied science. Without appreciating this similarity, ethical theory and ethical thinking become artificially separated from the overall intellectual activity of medicine.

Schema 1: Elements in the Evaluation of Factual Claims, Judgements and Beliefs

(1) Recognition of claims to know.

(2) Identification of sources or grounds for claims to know.

(3) Classification of claims to know.

(4) Appreciation that for practical purposes any claim to knowledge can be viewed as containing elements of data and elements of reasoning.

(5) Appreciation of the complexity of data:

  (a) ability to recognize the degree of theory-ladenness of data,

  (b) appreciation of the importance of reproducibility (reliability) of observations.

(6) Appreciation of good reasoning, with special emphasis on statistical reasoning.

(7) Ability to think critically using data and reasoning.

(8) Recognition that contradictory statements and/or unanticipated results are a signal to re-evaluate and think critically anew.

(9) Ability to evaluate and choose between mutually exclusive knowledge claims with the possibility of doubting all of the available alternatives.

(10) Understanding of the concept of warranted assertability: appreciation of the limited nature of our knowledge, the inherent limits on certainty, and the complexity behind claiming to know something.

Elaboration of Schema 1

(1) Recognition of claims to know. The everyday medical world is filled with claims and counter-claims, many of which are not explicitly recognized. These claims are in a sense layered on one another. The evaluation of the most manifest claim may hinge on the validity of a less explicit one. Consider what for a clinician is a simple and straightforward statement—'Mr X's congestive heart failure has worsened under the stresses of infection and hypoxemia' (reduced oxygenation of the blood). The clinical setting is that of an elderly man with previously well controlled congestive heart failure (CHF) who now has pneumonia and a fever. Many different types of factual claims may be found within the initial diagnostic statement. (a) There is a physiologic diagnosis of CHF. CHF is a theoretical construct that presumes an imbalance in a variety of intimately interconnected bodily subsystems and states (e.g. the ventricles of the heart, the tendency of the kidneys to retain salt and fluid, etc.). Among other things, the term 'theoretical construct' indicates that there isn't a specific 'thing' called CHF that can be directly observed like a rash or tumour. Indeed, without a proper theoretical background, CHF is as mysterious and elusive as Galen's humours. (b) In

the modern medical world, pneumonia often seems a simple observation by virtue of the appearance of an infiltrate on chest x-ray and well established correlation with morbid anatomy. However, diagnoses such as CHF and pneumonia are conclusions derived from a variety of direct observations and laboratory data. (c) The use of laboratory data presumes diligence on the part of the clinical laboratory and the validity of a variety of different types of measurements. (d) Many 'simple observations' are already interpretations selected from a virtually infinite choice of sense impressions. Thus one clinician sees shortness of breath while another focuses on anxiety.

(2) Identification of sources or grounds for a claim to know. The doctor who embraces such a multiplicity of factual claims may have different grounds for his different beliefs. (a) He or she may regard a statement about a high fever as a simple observation, even though the thermometer is an instrument with a long and intricate history. The notion of exploiting the expansile properties of materials to create a reliable temperature scale has become so accepted that many of the implied theoretical and factual claims are no longer recognized. (b) For a medical student the relationship of a rising level of urea in the blood (BUN) to worsening congestive failure may be a fact learned from a respected teacher. For an experienced clinician and/or researcher this relationship may have been confirmed many times in a variety of clinical and experimental settings. (c) The decision to use a specific antibiotic for a specific organism may be entirely based on the latest literature and may not be a matter of personal experience. Often a crucial step in analysis comes with the realization that the grounds for a belief are not adequate. Such a realization does not necessarily mean that a belief is false. In a field such as medicine where we base decisions on factual material spanning a wide range of subject matter, we must often depend on some appeal to authority. At such times an evaluation of the authority may be at the centre of our critical thinking.

(3) Classification of claims to know. The process of explicating a claim to knowledge requires being able to classify it. Consider the following examples. (a) A factual claim may represent a simple observation, e.g. 'patient X is SOB'. (b) A claim may represent some statement of regularity based on personal experience, e.g. 'whenever I have adopted treatment Y for respiratory insufficiency I have seen significant improvement'. (c) A claim may be a particular law, such as 'in congestive heart failure there is a tendency to retain salt and water' or 'when the pO_2 of arterial blood falls below 40mm (of water) one sees a variety of organ system failure'. These laws would be comparable to a particular law in physics such as the ideal gas law ($PV \propto T$). (d) A claim may represent a more general law, such as 'a living organism must have some mechanism for converting energy into a biologically useful form'. This might be compared with a law of thermodynamics. In most of medicine and applied science, general laws provide an overall view of the world but particular laws are critical to accomplishing our daily tasks. The significance of discarding a simple observation as incorrect or treating a personal success as mere coincidence is very different from discounting a particular or general law. By understanding the implications of our factual claims, we acquire some guide to the likely correctness or incorrectness of our individual beliefs. Much quackery, deceit, and foolishness can be readily and clearly identified by the magnitude of the scientific principles being contradicted.

(4) Appreciation that any factual claim (claim to knowledge) involves an element of data and an element of reasoning. From a practical point of view, some simple observations such as 'patient X is breathing at 30 respirations per minute' may be regarded as matters of pure observation. However, most of our statements such as 'patient X is short of breath' are more complex claims. X may be intentionally hyperventilating or may be hyperventilating to correct for a metabolic imbalance such as diabetic ketoacidosis. 'Shortness of breath' already implies an evaluation of the basic observation. Consider the deceptively simple claim 'X has a temperature of 101°F'. This statement is more complex than the simple observation that when a thermometer is placed in a patient's mouth for two minutes an opaque column is seen extending to the line marked '101'. The statement 'X has a temperature of 101°F' contains multiple theoretical constructs. Assume that the basic notions of temperature and measurement with a thermometer are clear (see 5b below). When we refer to the temperature of a person we are usually concerned with a 'core temperature'. This may be correlated with an oral temperature, but we presumably know that an oral temperature is unreliable in a patient who is hyperventilating or who has just consumed a cup of hot tea. Similarly, we are distrustful of axillary temperatures. Thus, while the initial statement 'X has a temperature of 101°F' appears to be a simple observation, it contains a host of accompanying assumption and provisos.

(5) Appreciation of the complexity of data. (5a) The ability to recognize the degree of theory-ladenness of data. There is a practical distinction to be made between an observation such as 'patient X is short of breath' and a more refined piece of data such as 'This waveform on the oscilloscope screen represents an action potential mediated by an increased flux of sodium ions'. This practical distinction is not that one claim is more reliable, but rather that one is more 'theory-laden'. So though I may doubt a student's report of shortness of breath and have confidence in the interpretation of the oscilloscope screen, nevertheless, it is easier to imagine that we should alter our explanation of a particular waveform than that we should decide that a patient with severe CHF was not really short of breath.

(5b) The importance of reproducibility. The term 'data' implies some degree of reproducibility of all relevant observations. For example, when we say that an oral temperature is 101°F, we imply that if we immediately repeat our measurement using the same thermometer for the same duration of time we will again see a column extending to the line marked '101'. On the other hand, if we possessed three different thermometers and each gave a different reading, and if there were a difference in the result when the same thermometer was used twice in succession, then there would not be any data labelled 'oral temperature'. (It is easy to imagine an unreliable thermometer. If the expansile material were such that it lost heat rapidly and varied greatly with small changes in temperature, then any delay in reading the thermometer would significantly alter the result. In poorly lit areas and at night it might be impossible to obtain a reproducible reading.) Because a variety of assumptions about the world accompanies even the simplest of data, as data become more complex the possibilities for nonreproducibility (unreliability) multiply.

There are many ways that unreliability may slip into what is called data. For example, a clinical investigator when conducting an open trial may tend to overstate improvement with each individual and create a systematic bias within the treated group. The treated patient may overstate his symptomatic improvement as a reflection of the 'placebo effect' or a reflection of his desires to be well and to please his doctor. The investigator may magnify symptoms within the control group. When such biases occur it is not that the data are deficient or 'spurious' but rather that there really are no data at all. Thus an evaluation of reliability and reproducibility of data is a critical step in evaluating factual claims.

(6) Appreciation of good reasoning, with special emphasis on statistical reasoning. This section will consist of an example of poor and then of good reasoning. An example of the former, common in the neurologic literature, concerns the claim that Parkinson's disease is associated with a high incidence of depression. The statement is true but the implication drawn is that the neurologic substrate of this illness predisposes to an incidence of depression far greater than would otherwise be anticipated in persons struggling with a progressive and debilitating illness. Here is an elementary issue of experimental design, i.e. the choice of an appropriate control population for comparison. This criticism should not be mistaken as support for the opposite conclusion. There is little in the way of a conclusion that can be drawn from the data, though the data are good, i.e. patients with Parkinson's disease do indeed have a higher incidence of depression than age-matched controls.

As an example of good reasoning, consider the justification commonly given when a physician ignores a 'single, minor' abnormality in a battery of blood tests. The physician may feel that he is being too casual and often says that one cannot pursue everything. The guiding intuition is that one can get away with ignoring small deviations from what is called the normal range and this intuition is backed by experience. But it is also backed by good reasoning. If 'normal' is defined as two standard deviations from the mean, then once 12 independent tests are drawn, the odds are better than 1:1 that at least one value will come back abnormal. The good physician's practice is identical with the statistician's conclusion. When a value is 3 or more SD from the mean ('abnormal enough') there may be a compelling reason to investigate further. Thus the decision is not a matter of cost-effectiveness or casualness in the face of a minor abnormality. The laboratory data are correct and there is no true 'abnormality' to investigate. The good physician's "intuition" is simply superior to what he often offers as a justification. Furthermore, medical education is defective when we casually attribute good judgement to experience and fail to examine why the "experienced" physician is so often correct.

(7) Thinking critically using data and reasoning. Here we are concerned with decision-making by the physician in his role as applied scientist. To illustrate the critical evaluation of data and reasoning we will examine a specific controversy—the role of carotid endarterectomy (surgical repair of the carotid artery) in the treatment of transient ischemic attacks (TIAs). A TIA is transient neurologic impairment due to a temporary decrease in blood flow to the brain. Carotid endarterectomy is now one of the most common major surgical procedures in the United States.

Some percentage of TIAs as well as stroke is related to the presence of atherosclerotic plaques in the carotid arteries. These plaques may ulcerate (fragment) permitting dislodged particles to occlude smaller vessels transiently or permanently. Since the presence of plaques is much more common than the occurrence of TIAs and/or stroke it is clear that there are other causal factors about which we are less certain. The intuition underlying carotid endarterectomy is twofold—(1) removal of the plaque that ulcerates ought to reduce the incidence of stroke, and (2) when plaque formation is extensive enough to reduce blood flow, removal of the obstruction ought to improve neurologic function. The reasonableness of these presuppositions depends on our model of cerebral blood flow, a topic that cannot now be considered. However, since surgery has been used extensively, clinical data are available and, therefore, clinical decisions do not hinge solely on the reasonableness of our initial pathophysiologic assumptions.

As discussed earlier, each medical decision involves numerous beliefs or conjectures. The use of a treatment 'T' for a disease, symptom or risk factor 'D', presumes some knowledge of the natural history of 'D', some knowledge of the altered history of 'D' with the intervention 'T', and some knowledge of the complications of 'T'. In seeking to understand the proper role of carotid endarterectomy our therapeutic claim needs to be clearly stated. What is being treated? Certainly not TIAs which, though distressing, are by definition transient. Therefore it behoves us to be cautious in adopting an expensive treatment with some mortality and morbidity. The claim for surgery is, and indeed could only be, that it acts as a prophylactic against subsequent stroke. Thus the next question must be what is the natural history of TIAs in the subpopulation where this symptom appears to be related to carotid disease. In the recent past the standard figure in the literature was that 30–50% of persons with TIAs would develop stroke within three to five years [3, 4]. While this figure is too high [5, 6] it is difficult to challenge simply from personal experience because of the follow-up period required, the numerous subgroups contained within the general category of TIA, and the lack of an available control population now that most patients receive some medical or surgical treatment. With medical treatment using antiplatlet agents, the 3–5 year incident of stroke following the onset of TIAs is about 15% [7]. With this altered natural history of TIA, a change must be made in our view of an acceptable surgical morbidity. The perioperative mortality and morbidity (complications of radiologic tests, perioperative stroke, etc.) is often claimed to range from 1–3% [8]. This claim is strong enough to permit considerable use of personal experience and any neurologist at a large teaching hospital has available to himself the data to make an estimate of the complication rate of his surgeons. Certainly for most of us at good medical centres with good vascular surgeons the 1–3% figure is a fantasy and we are all aware of a much higher incidence [9, 10]. Thus, depending on the nature of a claim and the quality of the data available, it may be possible to reach powerful conclusions based on personal experience. In particular, we may be able to disconfirm the positive claims of others.

Contrast this discussion of surgery with the problem of supporting the affirmative claim that in men with TIAs small doses of aspirin significantly reduce the incidence of subsequent stroke. Since the incidence of complications of small doses of aspirin is low, we cannot easily reach the negative conclusion that the natural history of the illness is better than that of the illness modified by treatment. We now require a study with an adequate number of participants, an adequate control population, and an appropriate follow-up period. The confirmation of the positive conclusion is beyond the reach of the personal experience of an individual physician.

Our concern here is not whether endarterectomy is appropriate in selected cases, but rather that decisions regarding treatment or further diagnostic studies involve presumptions that can be critically evaluated and tested. While it is difficult to validate positive claims or theories on the basis of personal experience, properly collected and analyzed personal experience (often summarily dismissed as 'anecdotal') is the constant data available to critically evaluate and reject many unwarranted assertions. An understanding of the correct and incorrect use of personal experience is part of a sophisticated approach to the evaluation of data and is a crucial element in enabling physicians to think critically in the clinical setting. Such critical thinking involves:

(a) clearly delineating what is either explicitly claimed or implicitly assumed,
(b) deciding whether the supporting data is reasonable or suspect,
(c) deciding whether the data collected supports the contentions being made, i.e. whether the reasoning is good or faulty, and
(d) recognizing what validity personal experience may have in one's accepting or rejecting the data presented and the conclusions reached.

(8) Recognizing contradictory statements and/or unanticipated results as a signal to re-evaluate and think critically anew. The recognition of contradiction and unanticipated results is central to the work of the applied scientist. Progress and the avoidance of error demand a positive attitude toward disconfirming standard practice. For the clinician, this effort involves the careful examination of the data and argument supporting the diagnostic, therapeutic, and prognostic claims that constitute standard practice, as well as the thoughtful consideration of personal experience. As discussed above, such experience may enable the physician to establish negative (disconfirming) conclusions in relation to the positive claims of standard practice. In applied science, the unsuccessful attempt to disconfirm our judgements is an important aspect of validation.

(9) Ability to evaluate and choose between claims with the possibility of rejecting the alternatives. In critically evaluating claims or decisions we may come to recognize (a) that the available data is inadequate to justify any action (decision) or (b) that the reasoning employed by ourselves or others is faulty. Such negative conclusions warrant further examination. In a case presenting diagnostic problems, where each of several possible diagnoses would lead to a different treatment, the desire to act (treat) may be checked by the realization that the diagnostic work is not yet adequate. In another setting, the diagnosis may be clear but we may lack confidence in the data or arguments presented in support of any particular treatment. It is difficult to confront an ill person and not have a treatment to offer. But there is little to be said for the illusion of efficacy to assuage the physician's discomfort on account of his limitations. Rather we must recognize how intense this discomfort is and how our emotional responses may impair our judgment. It is important to appreciate that in such contexts the decision not to act is itself a powerful and positive response. (It is worth adding that while the illusion of efficacy cannot be justified by a gain in the physician's personal comfort, it may be required by a patient to withstand the stress of illness. Thus, the physician may need to deal with illusion in ministering to the ill, but must not become confused in his role as applied scientist.)

(10) Understanding the concept of warranted assertability and the inherent limits on certainty. The use of the term 'warranted assertability' emphasizes the background of search and criticism that supports all valid belief and action within applied science. We do not possess the 'truth' or understand 'reality'. Rather, the data available, the level of

our technical abilities, and the quality of our reasoning allow us to assert 'A' in preference to 'B'. The assertion of 'A' as opposed to 'B' may be deceptive, for A and B may not exhaust the possibilities. Indeed, in medicine, the need to make a decision may lead us to affirm A where under other circumstances we would simply opt to withhold judgement.

Ultimately, the standards of critical thought in the clinical science that guides good medical practice are similar to those in other branches of pure and applied science. To appreciate this similarity it is necessary to see the rational, critical core in clinical thought. To do this, the distinction between clinical science and clinical practice must be clearly understood. Clinical practice requires that the physician make decisions. To withhold a treatment because its efficacy is not yet proven is functionally the same as to withhold a treatment because of a belief that it is ineffective. While in other branches of pure and applied science it is often possible to postpone a decision pending further analysis or research, in medicine this is not usually the case. If one confuses the activity of critical thinking in clinical science with the unavoidable need to make decisions in clinical practice, then the similarity between clinical and other applied sciences becomes obscured. To be valid, a clinical decision must be able to withstand the critical evaluation of available data (including personal experience) and theory. If the data is inadequate or a theory incomplete, a decision will still need to be made. In such cases a scientific practitioner will recognize the tentative nature of the justification. He must be able to tolerate the contrast between this uncertainty and the importance (and perhaps finality) of the actual decision for the individual patient. In the future the practitioner may discover that the patient would have been better served by another choice. However, the correctness of a decision can only be judged in the light of its justification at the time that it is made. The temptation for all physicians is to seek to justify whatever it is that they have done. The critical physician continues to question his decision, in essence seeking to disconfirm his justification [11].

Schema 2: Elements of Moral Reasoning in Medical Encounters

(1) Recognition of moral relationships.

(2) Identification of moral issues, the dramatic and the ordinary.

(3) Classification of moral issues.

(4) Appreciation that every medical encounter involves one or more than one central moral issue.

(5) Appreciation of the complexity of moral choice: recognizing that under specific circumstances highly valued moral principles may conflict.

(6) Ability to think theoretically about moral issues.

(7) Ability to think theoretically about moral conflicts.

(8) Recognition that contradictory moral claims or discrepancies between moral claims and actions are signals to re-evaluate and think critically anew.

(9) Adjudication of moral issues and conflicts.

(10) Understanding and tolerating the fact that despite our best efforts at adjudication, some degree of ambiguity and uncertainty is inevitable.

Elaboration of Schema 2

(1) Recognition of moral relationships. The medical world is filled with a variety of

important moral relationships, each involving some set of duties as well as rights or prerogatives. Consider the following incomplete list:

(a) family—patient (who may be either competent, temporarily incompetent or demented adult; or a child);

(b) physician—patient;

(c) physician—family of patient;

(d) physician—fellow physicians, e.g. as a consultant;

(e) physician—nurse;

(f) physician (as teacher)—house officers and students;

(g) nurse—patient;

(h) medical student (as clinical clerk)—patient.

While medical behaviour may proceed correctly simply with the tacit acknowledgement of moral relationships, critical thinking about ethics in actual medical encounters requires a more explicit recognition of them. For example, when a physician speaks first with the spouse or children of an ill patient, he may be assuming that the family member recognizes a variety of duties to the patient and may also believe that he has acquired certain responsibilities to the family. In the relationship of physician to nurse, a doctor's orders may require hours of labour or commit a nurse to actions that might be regarded as morally questionable. Perhaps the doctor has decided not to order pain medication for a patient whom a nurse believes to be suffering. It can be argued that the relationship between physician and nurse leaves the doctor with a 'duty' as a 'superior' within the hierarchy of the hospital. The nurse's willingness to follow orders presumes the physician's serious effort to give the correct ones. Some might argue that the physician-nurse relationship is purely a contractual one, i.e. the hospital employs the nurse and the doctor has been delegated a certain authority by virtue of a staff position. However, if a nurse recognizes a moral responsibility to a patient, then this simple contractual model for the nurse-physician relationship is unacceptable. The failure to recognize the moral nature of such relationships as doctor to nurse and nurse to patient obscures the moral dimension of the medical world.

(2) Recognition of moral issues. As with moral relationships, moral issues abound within the medical setting. Should one attempt to resuscitate a patient, suggest to the family of a patient that they embark on a course of treatment that they cannot afford, tell the truth to a patient over the objections of the family, coax a Jehovah's witness to undergo a transfusion that is contrary to a deeply held religious belief, treat patients against their will, discuss all potential complications of a contemplated therapy, use patients as research subjects without their explicit consent, reduce one's charges to a poor patient, etc.? The recognition that medical decisions invariably involve moral judgements is central to understanding what actually occurs within medical practice.

(3) Classification of moral issues. The physician must recognize general categories of moral issues so as to bring some order to a bewildering array of moral decisions. Proper categorization allows one to apply broader perspectives to specific situations. For example, the question of obtaining informed consent, whether to speak first with a patient or the family, and treatment against the objection of a patient, all relate to the broader issue of autonomy, i.e. the possibility of individuals acting according to their own choices. Our concerns with autonomy may be influenced by the use of this

concept in a variety of nonmedical contexts such as law, religion, and philosophy. The question of whether the physician should act according to what he believes to be the best interest of the patient, perhaps in opposition to a patient's apparent wishes, involves the issue of paternalism. Though commonly viewed as being opposed to autonomy, paternalistic action is not necessarily in conflict with respect for autonomy. We expect parents to make decisions for a young child and we expect a psychiatrist to recognize that the expression of suicidal intent in a severely depressed patient is not necessarily an exercise of the patient's autonomy. Other broad moral categories that apply to specific medical encounters include the principle of beneficence, the notion of the sanctity of life and questions of social justice.

(4) Appreciation of the central moral issue in a situation. Medical encounters are often structured by implicit or explicit decisions concerning a moral issue. In such circumstances the clarification of a 'medical' decision may depend on the clear identification of a moral concern. A common example is the dissension that may arise over a decision not to resuscitate a terminally ill person. Some staff members may believe that resuscitation violates a patient's "right" to die with dignity or that resuscitation involves causing unnecessary pain, while others may think that the decision not to resuscitate is too often a matter of convenience for the physician or the family and fails to honour the sanctity of life. While these concerns may reflect aspects of the actual circumstances, it may also be the case that the decision has not been discussed with the patient. Depending on how highly we value autonomy, the clear indication of a preference on the part of the patient might override other considerations.

The above example warrants further examination. Medical decisions often require the co-operation of many individuals. These individuals will need to be confident that they have acted properly and reasonably. It can be argued that the physician, the family and perhaps even the patient have a duty to make clear to all who follow orders (nurses, house officers, students, etc.) that such decisions are being thoughtfully made. Some would describe the process of reassuring staff as purely a matter of good administrative skills, a good tactic to enlist co-operation and maintain morale. However, this tendency to reduce (and thus devalue) moral issues to matters of social skills is misleading. In many circumstances, communication is a moral duty.

(5) Appreciation of the conflict between different moral values in a specific situation. Not all problems can be neatly resolved by clarification and classification. In the medical environment important rules and principles often come into conflict, e.g. 'tell the truth' vs. 'do no unnecessary harm'; 'always attempt to save and prolong life' vs. 'comfort the ill'; 'always treat an individual as an end in himself' vs. some ill-defined but nevertheless recognized obligation to advance the science of medicine. It should be noted that some principles, though stated in absolute terms, are general guidelines rather than absolute rules, that sometimes principles in conflict can be ranked (thus most people would agree that the principle 'thou shalt not kill' would take precedence over the principle 'thou shalt not lie') and that the ordering of some principles may vary between different social groups and between individuals within the same group. Obviously difficulties may arise when, for example, a patient and doctor have substantial differences in their orderings.

(6) Thinking theoretically about central moral issues. The ability to identify moral issues within specific medical encounters and then classify such issues under broader rubrics (such as informed consent in relation to 'autonomy') enables a physician to use the insights of other disciplines. Thus legal, religious, philosophical and historical perspectives may enrich a physician's approach to a specific problem. However, classification is only one aspect of theoretical (abstract) thinking. More is required to explore the ramifications and complexity of moral decisions adequately within the medical setting. For example, much of the importance attached to informed consent stems from the value we place on autonomy. However, careful consideration of informed consent involves more than just an appreciation of the principle of autonomy. We require some understanding of what constitutes being 'informed'. How much is a patient able or willing to understand? What about the passive individual who asks only 'what should I do?' or a patient so overwhelmed by fear or exhausted by illness that he needs or requests others to decide for him? How insistent should a physician be in informing such patients? At what point should a physician decide that a patient has been told enough? If informed consent (autonomy) is so important, should it take precedence over other aspects of patient care? Or should we interpret a patient's request that the doctor make a decision as an autonomous act delegating certain responsibilities to the physician? In the case of a child or a temporarily incompetent adult, how shall we identify the surrogate decision-maker and should we honour the surrogate's decision if we believe it to be based on incorrect factual beliefs? At the heart of informed consent there remains an element of paternalism. The clear formulation and consideration of such issues require an ability to think abstractly about moral issues separately from the context of individual decision-making.

(7) Thinking theoretically about moral conflicts. The ability to think theoretically may enable a physician to resolve at least some of the conflicts encountered in medical practice. For example, if a severely depressed person refused a lifesaving medical treatment, this refusal might be overridden if the medical judgement was that the severity of the depression made it impossible to consider such refusal as emanating from an autonomous agent. However, in most circumstances, moral choices are not so clearly resolved by a scientific judgement. And in the case of this hypothetical depressed patient, the resolution of one issue brings another to the fore, i.e. that of the appropriate surrogate decision-maker.

A potential conflict now receiving considerable attention is the role of the doctor as a dispenser of a scarce resource. When health care is broadly defined to include nursing homes, home health aides, as well as advanced technologies, it appears that the cost exceeds the willingness or ability of society to guarantee such services to all individuals. In thinking about the distribution of health care we may consider issues of social justice as well as historical and sociological 'realities' such as the advantages accorded to individuals because of wealth or social class. We may see discrepancies based on wealth as either a moral travesty or as a reasonable and proper method of distributing services. With these considerations in mind, what should be the medical profession's role in tailoring and administering the system of allocation? What should be the behaviour of a physician if society asks him to limit his care for a patient rather than to simply do the best job that he can? Also, if medical resources are limited, then unneeded studies or treatment for one person may mean the loss of necessary care for another. Excess and waste acquire additional moral significance. An intelligent examination of such concerns requires one's being able to think more abstractly about moral issues and conflicts.

(8) Recognition that contradictory moral claims or discrepancies between moral claims and actions are signals to re-evaluate and think critically anew. While this step may seem reasonable in light of our preceding discussion, several points should be emphasised. First, the search for contradiction and inconsistency is not an expression of skepticism or cynicism. As discussed earlier, in applied science the unsuccessful attempt to disconfirm our judgements is a crucial aspect of validation. The purpose of moral analysis (critical thinking) is not to point an accusatory finger at the failures of those around us. Rather it is a prelude to making decisions and a means of reviewing and revising decisions that have already been made. This process of explicit review and revision provides for good decision-making and continuing moral education. Secondly, in applied ethics, actions as well as expressed moral beliefs must be viewed as statements of moral principles. A justifiable action implies an underlying reasonable moral claim. In many instances, wisdom and moral sensitivity may be reflected in carefully chosen action while the words used to explain and justify may be inadequate. Conversely, the expression of high principles may conflict with actual behaviour. Third, critical thinking inevitably enhances the intensity of moral analysis. Actions must be judged against goals and goal choices are moral decisions. Contradictions are searched for rather than overlooked, and, when uncovered, are discussed rather than disregarded. The refusal to examine inconsistent moral positions should seem as great a deficit as indifference to contradictory factual claims. The physician must be able and willing to discuss moral judgements in the same way that he should be able and willing to discuss the rational (scientific) grounds for his diagnoses and treatments.

(9) Adjudication of moral issues and conflict. By adjudication we mean the actual making of decisions as opposed to the analysis of moral facts. This process of adjudication is distinct from, though dependent upon, earlier steps. If moral judgements are embedded in every medical decision, then in circumstances where highly valued moral principles conflict, a decision becomes an adjudication. While there cannot be clear and unequivocal guidelines for adjudicating all conflicts, nevertheless, by carefully identifying what is at issue one may resolve many conflicts and avoid many egregious errors. Dominating this process of adjudication is the need to determine how moral principles or guidelines are to be applied in actual circumstances as well as the existence of a constant tension between utilitarian and deontological viewpoints. These two issues are often confused.

The utilitarian maintains that actions must be judged by their consequences alone. Three questions immediately arise. (1) Do we judge people after the fact by the actual consequences of their actions or rather by the intended consequences? (2) By what scale do we judge consequences? Is it to be pleasure or some other 'good'? Can the necessary utilitarian calculus be constructed? (3) Who is to be considered when we do the arithmetic? For the physician this simple notion of judging by consequences is problematic. For example, if the medical costs of a suffering terminal patient were exhausting a family's assets, a calculus based on pleasure might justify doing away with a patient at the request of the family and against the patient's expressed wishes. A refinement of this consequentialist approach is 'rule utilitarianism'. Here the argument is that the social order will be undermined and great suffering will result unless we are confident that certain moral rules will be obeyed. Thus rules like 'always try to save and prolong life' and 'do not lie', can be ranked according to their relative importance to the social order and should be followed because of the consequences of widespread disregard. Some argue that rule utilitarianism ultimately reduces to 'act utilitarianism' as the first position is commonly referred to.

The major alternative to utilitarianism is a deontological approach to ethics. Here the claim is that certain principles ought to be followed simply because they are right, regardless of their immediate consequences. The origin of principles such as 'thou shalt not kill (murder)', 'thou shalt not steal', etc., is most commonly attributed to God, but philosophers have claimed other sources as well, for example, reason (Kant) and 'natural rights' [12].

In the 'practical world' we tend to vacillate between these two positions. But, as suggested above, this vacillation conceals another difficulty, the problem of how to apply moral rules in actual circumstances. A major distinction between applied ethics in medicine and moral philosophy as a theoretical activity is that, in medicine, moral decisions are unavoidable. Often a physician cannot say that more time is required to study the moral complexity of a medical decision. A decision not to act because of uncertainty carries the same medical consequences as the decision not to act because an action is improper. Thus, if the action, A, in question is that of performing a lifesaving treatment against a person's expressed wishes, and if we are uncertain of the patient's competency, the decision not to act because of this uncertainty has the same impact as affirming the patient's competency. Here a decision not to act because of uncertainty implies that respect for autonomy overrules most other considerations. The burden of proof thus falls on those who would declare a person incompetent. However, if we value saving life above autonomy we will simply act regardless of the patient's expressed wishes. But if we value both principles highly, how will this be reflected in our final determination? If we believe that one principle, P1 (always act to sustain life), is more important than another, P2 (always respect autonomy), does this mean that we always follow P1 before we consider P2 or do circumstances alter the relative weight in a particular case? Perhaps the available treatment is painful and often not effective. Perhaps an alternative approach ameliorates suffering without affecting survival. Under such circumstances we may not want to equate the failure to treat as disregard for the principle P1. Along a similar vein, if P1 were at all times our overriding concern, then the use of general anaesthesia with its small associated risk to life would always be unacceptable for any cosmetic surgery. Thus a badly scarred child might be deprived of a more normal childhood if he/she were unable to co-operate sufficiently to permit the use of local anaesthesia.

Our concern in applied ethics is not simply with the construction of a consistent argument. We must understand the implications of the ethical principles we invoke to guide our decisions. In applied ethics, while inconsistency and contradiction alert us to error, consistency gives no guarantee of being correct. The application of ethical principles requires a consideration of circumstances and consequences. This claim should not be mistaken for a consequentialist construction of the entire endeavour or as vacillation between the utilitarian and deontological perspectives. We refer to this process of application of ethical principles as adjudication, recognizing that such interesting and difficult problems involve circumstances where highly valued moral principles conflict and implying that in practical affairs, regardless of how precisely we formulate guidelines, decisions must be arrived at case by case.

(10) Recognition of the inevitability of ambiguity and uncertainty despite our best efforts at adjudication. This refers to a necessary and broader intellectual perspective without which it is difficult to apply the 'intellectual skills' discussed above. Conflict and uncertainty generate both psychological discomfort in individuals and disagreement among staff. A common response to conflict is denial and obfuscation. The price of critical reasoning includes the recognition of uncertainty and conflicts, and the inability to tolerate this unpleasantness makes critical thinking difficult and at times impossible. Therefore, physicians need to recognize that moral conflict and ambiguity will characterize many medical encounters and that uncertainty about decisions is unavoidable. Uncertainty may be the product of careful analysis rather than a reflection of intellectual inadequacy. While good moral reasoning cannot guarantee the best decision, it will aid in avoiding the worst. In a world where alternatives are limited, avoiding the worst possibilities increases the probability of making the best choice.

Summary

As this has been a long essay ranging over many topics it will be worthwhile to close with a brief review of our major points. (a) We have outlined the elements of good thinking in applied science and applied ethics. Because this requires frequent review and re-evaluation of decisions after they have been made and acted upon, we have used the term 'critical thinking'. (b) We have argued, though not in great detail, that there is substantial similarity between good thinking in clinical (applied) science and the theoretical sciences. (c) We have demonstrated a remarkable similarity between good thinking in applied science and applied ethics. This perhaps unexpected similarity arises from the application of reason to the actual world. In applied science and applied ethics, the need for action often requires choosing from a limited number of alternatives. These choices then remain to be re-evaluated.

Daniel A. Moros, Department of Neurology, Mount Sinai Medical School, 1 Gustave Levy Place, N.Y., N.Y. 10029, USA; Rosamond Rhodes, Department of Philosophy, Hunter College, City University of New York, 695 Park Ave, N.Y., N.Y. 10021, USA; Bernard Baumrin, Department of Philosophy, The Graduate School and Lehman College, City University of New York, 33 W. 42nd St., N.Y., N.Y. 10036, USA; & James J. Strain, Department of Psychiatry, Mount Sinai Medical School, 1 Gustave Levy Place, N.Y., N.Y. 10029, USA.

NOTES

[1] This subject has been discussed previously by Raanan Gillon (1981) in his Johne Locke Lecture published in the *British Medical Journal*, 283, pp. 1633-1639.
[2] Ibid., p. 1638.
[3] J. P. WHISNANT, N. MATSUMOTO & L. R. ELVEBACH (1973) Transient cerebral ischemic attacks in a community, *Mayo Clin Proc*, 48, pp. 194-8.
[4] J. ACHESON & E. C. HUTCHINSON (1971) The natural history of 'focal cerebral vascular disease', *Quarterly Journal of Medicine*, 40, pp. 15-23.
[5] ZIEGLER, P. K. & HASSANEIN, R. S. (1973) Prognosis in patients with transient ischemic attacks, *Stroke*, 4, pp. 666-673.

[6] A. CAROLEI *et al.* (1986) Cumulative Italian study on reversible cerebral ischemic attacks (RIAs): 4-year follow-up of 712 patients, *Neurology 36: Suppl.* 1, p. 141.

[7] H. J. M. BARNETT *et al.* (1978) A randomized trial of aspirin and sulfinpyrazone in threatened stroke: the Canadian co-operative study group, *New England Journal of Medicine*, 299, pp. 53–59.

[8] J. E. THOMPSON, D. J. AUSTIN & R. D. PATMAN (1970) Carotid endarterectomy for cerebrovascular insufficiency: long term results in 592 patients followed up to thirteen years, *Annals of Surgery*, 172, pp. 663–679.

[9] J. D. EASTON & D. G. SHERMAN (1977) Stroke and mortality rate in carotid endarterectomy: 228 consecutive operations, *Stroke*, 8, pp. 565–8.

[10] T. BROTT & K. THALINGER (1984) The practice of carotid endarterectomy in a large metropolitan area, *Stroke*, 15, pp. 950–5.

[11] This similarity may be further highlighted by reviewing some arguments of Karl Popper. Popper sees the activity of science as making conjectures (i.e. factual claims) and then carefully submitting them to experimental tests in an effort to disprove them. One function of logical argument is to uncover the implications of a claim, thereby expanding our ability to act upon the world and to test the (disconfirm) our belief. He maintains that our acceptance of a fact (warranted assertability in Dewey's terms) hinges on our failure to disprove. Popper argues that the scientific tradition, as do other traditions that generate beliefs, makes conjectures from experience. However, the scientific tradition also contains a critical attitude. Popper writes that "the scientific tradition is distinguished from the pre-scientific tradition in having two layers. Like the latter, it passes on its theories; but it also passes on a critical attitude towards them. The theories are passed on, not as dogmas, but rather with the challenge to discuss them and improve upon them." (1972) *Conjectures and Refutations*, p. 50 (4th Edn) (London, Routledge and Kegan Paul).

[12] Other standard views are egoism, subjectivism and relativism.

23

Public Bodies, Private Selves

SANDRA E. MARSHALL

ABSTRACT *A patient whose case notes had been used, without her permission, during a disciplinary inquiry on the conduct of Wendy Savage (her obstetrician) complained that this was a breach of confidentiality. Her complaint cannot be understood as based on a concern about the possible adverse consequences of this use of the notes: rather, her concern was just with the fact that medical information about her had been made known to others.*

My concern is with the meaning and status of the right to privacy, to which the Savage patient appealed. Such a right cannot be reduced to a property right, since this cannot capture what concerned the Savage patient. A proper understanding of what lies behind her complaint requires us to recognise the way in which facts about oneself—in this case facts about one's body—are intimately bound up with one's self, with one's identity, and thus with one's autonomy. What kinds of fact, and thus what conception of the self, are involved in such a conception of privacy need not everywhere be the same; the crucial point is that privacy and the self are concepts which, whatever their particular content, are internally related [1].

Do patients have a right that their medical records be kept confidential? A recent case in the United Kingdom brings this issue into clear focus and reveals the tensions which can arise between patients and their physicians when medical confidentiality and the public interest seem to be in conflict.

This case involved a disciplinary inquiry by the Health Service into the conduct of an obstetrician, Mrs Wendy Savage. During this inquiry one of Mrs Savage's patients attempted to prevent Tower Hamlets health authority from using her medical records in the course of its case against Mrs Savage. The patient strongly objected to the fact that these records, containing details of her pregnancy and the birth of her twins, were used without her permission. In her letter to the health authority (which was not read out to the inquiry) the patient says that she was "disturbed and distressed at the breach of the law of confidence".

> It is totally unacceptable to me that my notes be used, even with my name disguised, because it will be perfectly obvious to friends and neighbours who I am, and also because I have the highest esteem for Mrs Savage and the care she gave me and my children. It cannot be correct for you to use my notes and my own personal, intimate experiences against her, when I myself have absolutely no complaint to make.

To this counsel for the authority replied that,

> Her notes are the property of the department. We, as the health authority, have the custody and use of them. There is no question of this patient or that

saying they are not prepared to have the facts examined. They do not have the knowledge about whether this or that is right or wrong [2].

I shall henceforward refer to this patient as 'the Savage patient'.

This episode raises a number of issues about the nature of the relation between patient and physician, particularly within a system of socialised medicine. The most general question is: to whom do medical personnel have ultimate responsibility—the patient, or the wider institution and beyond that society as a whole? This is not however going to be my starting point, though the issue I wish to discuss is relevant to this general one. The patient clearly believed that she had some right to confidentiality which constrained the health authority as well as her own physician; and that in using her medical notes as it did the authority had violated that right. I am not here concerned with the question of whether any such right is in fact, or should be, enshrined in English law; my concern is rather with what such a right to confidentiality amounts to [3].

It is unclear whether the authority admitted either that there is such a right or that it was under any obligation to respect it. The patient's reference to her name having been disguised suggests that the authority did acknowledge such a right, and claimed to have respected it: for it suggests that she was told that there was no breach of confidence because no one could know to whom the medical notes referred. But, as she herself points out, this was not likely to be the case; people are recognisable not just through their names, but through many other things about them. So if the question of whether confidentiality has been breached depends upon whether others can *in fact* identify you as the subject of the facts which are made public, and if, as this patient claims, others could easily identify her, then there will have been a breach of confidentiality. If, however, medical files are made public with the patient's name disguised, and no one in fact connects the file with the patient, then it will seem that confidentiality has not been breached, and the patient would have no ground for complaint. I shall argue that this account of the matter would not satisfy the Savage patient; this is not all that the requirement for confidentiality amounts to.

Before embarking on this discussion I should mention a second sort of question to which this case draws our attention. It might be that the authority could admit to a breach of confidentiality, but go on to argue that such a breach was justified in the circumstances, and that everything had been done to minimise the effects of such a breach. The issue then would be, not whether there is such a thing as a right to confidentiality, but how far that right extends. Such an individual right as this is bound to conflict, at least sometimes, with the interests and rights of other individuals and with collective interests. Unless we are to argue that the right to confidentiality is absolute and inviolable, we shall need to be clear about the circumstances in which a physician is justified in breaching confidentiality. That this is an important issue is obvious: we need only think of the situation of AIDS sufferers and their physicians to see what is at issue here. Somehow the practical problems will have to be resolved; and it may even be the case that philosophers will have something helpful to say. This is not, however, the issue which I am concerned to discuss. There is not a lot of point, I suggest, in discussing the extent of any individual or collective right until we are clear what that right amounts to. The question of confidentiality involves quite deep philosophical concerns; and in a discussion of confidentiality these wider issues can be given some context and focus.

Why should we be concerned that medical facts about us, kept by our physicians and hospitals, be kept confidential? One answer to this, which might seem the most obvious, is that information about us may concern matters which we just do not wish others to know about, because it reflects badly on us; or because, even if it does not do that directly, it is such that it could be made use of by others to our detriment. It is not hard to think of all sorts of cases in which information, innocent in itself, could be used to one's detriment: information for instance about past venereal disease or past mental illness. Since these harmful consequences are not always predictable, we might argue that no information should be revealed by medical personnel without permission of the patient. At least then the responsibility will be the patient's own.

Two things are immediately obvious about this account of the matter. First, it suggests that what is at the bottom of a demand for confidentiality is the simple right not to suffer a variety of consequential harms; and thus that what we have is here a derivative right, not one which stands on its own. Secondly, and this is what will concern me most for the moment, even if a concern with the consequences of revealing information is what partly underlies the demand for confidentiality, this cannot be the whole story. The arguments offered by the Savage patient make this quite clear. What upset her was not that someone might use this information to her detriment. It is difficult to see how in the circumstances the details of the birth of her children could be so used, but I dare say if we were inclined to be sufficiently inventive we could come up with a plausible story. This is not necessary, however, since what clearly concerns her is not that enemies will discover that the information used in the hearing is about her, but that her friends and neighbours will know it. What concerns her is not that the information will reflect badly on her but just that they will know it. The sheer fact of others, even if they are friends and neighbours, knowing the facts about her "own personal, and intimate experience" is what is disturbing. What she wishes is that this information remain private just because it is information about her. Indeed I will suggest later that the crux of the matter is not whether anyone would recognise that the information is in fact about the Savage patient, but just that someone knows the facts at all. What we need is an account of confidentiality which will capture some of these ideas.

It seems from this that our concern with confidentiality in medicine is an aspect of our concern with privacy. What lies behind, but not at all deeply hidden, our demand that medical records be kept confidential is the demand that our right to privacy be respected. It is the nature of this right and why it is important to us, which needs to be examined. Let me make clear before proceeding with this, however, that the question I wish to ask here should not be taken in any complicated, ontological sense: I am not concerned, that is, with the sense in which we may be said to have any rights at all; nor with whether the right to privacy is a basic human right. These questions I leave entirely alone, although it might be that what I say would point in one direction rather than another. My concern is much more limited—it is with how far there is a right to privacy as such, and how far this right may be seen as deriving from other rights or to be simply collapsible into a cluster of other rights (for instance, most notably, property rights). This is not the place to attempt a general or complete account of everything that might fall within the scope of a 'right to privacy': rather, my main concern is with the notion of privacy which might underpin the Savage patient's complaint.

In 1890 Samuel D. Warren and Louis D. Brandeis argued there is a right to privacy and that this right is enshrined in the law of the United States. They claimed that,

> The principle which protects personal writings and all other personal pro-
> ductions, not against theft and physical appropriation but against publication

in any form, is in reality not the principle of private property, but that of an inviolable personality [4].

Much argument has been directed against this view. Among the more recent argument against there being any right to privacy as such are those offered by Judith Jarvis Thomson [5]; and I shall taken Thomson's arguments as standing for a general kind of argument to the effect that there is no specific right to privacy. (From this it should be clear that I am not concerned at all with the question of whether in fact there is any such right enshrined in the American or any other constitution.)

Thomson uses a series of rather bizarre examples which, she claims, will show

> that the right to privacy is itself a cluster of rights, and that it is not a distinct cluster of rights but itself intersects with the cluster of rights which the right over the person consists in and also with the cluster of rights which owning property consists in [6].

So, to take one of Thomson's bizarre examples, if you train an X-ray device on a person's wall-safe in which they keep a pornographic picture, then their right to privacy has been violated; but it will turn out that what this actually consists in is a property right, in this case the right that others shall not look at this picture. This right is, according to Thomson, one of the rights which go to make up ownership of the picture. It is in this way that the right to privacy will on her account collapse into property rights.

The rights which go to make up what she calls 'the right over the person' are described as 'un-grand rights', as contrasted with grand rights like the right to life, the right to liberty and so on. These 'un-grand rights' apparently consist in such things as the right not to have your hair cut off when you are asleep, or the right not to have your elbows painted green. A right which might be of more interest to most of us, I suppose, which would also fall into this category would be the right not to have your left knee stroked without your permission. I might be more inclined to call these rights, at least those listed by Thomson, frivolous rather than un-grand: but however one sees them, it will be clear that the right which the Savage patient claims does not fall into either of the categories of rights from which Thomson claims any right to privacy must be derived. Indeed she makes this much plain when she says

> . . . it seems to me that none of us has a right over any fact to the effect that it shall not be known by others. You may violate a man's right to privacy by looking at him or listening to him; there is no such thing as violating a man's right to privacy simply by knowing something about him [7].

But this is just what the Savage patient's claim comes to, since she does not argue that her Thomsonian 'right over the person', nor indeed any property right, has been violated, but just that people are now in a position to know things about her. I will argue later that there is a sense in which her person has been violated; but this is a sense which Thomson's account cannot capture. It is perhaps worth noting here that one way of interpreting the health authority's response to the Savage patient's objection is in terms of an argument which is indeed about property rights. The authority seems to take the view that it is the *medical records* themselves which constitute the property in question, and then to argue that these belong to the authority and not to the patient—so that the patient therefore has no right to them. A similar view is taken, or so it would appear, by the British Medical Association, which recently decided that patients should not have any right of access to the information held in the medical records kept by their physicians because the records were the property of the physicians or ultimately the Department of Health and Social Security [8]. Although this is not an issue which I shall tackle directly here, I think that it will become clear that there is a connection between the right of patients to information about themselves and the idea of privacy.

Thomson's argument to the effect that the right to privacy is a 'derivative' one can be criticised simply on the grounds that even if she has shown that there is an overlap, in some cases, between the right to privacy and property rights (I am inclined to think that she takes the right over the person to be a form of property right), she has not shown that the right to privacy is derivative, i.e. that these other rights are somehow prior; from the cases she considers it would be just as plausible to argue that the property rights are themselves derived from the right to privacy. My main objection to her argument is, however, that her account does not make any room at all for the sort of right which I have suggested is claimed by the Savage patient.

Why should an account of the right to privacy capture this claim? Might it not be argued that if the account is correct then it will just show that the Savage patient was wrong to suppose that she had any such right? This response will not do. To begin with, the case which Thomson makes for her account of privacy rests on the use of singularly bizarre examples, whereas the Savage patient's case is not in anyway bizarre, but is an example of a whole class of cases which are perfectly ordinary and which reflect a very ordinary sense of things which we would claim are just not anyone else's business. As James Rachels puts it in his reply to Thomson's paper,

> We have a 'sense of privacy' which is violated in such affairs, and this sense of privacy cannot be adequately explained merely in terms of our fear of being embarrassed or disadvantaged in one of these obvious ways. An adequate account of privacy should help us to understand what makes something 'someone's business' and why intrusions into things that are 'none of your business' are as such, offensive [9].

Rachels' account of privacy starts from the question of why privacy is important to us. His answer, in common with the one given by Charles Fried [10], is that privacy is important to us because without it all sorts of human relationships would be impossible. These relationships of friendship, love and trust are ones in which we give something of ourselves to the other person. They are relationships within which another person is allowed to come to know things about us, to share a degree of intimacy, from which others are excluded. If there were no such private information for us to give to those whom we choose as our friends and lovers, then there could be no such special relationships. There is at first sight a certain plausibility to this argument. There are, as we will see later, difficulties in trying to imagine a society in which there is no such thing as privacy, without going in for the kind of science fiction which would sit unhappily with my earlier strictures on Thomson's examples: but there are many communities, for instance prison communities, in which there is at least very little in the way of privacy; and in which we might see that certain kinds of close and exclusive friendship are no longer possible. Think too of how often among children the very 'special friend' is the one with whom some secret about themselves is shared. Certainly it is true that those to whom we are closest are those who know things about us, things which we are prepared to reveal to them but not to others.

However, the account which Fried and Rachels give of this cannot be entirely right; what is wrong with it is shown in this remark by Fried:

> ... intimacy is the sharing of information about one's actions, beliefs or emotions which one does not share with all, and which one has the right not to share with anyone. By conferring this right, privacy creates the moral capital which we spend on friendship and love [11].

One might say here that if this is the way you see friendship and love then you will soon go bankrupt. The idea that friendship might be based on the amount of information invested in it surely puts the whole business the wrong way round. It is just because someone is my friend that I am prepared to reveal things about myself that I do not reveal to others; I do not make someone my friend according to the amount of information I am prepared to give them. I do not, as it were, trade off information for friendship. This is, of course, just what children sometimes do; the child may indeed say "Tell me a secret and I'll be your best friend": but that is surely something which we might hope the child will grow out of.

No doubt privacy is connected to the possibility of certain kinds of human relationships: but the connection cannot be as Rachels and Fried portray it. Privacy is not important to us because it allows us to trade off information and thus create different kinds of relationship—even though I have agreed that certain kinds of relationship would not be possible without privacy, that is without there being some things about me which are not available to everyone and over which I have control. What matters here is the way in which these facts are about me, the way in which they are a part of my *self*. Privacy is important because it has to do with the drawing of the boundary around my self, and thus with the separation of my self as mine from others. It is, that is to say, crucially connected with my identity, with my existence as an autonomous individual, and with the possibility of my seeing myself in this way. Some things about me, my thoughts, feelings, desires, joys, sufferings and so on are in an important way *mine*. Here there is the logical point that they cannot be anyone else's: someone may have the same pain as I do, but cannot have my pain; this is part of the grammar of 'the same pain'. But this is more than a matter of logic, since it is necessary for me to acknowledge them as mine not just in that I am aware of them as objects of consciousness, but in that it is through them that I develop a sense of self-hood. They go to make up what I am, my personality, my self. Brandeis and Samuel were right to say that the principle behind the right to privacy is "that of an inviolate personality". The trouble with the way Fried and Rachels put the matter is that they make this 'personality' look like an item of property which can indeed be traded for some good like friendship.

Selves or persons (I do not think the terminology is vitally important here) are not born, however. As Jeffrey Reiman points out, the self in the sense relevant here is a social creation; it is a moral self which does not spring into being fully formed at the moment of birth—or at any other moment, for that matter [12]. Our selves develop in and through the language and life of the communities in which we live; the solitary creature forever pacing the confines of a desert island onto which it has been dropped by countless philosophers is not the ultimate private person. This is no place to explore the entrails of the Private Language Argument, but it does reverberate here. That solitary creature, the one and only solipsist, is not a person. Solipsism is not a state of total privacy, if indeed it is any state at all; but this claim must rest upon the arguments about solipsism—which are no doubt very familiar. Our sense of self is given only through our community with others. If there are no others then there is no "me" either. The thoughts and feelings which are mine must be recognised as mine by others if *I* am to have any sense of them as mine, and thus any sense of my self. The loss of what is mine, the fact of such things becoming public, when I gave no permission and thus have no control, involves then a loss of self. The self here has been appropriated by another and thus ceases to be mine. Here again I should emphasise the concern is not merely that someone else might manipulate me by using the knowledge they now have and that this might turn out to be to my detriment. What I am suggesting here perhaps comes closer to the account which Sartre gives of what he calls "the look of the other" [13]. The other's look is the way in which that other appropriates myself, and in doing so turns me into a mere thing. (Let me be clear at this point that, although my view here bears some relation to the Sartrian view, I do not wish to appropriate for my view all the existentialist metaphysical baggage that goes with Sartre's; my own metaphysical baggage will be quite enough to be going on with.) My argument is then that our concern with privacy is a concern with the protection of the self.

There are many who do not need philosophical argument to recognise this fact; all those who wish, for whatever reason, to exercise control over others, to use them as public objects subject only to their own will, see that the way to achieve this is to bring about in those individuals a loss of this sense of self, to get them to see themselves as such public objects. One way of doing this is to subject them to a regime in which all privacy is lost. Regimes which subject individuals to constant observation and probing into thoughts and feelings have the effect of destroying a person. Such forms of torture are not unfamiliar, and they are used because they work; no clearer account of this could be found than that given by Bruno Bettelheim in *The Informed Heart* [14].

Even treatments which are not directly intended to have this effect, but which do involve the exposure of a person's body to public gaze, will have the effect, perhaps only temporary, of some denial of the right to self. A recent example of this can be found in descriptions given by women subjected to strip searches by the police:

> There were all these policemen standing around and they stared. I couldn't understand it. All these men could be my father. How could they allow this to happen to me? I couldn't accept it. I thought I could cope, I thought I was strong, but I've felt completely inadequate since—crazy like a zombie [15].

Now why not describe this as an infringement of the rights against the person which Thomson claims are one cluster of rights from which the right to privacy is derived? Here certainly is a case in which attacks have been made upon 'the person' in the sense in which Thomson uses 'person', but this sense does not correspond to the sense in which I have been talking about the self. Reiman's argument is important here: that the person or self which is given through our existence in a community is one which is prior to the 'person' in the sense in which Thomson uses it. In her sense the 'person' over which I have a right is analogous to an item of property: I have a right not to have my knee stroked because that knee is mine, I own it. But my self is not something that I own, it is what I am. For there to be property and 'the person' in Thomson's sense there first has to be a self. Now we may sometimes be misled by language into supposing that my self is something which is owned in the same way that any item of property is owned: we can after all talk quite properly of someone selling themselves, when we do not just mean that they have sold their hair to a wig-maker or their blood to a hospital. Some moral debates do indeed hinge upon which sense of 'selling oneself' is in question; for example part of the debate about surrogate motherhood is about just this, whether selling or renting a womb is selling part of yourself in the way in which selling your hair is, or whether it is selling yourself where that is closer to the sense of 'selling your soul'—if not to the devil then at least in some sense which involves the loss of the moral self. But when we talk of 'selling oneself' or of 'owning oneself' in such cases, we shall be misled if we suppose that 'own' has the same use here as it has when we talk of owning a coat or a pair of shoes. My self is indeed 'mine' and no one else's: but it would make no sense for someone to ask if they could have a part share in it or inherit it, or have it at a discount. To steal a woman's soul is not at all the same as to steal her suitcase. To whom would the stolen soul be returned when found?

Some of the arguments about prostitution may serve to make the point here. One argument levelled against prostitution is precisely that in the business of buying and selling women's bodies those bodies are treated as items of property. The women then become mere items of property and the self is destroyed. That this is a loss which can be seen and experienced is shown in many of the accounts of prostitution, particularly those of the great feminist campaigners of the nineteenth century like Josephine Butler [16]. Of course seeing the matter in this way does presuppose the conception of the self as embodied. It would be interesting, perhaps, to see how far a thoroughgoing Cartesian could really object to prostitution.

Where we draw the boundary round the self, what is private and what is not, is what is likely to be in contention in many of the disputes about the infringement of the right to privacy. The account I have sketched of what might be called the 'metaphysical' self will not, and is not intended to, settle this kind of issue. The argument so far is only that the concept of the self and the concept of privacy belong together. The emphasis on the development of the self within a community rather than being a given from which the comunity is then constructed should make it clear that the content of the self cannot be given *a priori*.

Clearly not everything about an individual is part of the self in the sense in which I have been using it. But it is clear too that different communities may draw the boundaries in different places; there is no reason why we should assume that the sense of self will be everywhere the same. It is quite possible, for example, that the boundaries of the self could extend beyond the physical body to other objects. Such objects would then be part of the self; loss of them would be loss, or partial loss, of the self. Here they may be affinities with Hegel's account of the property relation, according to which property is the embodiment of the personality or the externalisation of the will [17]. Seen from such a perspective my earlier suggestion that property rights might be derived from the right to privacy would be vindicated since the self, and with it the idea of privacy, is now shown to be the prior notion in terms of which the concept of property is articulated. In demanding that our property be protected we are demanding that our selves be protected, and the concern with privacy is a concern for the self.

One upshot of these arguments might now seem to be not just that the concept of the self and the idea of privacy are inseparable, but that the same is true of the concept of community and the self; for there to be a community there must be selves, and thus in any community there must also be a distinction between the public and the private however that distinction is drawn. But perhaps it *is* possible to imagine a community in which there was no privacy at all, in which case, according to my argument, here would be a community in which there were no selves or persons in the sense in which I have been speaking of them. It would be a community in which everything was public—or rather in which there was no distinction between a public and private domain; in which bodies were not mine or yours, in which all thoughts and feelings were available always to everyone.

Now I said that perhaps such a community might be imagined: but so far I have gone no way towards imagining it; I have not, that is, shown anything at all about how things go on in that community—I have not shown it to be a community at all. It may well be that, lacking the imaginative powers necessary for such an exercise, I am too ready to conclude that such a thing cannot be done: but all the same this is what I am inclined to say. Part of the problem is that it is very difficult to see what it is that has to be imagined, since the people we imagine here cannot be just like us only with the privacy knocked out. We might start perhaps with an example of a community with less privacy than we have, for instance a prison community, and try extending it to our whole community: but, although we might well find such a community uncongenial, this clearly will not support the argument, since all that will have happened is that some of the things which we take to be private will not be. It need not be that there are no areas or privacy; after all even in the inadequate prisons which we have it is still possible for prisoners to keep their thoughts to themselves. If we imagine the extension of the prison community all we shall have imagined is a community with different concepts of self and privacy, not one in which all sense of self is lost. There are in any case plenty of anthropological examples of communities which are informed by different concepts of self and privacy.

The prisoner, I suggested, will still at least be able to keep her thoughts to herself and in that way retain a sense of self. Perhaps then we should try to imagine a community in which not only are individuals always seen by one another but their thoughts are always available too. There are novels in which such possibilities are developed, such as Salman Rushdie's *Midnight's Children* [18]: but in this case the children who are able to experience one another's thoughts directly are able to control this access, to switch on and off, and they are already given their identities prior to developing this capacity. What we need to imagine is a community in which everyone has access to the thoughts of everyone else; and this has to be not something which is acquired, but something which is there from the beginning. My suggestion is that now it is very difficult to give any coherent content to this community, i.e. to see it as a community at all. To begin with it is not clear how any conception of self and others could develop at all, since it is not clear how the thoughts are to be distinguished as mine or another's. How can any individual come to develop a sense of self? One might say here that what we are trying to imagine is something like the reverse of the solipsist view, for now we are trying to imagine a community which consists only of others. This will make no more sense than a world which consists of myself. I am inclined to say here that it is no longer clear what we are to imagine, though we may need to go further in this attempt at imagining than I have time to do here.

Where does all this leave the Savage patient and her demand that the facts about her pregnancy be kept confidential? After all, it might be said, she was not subjected to any invasion of her thoughts, what was made known about her were facts about her body, about her health. Surely this cannot involve the kind of invasion of self that I have been talking about? So far I have been concerned to argue that the right to privacy is important to our status as persons or selves, in that if we are to have some sense of our selves there must be some things which are recognised as ours, in the sense that these will form the content of the idea of self. If we are to have control over our selves, to be autonomous, then these are the things over which we must have control; and these may include facts about us. To respect privacy will be one of the ways in which we show respect for one another as persons.

But, as I have already said, the account of the 'metaphysical' self which I have offered can accommodate a range of contents; it does not specify any one in particular. Suppose it were agreed that we do have an underivative right that some things about us should not be known by others unless we agree to it: what argument is there to show that the things the Savage patient is concerned with, those "personal, intimate experiences" of pregnancy, fall into this category of things which go to make up the self? What reason is there for any claim that patients have a right to confidentiality in medicine beyond the right that they shall not suffer consequential harms through their medical records being deemed public property?

Physicians may be in a position which few other people are ever in, namely to discover things about us which we cannot discover for ourselves. These facts will concern our health and our health, I would suggest, is indeed a facet of our selves which is quite fundamental. It is so just because, unless we are perhaps Platonists of a radical kind, our bodies are essential aspects of our selves. Our bodies are not mere objects which we own like pieces of property; we do not inhabit our bodies as we inhabit our houses: the facts about our health are facts essentially about *us*, and it should therefore be we who determine who shall know about this aspect of ourselves. The right we have to expect confidentiality from our doctors is the same right that we have to expect it from anyone else. If I learn that my friend has lung cancer, she could rightly protest if I go around telling others of this when she herself does not. This is not just because some bad consequence might follow from my revelations; it might well be the case that only good consequences follow. My friend's protestations stem from the fact that her health is a facet of her self and a private matter. She is right to say that this just is none of my or anyone else's business unless she chooses to make it so.

But we need to be a bit clearer about how far this argument is to be taken, since it surely cannot be the case that every single fact about health is private in the way I have described. To begin with, it is not easy to see how something can be private unless there is some way in which it can be kept from others. A person with a broken leg can hardly suppose that this is a matter of fact which others have no right to know. How could they avoid knowing it when they are faced with the leg in a plaster cast? The point is, however, that it is up to the person with the broken leg whether she goes out and subjects her leg to the public gaze. If she chooses not to, then her privacy is invaded if I tell others about it. How far we can go here will depend upon how we see our bodies and ourselves, and the only way to discover where the boundaries are drawn is to consider examples of many different kinds. Our concept of health, both physical and mental, is very complex, the topic for another paper.

Complex though the concept of health is, I think it would be difficult to deny that pregnancy and birth are experiences in which a woman's self is deeply involved. It may indeed be very difficult to imagine it otherwise; not that this should be taken as suggesting that the *way* in which the self is involved will be everywhere the same. But the Savage patient was right to expect that the intimate details of her pregnancy should not be revealed to others, whoever they were, unless she agreed to such a revelation. Indeed no other person had the right to even know that she was pregnant unless she wished them to know it. Her sense of grievance is further heightened by the fact that in revealing the facts about her pregnancy to build up a case against someone against whom she had no complaint, the Health Authority was treating her in her very self not as a person but as a public object; her right to respect as a person had been violated. Doesn't that just show then that her right to privacy is derived from a more general right to be respected as a person? I can see no reason why it should be put in this way, rather than saying that the respect which should be accorded a person's privacy is just one of the forms which respect for persons takes.

I said at the beginning that the question of where a physician's responsibility lies, how much to the patient and how much to the wider community, is raised by the discussions about confidentiality. It might be thought that my claims about privacy have the implication that the claims of the patient are stronger than those of the community. This would be a confusion. My argument has been concerned with the idea that there is a right to privacy which demands the respect of everyone. It does not follow from this that physicians may not sometimes have no choice but to infringe that right. What does follow is that patients should be consulted in these matters; and it may be rather that we should, as patients, be prepared to waive the right to confidentiality in some cases. If a person is diagnosed as having a disease like AIDS, which is capable of being passed on to others in particular circumstances, then it seems clear, to me at any rate, that such a person should be prepared to let others know that she has such a disease. In extreme cases in which a patient will not waive her right of her own accord, perhaps a physician would be justified in violating the patient's right to confidentiality: but these are extreme circumstance, and nothing of the sort was at stake in the Savage case. The limits to be placed on social utility must be very strict indeed. Exactly what those limits are I do not know, but one thing is clear to me: whatever limits are to be set, the setting of them cannot be left to the health authorities; as the Tower Hamlets authority showed, "They do not have the knowledge about whether this or that is right or wrong".

Sandra E. Marshall, Department of Philosophy, University of Stirling, Stirling FK9 4LA, United Kingdom.

NOTES

[1] Earlier versions of this paper were read at the Centre for Philosophy and Public Affairs, St Andrews and the Universities of Stirling and Glasgow. I am grateful to all those who discussed it with me and in particular to Antony Duff, Stanley Kleinberg and Alan Millar.

[2] The quotations here are from the report of the case in *The Guardian*, 5 February, 1986.

[3] Throughout this paper I shall be concerned with the right to medical confidentiality. By this I shall mean the right of a patient not to have medical information revealed without consent. Issues concerning confidentiality are not, of course, limited to such cases as these, where what is in question is the confidentiality of the facts about a person's private affairs, nor do breaches of confidence always involve the revealing of such private information. My concern in this paper, however, is not with confidentiality in general (indeed, I am not sure how much can usefully be said about it *in general*) but with the particular kind of confidentiality which concerns the Savage patient, and its relation to notions of privacy.

[4] SAMUEL D. WARREN & LOUIS D. BRANDEIS (1890-1) The right to privacy, 4, *Harvard Law Review*, 193, p. 205.

[5] JUDITH JARVIS THOMSON (1975) The right to privacy, 4, *Philosophy & Public Affairs*, p. 295.

[6] op. cit., p. 306.

[7] op. cit., p. 307.

[8] cf. (1986) 293 *British Medical Journal*, pp. 78–82.

[9] JAMES RACHELS (1975) Why privacy is important, 4 *Philosophy & Public Affairs*, 323, p. 325.

[10] CHARLES FRIED (1967-8) Privacy, 77, *Yale Law Journal*, p. 475.

[11] FRIED, op. cit., p. 484.

[12] JEFFREY H. REIMAN (1976) Privacy, intimacy and personhood, 6, *Philosophy & Public Affairs*, p. 26.

[13] JEAN PAUL SARTRE *Being and Nothingness*, p. 252ff. (Trans. Hazel Barnes) (London, Methuen).

[14] BRUNO BETTELHEIM (1986) *The Informed Heart* (London, Penguin).

[15] Quoted in *The Observer*, 27 July, 1986.

[16] cf. MARGARET FORSTER (1986) *Significant Sisters* (London, Penguin).

[17] For my understanding of HEGEL I am indebted more than somewhat to DUDLEY KNOWLES' paper HEGEL on property and personality, (1983) 33, *The Philosophical Quarterly*, pp. 46–64.

[18] SALMAN RUSHDIE (1982) *Midnight's Children* (London, Pan).

24

Donation, Surrogacy and Adoption

EDGAR PAGE

ABSTRACT   *The Warnock Report fails to reveal an important underlying principle concerning the donation and transference of gametes and embryos. This principle contrasts sharply with the principle that children are non-transferable. Consideration of where to place the line between transferable embryos and non-transferable fetuses, or children, yields a conception of surrogacy that would set it apart from adoption. The paper argues for a coherent system of surrogacy supported by regulative institutions in which surrogacy is seen to facilitate an acceptable form of parenthood.*

Much of the discussion in this paper connects with certain aspects of the Report of the Warnock *Committee of Inquiry into Human Fertilisation and Embryology* [1]. However, that report contains recommendations aimed at suppressing all forms of surrogacy. It will become obvious that I am opposed to the broad condemnation of surrogacy that these recommendations imply, but I shall not argue directly against them in this paper. I am not really concerned here with the rights and wrongs of surrogacy.

There is a sense in which I shall advance a theory of surrogacy, although not a moral theory. I am inclined to think that we need a theory if we are to understand the problems that surrogacy will inevitably generate. This theory would need to show the relation between surrogacy and adoption, for example. Towards the end of the paper I shall make some remarks on this. However, to begin with I make an indirect approach through the question: who are a child's parents?

Normally we have no difficulty in saying who a child's parents are. The traditional view is that they are its natural parents—or for clarity, its genetic parents. This view has receded somewhat in recent years—partly, perhaps, because of the growth of adoption since the 1920s. There is now a question of whether the traditional view will receive further battering as a result of new techniques in reproduction. The Warnock Committee dealt with certain aspects of this and my discussion will relate to some of the views and recommendations that the Committee puts forward.

The donation of gametes and embryos for use in reproduction sets up tensions concerning who should be considered the child's parents. For example, sperm donation in the practice of AID raises questions about who is the child's father. In most cases, probably, AID is supplied to women whose husbands consent to the use of it and who want to take the resulting child as their own. Yet an AID child is illegitimate, technically, under the present law. The husband is not recognised as the child's legal father and cannot legally be entered as the father when the child is registered. Furthermore, a sperm donor, who usually remains anonymous, could legally be made liable for the maintenance of the child. He could also apply to a court for custody or access. To this extent he is considered to be the child's father.

Most people would now think that all of this is unjust and the Warnock Committee seeks to remedy these injustices. It recommends changes in the law to the effect that the husband of a woman who receives AID, if he consents to it, should be the (legal) father of the child and should be entered as such at registration of the child, that the donor should have no rights or duties in respect of the child and that the child should be legitimate.

AID has raised the question of who is the child's father. This question is now sharpened by the fact that *in vitro* fertilisation and other new techniques have made egg and embryo donation possible and raise the question: who is the child's *mother?* As the Warnock Report says, "Egg [or embryo] donation produces for the first time the circumstances in which the genetic mother (the woman who donates the egg), is a different person from the woman who gives birth to the child" (6.8). A woman who gives birth to a child by egg or embryo donation is not genetically related to the child although it may be the progeny of her husband. Now clearly, the intention of the woman who bears the child, and her husband, is that the child should be theirs. But if the egg donor, who is the genetic mother of the child, claims that the child is hers, or if there is an issue concerning inheritance or citizenship that turns on the question of who is the child's mother, how could the problem be solved?

In the Warnock Report the problem is dealt with as follows. First, where an egg or an embryo is donated it is argued that, "the donation should be treated as absolute" and that the donors should have no rights and duties with respect to the child. Secondly, it is recommended that, "the woman giving birth" to the child should be regarded as the mother. There are, then, two factors to be taken into account: on the one hand, the fact that the egg or embryo has been donated and, on the other hand, the fact that the woman who receives it is the woman who gives birth to the child. It should be noticed, however, that the fact of donation is assigned only negative importance. That is, the sole importance of donation is that the donor loses all rights and duties in respect of the child. The embryo, or at any rate the resulting child, belongs to the recipient because she gestates and gives birth to the child and *not* because the egg or embryo was donated to her. The embryo is (physically) transferred to her uterus, but there is no hint in Warnock that the reason it now belongs to her is that the rights and duties of ownership, which the donor surrenders, are transferred to her.

This is more apparent when we come to the Committee's discussion of how surrogacy could raise the "stark issue" as to whether "the genetic mother or the carrying mother is the true mother". The main difficulty here is "the possible case where the egg or embryo has *not* been donated but has been provided by the commissioning mother or parents with the intention that they should bring up the resulting child" (8.20). We are to imagine then a case where a woman undertakes to have an embryo transferred to her uterus so that she can gestate it for the commissioning parents. I shall call this 'gestatory' surrogacy [2]—so a gestatory surrogate gestates an embryo that is not genetically related to her. Faced with this case the Committee argues that the legislation already recommended, to deal with cases where the egg or embryo has been donated, should be drawn "sufficiently widely" to cover it. That is, the principle that the true mother is the woman who gives birth to the child is to be applied here on an *ad hoc* basis. This is required, it is argued, "for the avoidance of doubt" as to who the true mother is. It is acknowledged that this ruling could result in injustices to the child that lives with the commissioning parents, who are its genetic parents, rather than with the woman who gave birth to it and who would be its legal mother; but there is no mention of any possible injustice to the commissioning couple.

This strikes me as being entirely unreasonable and I suspect that others, like me, will be unable to accept it [3]. Even those who agree with the Committee's overall condemnation of surrogacy may feel that this is an unsatifactory *ad hoc* ruling. When the woman who gestates the child receives the embryo by donation, she has a strong claim to the child *because* the embryo was donated to her. But surely if the embryo transferred to her uterus was *not* donated to her, her claim to the child would not be the same, especially if those who supplied the embryo did so on the explicit understanding that the resulting child would be returned to them and if they would not have supplied the embryo otherwise.

Imagine that the couple who want the child are childless; that by normal standards they are fit people to start a family; that they can produce their own viable gametes but, for compelling medical reasons, the wife cannot undergo pregnancy; that other possible solutions to their childlessness, such as adoption, are not open to them; and that in any case they are strongly motivated to have a child that is their own genetic offspring. A strong case could be made for saying that if a child from their genetic materials could be brought into existence, they should be helped. So, if another woman who already has children of her own wants to help this couple by gestating their embryo for them, on the strict understanding that the child is theirs and will be handed over to them at birth, should she not be allowed to do so? And if she does have a child for them with this explicit understanding, does that couple not have a claim to the child?

I shall not discuss the wider ethical issues here. My concern is the narrower question of who has a claim to the child and the importance for this question of the fact that in this case the genetic parents patently do *not* donate their embryo to the surrogate gestator. This fact is more important than tends to be recognised. And conversely, when an egg or embryo *is* by donation, this too is more important than is generally recognised and certainly more important than is suggested by the Warnock recommendation that legislation designed for cases involving donation should be applicable to cases that do not involve donation.

It is natural to take the donation of an egg or embryo to involve the surrender and transfer of all the rights and duties in respect of the child that would otherwise be the donor's as the child's genetic parents. A donation is a gift and if you give something away any rights and duties you have in respect of that thing are lost and transferred to the person to whom it has been given. If you give away a building you would normally expect to lose your right of access to it along with whatever liability you had to maintain it. The new owner would acquire this right and liability. Of course, a gift transaction need not be a direct transfer of rights and duties from one person to another. It might involve intermediaries, so that the donor and the recipient do not know each other. This is commonly the case in donations of genetic materials where, in any case, donors usually remain anonymous.

It is reasonable to say that AI donors relinquish their rights and duties in respect of the sperm they donate. Can we say that these rights and duties are transferred to the recipient of the sperm? In many cases where rights and duties are transferred it is possible to account for the fact that the recipient has those rights and duties by saying they were transferred to her. But we cannot account for the fact that an AID mother has parental rights and duties by saying that they are *transferred* to her. She has those rights and duties in virtue of being herself the genetic mother of the child.

However, the fact that she has them in her own right does not mean that her acceptance of the sperm donation did not involve the transference of rights and duties to her. It is rather that the transfer of the rights and duties to her could make no difference to her position.

If the woman is unmarried she would hold these rights and duties exclusively. If she is married, though, there is a question of whether the rights and duties of the donor could be considered to be transferred to her husband, or to her and her husband jointly. Imagine a social practice of AID in which the donated semen is first given to the husband of the woman to be inseminated, not to maintain a pretence that the woman is inseminated by her husband, but to symbolise that the donor's rights and duties are now transferred to him. It would be necessary for the husband to accept the semen and so to acknowledge transference of the rights and duties to him.

In our own society, when the husband consents, it is reasonable to suppose that the intention is that the rights and duties that the donor surrenders are transferred to the husband, or to the husband and wife jointly, so that they are both the parents of the child, even though under the present law the husband is not considered to be the father of the child.

Let us now return to the question as to who should be recognised as the mother of the child, the genetic mother or the gestator, when a woman is pregnant by embryo transfer, the embryo not being genetically related to her. This question is basically the same question as: which of the two women have the rights and duties of the mother? The woman who gestates the child could not have these rights as the child's genetic parent—she is not the genetic parent. Therefore, on my view, it will be a matter of whether the rights and duties have been transferred to her. And this will depend on whether the embryo that was physically transferred to her was donated, or not. In the case where the egg or embyro is donated the donor relinquishes her rights and duties in respect of it and they are transferred to the recipient. Therefore the gestator as the recipient is the mother of the child. But this is because the rights and duties are transferred to her and not because she gestates and gives birth to the child, as the Warnock Committee would have us believe.

In the case of gestatory surrogacy the genetic parents supply the embryo that is transferred to the womb of the surrogate but they do not voluntarily surrender and transfer their parental rights and duties. On the contrary, it is their explicit intention that they should retain them and have the child themselves. There is a clear agreement between them and the surrogate that the child will be returned to them when it is born. Therefore there could not be the same justification here for saying that the gestator is the child's mother as there is in the case where the embryo is donated. Of course, there is a strong temptation to describe the surrogate gestator in this case as the surrogate *mother* and to think of her as having entered into an agreement to give up *her* child to the commissioning couple. But this is to beg the question. The case has yet to be made for saying that the claims of the gestator override the claims of the commissioning parents who in this case wish to retain rather than surrender their rights and duties in respect of the embryo and resulting child. We cannot simply assume this. And to make an *ad hoc* ruling would seem to do an injustice to the commissioning couple.

In making its recommendations about sperm, egg and embryo donation the Committee draws on a mish-mash of considerations where we might have expected, or hoped for, a unifying principle. In connection with sperm donation they are concerned, and rightly so, that the child should not be regarded as illegitimate and that husbands should not be driven into falsifying the register, for example. In considering egg and embryo donation they appeal to the need to 'remove doubt' as to who the 'true mother' of the child is and they were swayed, perhaps, by a natural sentiment favouring the woman who gives birth to the child. The fact of donation itself is seen to be of some importance, but only negatively. Perhaps that made it easy for the Committee to dismiss the fact that in cases of gestatory surrogacy the embryo is clearly *not* donated.

I want to suggest that, in this, there is a failure to reveal the underlying principle—a matter of some importance in a report that aims to expose the principles underlying public policy. The principles involved here are, first, that genetic parents, as the producers of gametes, are the initial holders of parental rights and duties and, secondly, that these rights and duties can be surrendered and transferred by the donation of gametes and embryos [4]. Put simply it is the principle that gametes and embryos are transferable. This principle makes it possible at once to see why we agree with the Warnock Committee's recommendations concerning AID, and the donation of eggs and embryos and, also, why we want to reject the recommendation that the gestator, the woman who gives birth to the child, should be considered the mother in gestatory surrogacy. The principle allows us to see more clearly why donation of gametes or embryos is important, when it takes place, and why its absence is important in cases where it does not: that is, in gestatory surrogacy.

Let us now consider the more familiar form of surrogacy where a woman agrees to produce her own genetic child for a married couple who are unable to have a child themselves by the wife becoming pregnant. The most common case is where the surrogate mother is impregnated with sperm from the husband of the couple who want the child, usually by artificial insemination but sometimes by sexual intercourse. As it is plain that the surrogate mother in this case is the genetic mother of the child, it will be convenient to refer to this kind of surrogacy as 'genetic' surrogacy to distinguish it from gestatory surrogacy. But note that whereas a surrogate gestator is not the genetic mother of the child, a genetic surrogate does gestate.

In genetic surrogacy most people would think that the surrogate is the child's mother. And certainly that would be the position legally. Now much of the discussion of this kind of surrogacy centres on the agreement, or contract, drawn up between the surrogate and the commissioning couple. The question is whether an agreement or contract requiring the surrogate mother to give up her child should be binding. Should it be enforceable? The Warnock Report takes a very firm line here and recommends that legislation should be introduced to lay down by statute that no surrogacy agreement shall be enforceable. This would take the matter entirely out of the hands of the courts.

I am inclined to think that this would be a very rough sort of justice. In genetic surrogacy, for example, when the husband of the commissioning couple has supplied the sperm that fertilised the egg, it was obviously no part of his intention to donate his sperm to the surrogate. It certainly was not his intention or wish that he should relinquish all rights and duties in respect of the child and we might naturally think that, as the genetic father, he therefore has some rights. Under present law in England he is, of course, in the same position as the father of any illegitimate child. He could be made liable for the maintenance of the child and he could ask a court for custody or access. But recent cases have shown first that he is unlikely to be granted custody if the surrogate decides that she wants to keep the child and secondly that in any case there would be no easy way for him and his wife to adopt the child. Many people take the view that the agreement entered into by the surrogate mother could have no binding effect and should not be enforceable. But I would argue that because there was an agreement, it is unjust to treat the husband in this case as having no more claim to the child than the natural father of an illegitimate child resulting from a casual sexual relationship.

I shall not discuss the question as to whether the husband has a special claim as the *genetic* father in this case. Indeed, to do so could cause confusion. The main issue is whether the commissioning couple should have any claim to the child in virtue of the surrogacy agreement. This question does not hang on the fact that the husband of the commissioning couple is the genetic father of the child.

The issue of the agreement is clearest in the simplest of all forms of surrogacy —that is, where one married couple enters into an agreement to have a child for another married couple who, let us assume, are themselves unable to have a child. No new techniques are needed for this form of surrogacy. We can assume that the child would be conceived naturally by sexual intercourse. The surrogate couple supply all the functions for producing the child and are thus complete substitutes for the commissioning couple. Therefore I shall call this 'total' surrogacy. We can assume that the child is to be produced for the infertile commissioning couple from altruism. We can further assume that a formal agreement is drawn up but without involving any monetary considerations.

In any other circumstances we would certainly say that this child belongs to its natural parents. But in this case the natural parents entered into a surrogacy agreement to produce the child for the commissioning parents. If it were not for the agreement, we may suppose, the natural parents would not have had the child at all. Which couple therefore have a claim to the child?

If the commissioning parents have a claim to the child, in total surrogacy, it must be entirely because of the agreement drawn up between them and the surrogate couple. No other factors are relevant. Now the agreement is that when the child is born it will be handed over by its natural parents to the couple who want it. And the intention is that this would involve a transference of all the rights and duties of the natural parents in respect of the child to the commissioning parents. It is tantamount to an agreement that the child will be handed over to the commissioning couple for adoption.

This raises a special problem. In this country the law does not allow private adoptions or private arrangements for adoption. A child can only be adopted by an adoption order made by a court and no court would be likely to allow an agreement of the kind we have here to pre-empt the question of whether an adoption order should be made or not.

The Children Act 1975 [5] lays down explicitly that the child's parents must agree to the adoption, except in special circumstances which do not affect the issue here. Furthermore, agreement by the natural mother is "ineffective" if given less than six weeks after the child is born (12.6). It is also expressly laid down that parents cannot surrender or transfer their parental rights and duties in respect of a child. These rights and duties can only be removed or transferred by an order of the court. So it would appear plain that the surrogacy agreement could not be legally binding on the child's natural parents should they change their minds and decide that they want to keep the child.

This reveals a principle of fundamental importance for the present discussion—*the principle that children are not transferable by individual parents.* Only a court can effect the transfer of a child from one set of parents to another. This is not simply a feature of the law as it now stands. It underlies much of our thinking in these matters and it seems to lie behind some moral objections to surrogacy.

I shall not try to uncover the foundations of this principle. A number of relevant factors come readily to mind. For example, if people were free to divest themselves of their parental responsibilities, children would be put at risk. There is also the view that children are not simply objects and that to think of them as transferable in the way that objects are is to devalue them. However, whatever the reasons, I would expect most people to accept the principle so, for the remainder of the discussion, I shall assume that it is to be accepted.

Now acceptance of the principle that children *cannot* be transferred contrasts sharply with our acceptance of the the principle that gametes and embryos *can* be transferred. We have seen how the Warnock Committee accepts the donation of gametes and embryos and recommends changes in the law that would *in effect* make it possible for donors to divest themselves of their parental rights and duties and transfer them to the recipients of their genetic materials. This indicates a large difference in attitude to gametes and embryos, on the one hand, and to children, on the other. Clearly, there could be no acceptance of *child donation.*

It would seem to follow directly from the principle that children are not transferable by individuals that *genetic* surrogacy and *total* surrogacy agreements could not be regarded as binding or enforceable. However, I argued earlier that *gestatory* surrogacy could be accepted and that the agreement involved there could be considered binding. The difference is that in gestatory surrogacy the child belongs to the commissioning parents from the outset as they do not at any stage relinquish their rights and duties in respect of it. The commissioning couple in this case are (to be considered) the child's parents even though the surrogate provides the function of gestation. There is therefore no question of the child being transferred except in a purely physical sense and consequently gestatory surrogacy would not fall foul of the principle that children are not transferable.

Now it will seem odd that gestatory surrogacy should be allowed if we are to bar genetic surrogacy and total surrogacy. However, we need not leave the matter there. In the example of gestatory surrogacy that we considered above, the commissioning couple were able to supply an embryo from their own gametes for transfer to the uterus of the gestatory surrogate. But if gestatory surrogacy is permitted at all, there could be no objection to the commissioning couple supplying an embryo from an egg that was *donated* to them and fertilised by the husband's sperm. If the wife of the commissioning couple was both sterile and unable to undergo pregnancy this could be a solution to their childlessness. But now there is no reason why the gestatory surrogate should not be the same woman as the egg donor. If she were, unlike the normal gestatory surrogate, she would then be the genetic mother of the child she gestates. But she would not have the usual parental rights and duties in respect of the child because these rights and duties were transferred to the commissioning couple when she donated the egg. On the principles we have been following the child here would belong to the commissioning couple and the surrogacy agreement need not be viewed as violating the principle that children are not transferable.

We now seem to have got ourselves into an absurd position. We are saying that a surrogate could legitimately undertake to provide her own progeny for the commissioning parents providing that she first has the egg removed from her body so that she can donate it and then has the embryo from it transferred back to her uterus. But she could not legitimately undertake to provide her progeny for the commissioning couple by having the same egg fertilised in her body by artificial insemination.

To escape from this ridiculous position we need to bring into the account the idea that an egg or embryo could be donated without being removed from the woman's body. I shall call this *donation in utero* [6] to distinguish it from the donation of eggs or embryos that are outside the body. To be clear here we need to distinguish between the physical transference of an egg or embryo from one woman's body to another woman's body and the transfer of the ownership of an egg or embryo. The latter involves the transference of rights and duties in respect of the egg or embryo and the resulting child but not necessarily the movement of the egg or embryo physically from one person to another.

Let us suppose then that a woman agrees to make an egg donation *in utero* to the commissioning couple and also to perform the function of gestation for them. The egg is fertilised with sperm from the husband of the commissioning couple by artificial insemination. The child could then be considered to belong to the commissioning couple from the outset, thus removing all question of it being transferred to them by adoption at birth, or soon after. There would then be no breach of the principle that children are not transferable and therefore there could not be *that* reason for refusing the arrangement moral or legal recognition. A similar account can be given of total surrogacy. We simply suppose that the couple who are to produce the child enter into an agreement whereby the woman is to donate her egg *in utero* and her husband donates his sperm, or they donate the embryo *in utero* as soon as the egg is fertilised. The embryo and the child could then be regarded as belonging to the commissioning parents from the outset.

It is most unlikely that any surrogacy agreements have ever been drawn up in these terms. But is there any reason why they should not be? If there is not, would understanding genetic surrogacy in these terms make any significant difference to our attitudes to it? If eggs and embryos can be denoted or transferred at all, it is an important question whether they can be donated *in utero*. Is there any reason why it should not be possible? The mere fact that the egg or embryo is still in the woman's body is hardly enough in itself to show that it could not be donated or transferred in ownership to the commissioning couple. Obviously, someone could give away or sell a crop of apples without removing it from the orchard. The owner of a donkey could give away or sell a donkey foal while it is still *in utero*. Similarly, there is no incoherence in the idea that an egg or embryo in the body might be donated. In the end it is a question of whether the surrounding rules, conventions or laws allow anything to count as the donation *in utero* of an egg, or embryo, with a consequent transference of rights and duties in respect of it.

It is clear that nothing could count as the donation of a *child* because nothing is allowed to do so. We think there are good reasons for not allowing it. But our attitudes to gametes and embryos are different. Eggs and embryos can be donated when they are outside the womb. On this there is wide agreement. Furthermore, there appear to be no settled attitudes that would prohibit their donation *in utero*. Nor is there any clear reason why there should be.

Against what I am saying, it might be argued that during gestation the child cannot be regarded as belonging to anyone other than the gestator. It might be thought to be absurd or senseless to suppose as I am that it might belong to the commissioning couple. But in the normal situation in which a married couple have a child the child belongs to the father as well as and as much as to the mother during gestation. Of course the mother has rights that the father does not have at this stage. No doubt these have to do with the fact that pregnancy can affect the mother's health and could even threaten her life. In any case, a woman has a right to choose what should happen in and to her body. But this does not mean that the father is not the child's parent or that the child does not yet belong to him.

Now the commissioning couple could be considered to be the parents of the child during gestation just as the normal father is a parent at that time. They might have to accept that the surrogate is in a privileged position concerning certain decisions affecting the child. For example, she must be free to have an abortion if her life is in jeopardy. But that would not negate the idea that they are the child's parents.

If we had a coherent system or practice of surrogacy in which a woman could donate an egg or embryo *in utero*, certain problems would arise. If embryo donation *is* permissible but child donation is *not* permissible, there is a question of where the line is to be drawn. This connects with the issue of the status of the embryo as it arises in connection with abortion or fetal research, but it is not the same problem. For example, embryos might be considered to be transferable but neither abortable nor proper subjects for experimental research. On the other hand, it is not clear to me that if a fetus of a given age may be aborted then fetuses of that age are therefore transferable.

If we were concerned only with the donation of IVF embryos outside the body for transfer to a woman's uterus there would be less of a problem because embryos for transplantation are necessarily at an early stage in their development. But if embryos can be donated *in utero*, then the question of where to draw the line between transferable embryos and non-transferable children becomes an urgent matter. We saw that the principle of non-transferability of children requires that people should not be free to arrange adoptions privately. This principle would be seriously undermined if a woman could donate a seven month old fetus, say, to a couple who want a child.

It is doubtful whether this problem could be resolved by drawing a line in terms of the development of the embryo or fetus. Such a line would appear arbitrary and would be the subject of controversy. A clear line would be at birth, but if it were drawn there it would be impossible to defend. If children were transferable until they were born but were not transferable after birth, it would be difficult to see what practical point the rule could have. Children could be put at risk by parents anxious to rid themselves of their responsibilities. And allowing fetuses to be donated or transferred at seven or eight months would devalue children as much as allowing them to be transferred when they are born. Furthermore, although donation *in utero* cannot be excluded in principle, there would be practical difficulties in placing the line between conception and birth. For example, a woman who unexpectedly found herself pregnant would have a strictly limited time in which to decide whether to donate her fetus or not.

Perhaps the only rational and practically reasonable place to draw the line would be before conception or fertilisation. A clear and simple rule would be that embryos can only be transferred or donated by agreements entered into at a point clearly before conception. Such a rule would allow us to make a potentially valuable distinction between adoption and surrogacy—a distinction that is not normally made although it is one that could change our attitudes to surrogacy.

Surrogacy tends to be treated as a form of adoption because to achieve its aim, *under existing laws and modes of thought,* the commissioning couple must hope to be able to adopt the child from its legal mother, the surrogate mother, after it is born. The surrogacy agreement, or contract, inevitably appears to be aimed at committing the surrogate mother to giving up her child for adoption at birth or soon after. Clearly the agreement runs contrary to the rules for adoption. However, if we had laws that recognised agreements whereby before conception a woman donates her egg, or embryo, *in utero* the embryo would belong to the commissioning couple from the outset and the resulting child would be theirs. At no point then would there be a question of transferring the child.

It would be possible for the issue of surrogacy to be kept totally separate from adoption. Quite apart from any consideration of egg or embryo donation and transference of ownership, quite apart from the question as to the proper basis for the attribution, loss, acquisition or transfer of parental rights and duties, there would be positive advantages to be gained from treating the issue of surrogacy apart from adoption. Of course, there is the common factor that both surrogacy and adoption are ways for people to acquire children. But adoption is concerned with arrangements for *existing* children who need parents whereas surrogacy is concerned with the *production* of children for parents, or would-be parents, who want them.

Adoption as it exists in this country has to be understood in relation to a body of law and regulative institutions established largely by a succession of legislation since 1926. This legislation has little regard for the position, aspirations and interests of adoptive parents. The emphasis is entirely on the interests of the children. Of course it would be easy to think that the law regulating adoption should be concerned with the interests of children rather than the interests of adults because children are defenceless. But that is not quite the point. Adoption as it exists in this country is aimed at serving the needs of children who have the misfortunate not to have parents to care for them and bring them up. Adoption is instituted largely as a means of dealing with the social problem created by the existence of parentless or unwanted children. Perhaps the majority of adoptive parents want children for much the same sort of reason as most other parents have them. Infertile couples might see adoption as a solution to their own needs. But their needs are of secondary importance as far as institutionalised adoption is concerned. It is clearly laid down that the first concern of the adoption services must be the welfare of the child.

By comparison an institutionalised system of surrogacy would naturally have the interests of the commissioning parents as its first concern. Of course, everyone is rightly concerned that surrogacy should not put children at risk. But if surrogacy is to occur at all it must be seen as essentially aimed at meeting the needs of the commissioning parents. Unless their needs were allowed to be met there would be no surrogacy children. Surrogacy would not occur if the commissioning parents did not want the child.

When a child is given up by her parents for adoption, for whatever reason, it is likely to be seen by the adopted person as a form of rejection and to have an adverse effect on her. Under a system of surrogacy along the lines I have described, the child comes into being *only because it is wanted by its parents,* that is, by the commissioning parents. There is then the possibility that being a surrogacy child in a society with a suitable framework of institutions that kept surrogacy apart from adoption would have advantages over being an adopted child.

But perhaps the most important thing about a properly instituted system would be that in important ways parenthood by surrogacy would be much closer to normal parenthood than it is possible for adoptive parenthood to be. I have argued elsewhere, in a paper on 'Parental Rights' [7], that human parenthood is a distinctive form of activity that is desired for its own sake and stands among our basic values. I argued further that parenthood as we know and value it cannot be understood properly without taking into account the characteristic parental motive of creating another human being. This creative motive embraces both begetting and rearing the child. Adoptive parents necessarily forgo the begetting of the child. This is in no way a slur on adoptive parents, many of whom consciously aim to love and care for a child that has the misfortune to be parentless or even handicapped. But for those adoptive parents who seek adoption as a solution to their infertility it is bound to be second best to natural parenthood because of the absence of the procreative role.

By contrast it is plain that surrogacy allows this creative role to be there in varying degrees, depending on the particular form of surrogacy. But in all cases, under the concept of surrogacy that I have developed here, there is the fact that but for the commissioning parents the child would not have been brought into existence. That, it seems to me, is a singular fact that can easily be lost sight of if surrogacy is not clearly distinguished from adoption—at least, as it exists in our society.

Of course, a system of surrogacy could be open to abuse, especially if under it surrogacy was allowed to become commercialised. But that would be true of adoption or even natural procreation if there were no regulation of these practices by laws, social rules and conventions. Like adoption, surrogacy would need the benefit of institutions and regulation. This is not the place to detail the form that these regulative institutions might take. But, if the argument of this paper is right, they should be based on a notion of surrogacy as facilitating a close approximation to normal parenthood rather than as an unnatural and unwholesome substitute for it [8].

Edgar Page, Department of Philosophy, University of Hull, Hull HU6 7RX, United Kingdom.

NOTES

[1] Cf. *Report of the Committee of Inquiry into Human Fertilisation and Embryology*, Chairperson Dame Mary Warnock DBE, HMSO, 1984 Cmnd. 9314.

[2] Other terms are sometimes used. For example, Peter Singer & Deane Wells say 'full' surrogacy where I say 'gestatory' surrogacy and 'partial' surrogacy for what I shall call 'genetic' surrogacy below. They have no term for what I shall later call 'total' surrogacy. The terms I propose are clearer and more precise than those proposed by Singer and Wells. Cf. Peter Singer & Deane Wells, *The Reproduction Revolution* (Oxford, OUP), 1984.

[3] Two members of the Warnock Committee express their dissent from some of the views in the Report on the question of surrogacy in 'Expression of Dissent: A. Surrogacy' appended to the Report.

[4] These principles leave it an open question whether gametes and embryos are *owned* in the sense of being property. Mary Warnock would say they are not. I would argue that they are, but that is an issue to be pursued elsewhere. Cf. Mary Warnock (1983), In vitro fertilisation: the ethical issues (II), *The Philosophical Quarterly*, 33(132), pp. 245–6.

[5] Cf. FREEMAN, M.D.A. (1976) *The Children Act 1975—text with concise commentary* (London, Sweet & Maxwell).

[6] The term 'in utero' as I use it has a wider meaning than in current medical use. It might be rendered as 'in the belly' rather than as '(implanted) in the uterus'.

[7] Cf. PAGE, EDGAR (1984) Parental rights, *Journal of Applied Philosophy*, 1(2), pp. 187–203.
[8] This paper was written for the 1985 Conference of the Society for Applied Philosophy. It was also presented to the Philosophical Society, University of Hull. I am grateful to many, not least students, for valuable discussion of the paper, but I am especially indebted to David Haslett & Dilys Page for criticism and help with an earlier draft.

25

Gifts of Gametes: reflections about surrogacy —comment on Page

JENNIFER TRUSTED

In his paper 'Donation, surrogacy and adoption', Edgar Page is concerned with the social and legal problems arising from the fact that the ordinary method of human reproduction can now be supplemented: by AID and also by fertilization *in vitro* followed by implantation. Thus a woman may carry and bear a child who has not developed from the sperm of her husband or lover and/or has not developed from her own ovum.

New techniques have given hope to infertile couples who would previously have had to adopt. They may commission an embryo produced by others' gametes or they may be able to produce a child which is genetically related to at least one partner and possibly to both. Obviously some of these methods involve the help of a surrogate mother.

I think that Page is right to object to the suppression of all forms of surrogacy and I also think he is right to draw our attention to the inevitable lacunae and inadequacies of current laws, and to the particular problems that arise when the desires of commissioning parents (the infertile couples) conflict with the wishes of surrogate mothers. Who has the legal right to care for the child that has been born, and who indeed has the legal duty? Page is concerned with parental rights, rather than duties and, in this paper I shall consider just these.

Page proposes a legal solution to the problem of rights based on his view that gametes are negotiable goods in that they can be freely donated by those who produce them and that, once donated, ownership is transferred absolutely to the donee(s) so that donors cease to have any rights or obligations. He reminds us that in regard to AID current law is out of touch with common sense in that a husband who approves his wife's having AID is not the legal father of her child. He supports the Warnock Committee's recommendation that the law be changed:

> Most people would now think that all of this is unjust and the Warnock Committee seeks to remedy these injustices. It recommends changes in the law to the effect that the husband of a woman who receives AID, if he consents to it, should be the (legal) father of the child and should be entered as such at registration of the child, that the donor should have no rights or duties in respect of the child and that the child should be legitimate [1].

It seems that we do think of sperm as negotiable entities (they have always been relatively freely given!) and most of us are likely to incline to the view that a woman should be free to donate her ova if she so desires. Donating our gametes is in part analogous to donating our blood; both donations may be contrasted with donating a hand—we are *not* free to do this, for it is illegal to mutilate oneself or others.

However Page is advocating more than legal freedom to donate for he is saying that in donating we must abandon all claim to interest in the subsequent fate of the gametes. We are to be legally absolved of all responsibilities and we have also renounced all legal rights. These are transferred to the donee(s), just as if a sum of money or a house had been given.

Page's suggestion is interesting and stimulating and it leads him to object to the Warnock Committee's recommendation that a woman who gestates an embryo should *always* be the child's legal mother. He wishes to make a sharp distinction between the woman who has an embryo donated *to* her (she should indeed have legal rights as a mother) and the woman who gestates an embryo that has *not* been donated to her. Page says:

> When the woman who gestates the child receives the embryo by donation, she has a strong claim to the child *because* the embryo was donated to her. But surely if the embryo transferred to her uterus was *not* donated to her, her claim to the child would not be the same, especially if those who supplied the embryo did so on the explicit understanding that the resulting child would be returned to them and if they would not have supplied the embryo otherwise [2].

Page holds that rights over the child should be abnegated even when the surrogate mother provided her own ovum *if* she had previously agreed to donate the ovum to the commissioning couple. For Page the contract of donation is fundamental. He makes it quite clear that he is not referring solely to *in vitro* donation and fertilization. An ovum could have been donated *in utero*; and presumably sperm could be donated in sexual intercourse, as might occur in total surrogacy (see (3) below). He says:

> If eggs and embryo can be donated or transferred at all, it is an important question whether they can be donated *in utero*. ... The mere fact that the egg or embryo is still in the woman's body is hardly enough in itself to show that it could not be donated or transferred in ownership to the commissioning couple. Obviously, someone could give away or sell a crop of apples without removing it from the orchard. The owner of a donkey could give or sell a donkey foal while it is still *in utero*. Similarly, there is no incoherence in the idea that an egg or embryo in the body might be donated [3].

Since he does not want to advocate the transferring of children, Page proposes that, as a practical rule, embryos should not be transferable; only gametes could be donated and transferred. Then, provided there is a contract of donation before conception, a surrogate mother would have no rights or responsibilities towards her baby after its birth. Thus all the following kinds of surrogate mothers could have relinquished their rights:

(1) A woman who gestates an embryo developed from gametes provided by the commissioning couple.

(2) A woman who gestates an embryo developed from her own ovum—sperm being provided by the commissioning father through AID or through sexual intercourse.

(3) A woman who gestates an embryo which has neither gamete from the commissioning couple—possibly she has provided the ovum. Page calls this 'total surrogacy'.

My first objection arises because gametes are not like apples or fetal foals, they join to make embryos that are destined (bar accidents) to make human beings. We sell fruit (unripe and ripe) and we sell animals (*in utero* and when mature). Not only do we not sell people, we don't sell embryos and nor do we *sell* gametes. Any argument for a legal contract involving relinquishing rights after donation cannot be supported by analogies with contracts concerning goods that differ in such an important way.

The view that such donations should be accompanied by legal forfeit of rights is better supported by analogy with donations of other body tissues. I gave the example of blood donation and there are cases where living donors have supplied kidneys and other organs. Indeed I can surmise that medical techniques could advance enough for it to become possible to donate a hand or an eye. Then the law might be changed so that, for example, a parent could donate to her child. In all such cases it must follow that the donor has no further claim on the tissue or organ.

Then why can I not follow Page and agree with his view of the loss of rights of the surrogate mother? My inability stems from the fact that a surrogate mother is not simply acting as an incubator for another's embryo. This makes her situation very different from that of the man who donates his sperm *and* from that of the woman who donates (but does not gestate) her ovum or ova. For neither the man nor the woman make any further contribution to the development of the zygote into the child. *After they have donated they have played their part.* By contrast the surrogate mother provides material from her own body for the developing fetus; everything it gets comes from her blood via its placenta. She feels it grow and move. Fetus and mother react on each other: there may be blood changes in both (for example, the effect of the *Rhesus* factor) and diseases can pass from one to the other (the spirochete, for example). The growing fetus affects the mother's hormone balance and there are consequent physiological and psychological changes; a woman who carries a baby is being prepared to nurse it after its birth; for the nine months' development *in utero* does not result in an independent being. Therefore whether the surrogate mother donated her own ovum or accepted a tenant embryo, she has actually given part of herself over and above any germ tissue. Should she be legally required to part with this if she has made a prior arrangement to donate her ovum or to accept an embryo? I suggest that there are substantial objections to this and very good empirical reasons for making such arrangements legally invalid. Just as a mother cannot be compelled to part with a baby she has produced for adoption so a surrogate mother should not be compelled to part with the baby she has gestated. And this should be so despite any prior 'understanding'; such 'understandings' should not be legally enforceable.

In discussion Page has said that many women carry babies from whom they wish to part at birth. It may be that we could find volunteers of this sort for surrogacy. Commissioning couples would then not need legal rights but would not suffer disappointment. However, it is possible that the proportion of such women is low (we have after all to discount those who reject their baby and did not want to be pregnant, for these women will not volunteer for surrogacy). It is also possible that prospects for the baby are better if it is carried by a woman who does develop maternal instincts of care. We need empirical evidence but I do not think that the problems arising when a surrogate mother develops an interest in the child during gestation can simply be dismissed as irrelevant to the legal validity of a contract of donation prior to conception. The ties between surrogate mother and fetus are, I suggest, too close to allow them to be broken; we cannot make legal contracts about this kind of gift. An arrangement to gestate a human embryo is not analogous to an arrangement to look after someone else's car, or orchard, or puppy.

I appreciate that infertile commissioning couples will lack security but there is no *injustice* if they are aware at the outset that they cannot make a legal contract with a surrogate mother such that they have a right to take possession of the baby at birth. They will be in no worse position than those who seek to make an arrangement to adopt before birth.

Jennifer Trusted, 15 Victoria Park Road, Exeter, Devon EX2 4NT, United Kingdom.

NOTES

[1] PAGE, EDGAR, (1985) Donation, surrogacy and adoption, originally published in *Journal of Applied Philosophy*, 2, p. 162.
[2] Ibid., p. 163.
[3] Ibid., p. 168.

26

The Market for Bodily Parts:
Kant and duties to oneself

RUTH F. CHADWICK

ABSTRACT   *The demand for bodily parts such as organs is increasing, and individuals in certain circumstances are responding by offering parts of their bodies for sale. Is there anything wrong in this? Kant had arguments to suggest that there is, namely that we have duties towards our own bodies, among which is the duty not to sell parts of them. Kant's reasons for holding this view are examined, and found to depend on a notion of what is intrinsically degrading. Rom Harré's recent revision of Kant's argument, in terms of an obligation to preserve the body's organic integrity, is considered. Harré's view does not rule out all acts of selling, but he too ultimately depends on a test of what is intrinsically degrading. Both his view and Kant's are rejected in favour of a view which argues that it does make sense to speak of duties towards our own bodies, grounded in the duty to promote the flourishing of human beings, including ourselves. This provides a reason for opposing the sale of bodily parts, and the current trend towards the market ethic in health care provision.*

A penniless Italian awaiting trial for murder has offered to donate a kidney for transplant in exchange for a defence lawyer. Maurizio Bondini, aged 25, said in a letter to newspapers he could not afford counsel and believed a state-appointed lawyer could not defend him well enough. (*Guardian*, 11 January 1988)

The practice of selling one's organs for money is now a feature of contemporary life. Is there anything wrong in this? In particular, does the seller of the organ violate a moral duty to him or herself? In *Lectures on Ethics* Kant argues that we have duties towards our own bodies, and what he says gives rise to an argument that certain trends in modern medicine are wrong because the participants are not fulfilling these duties. In this paper I want to look at whether there is any sense in this notion of duties towards our own bodies, and its implications for medical ethics in the context of organ transplants.

A. Duties to the Self

First, we must face the problem that traditionally the idea that there are duties to oneself has caused something of a problem in moral philosophy. Several arguments have been advanced which suggest that speaking of such duties makes no sense. We need to look at whether they can be answered, and in particular, whether Kant had an answer to them.

1. *The Concept of Morality*

Some would say morality arises where the interests of different people conflict. The concept of morality would not be needed, on this view, in a world inhabited by a solitary individual. It would never get off the ground. Morality is concerned with how people treat *each other*.

For example, according to one well-known view morality arises as a response to certain features of the human condition, viz. human beings have unlimited wants and demands, but exist in a situation not only where there are limited resources but also where they themselves have limited sympathies. These limitations make them liable to regard the demands of others as being of less importance than their own. Morality is a device designed to counteract the natural tendency of human beings to selfishness, the tendency to be moved more by their own needs than by those of others [1].

Again, let us look at sociobiological explanations of morality. What has to be explained, according to the sociobiologists, is how it comes to be that human beings are apparently capable of altruism, which is defined in their theories as behaviour that as a matter of fact benefits individuals other than the agent. If what we have been told about the struggle for the survival of the fittest is true, why have all the altruists not died out? [2].

Both these views, in their different ways, take it as obvious that there is in general no deficiency in people's capacity to pursue their own interests, and no difficulty in understanding such a phenomenon. So there would be no *point* in speaking of a duty to ourselves. There would be a point in this only if it were necessary to exhort people to pursue their own good, but as it is they are doing so anyway.

If there *is* a problem it is one of failure to pursue enlightened, or long-term, as opposed to short-term self-interest. But if we say that we *ought* to pursue our long-term, as opposed to our short-term, self-interest, this 'ought' is construed, by the critics of duties to oneself, as prudential rather than moral. It still falls outside the concept of morality.

Kant is quite clear that duty to oneself is not to be confused with prudence, saying in the *Lectures on Ethics* that "The basis of such obligation is not to be found in the advantages we reap from doing our duty towards ourselves" [3]. Again, he says "In fact, the principle of self-regarding duties is a very different one, which has no connexion with our well-being or earthly happiness" [4]. On the contrary,

> Not favour but self-esteem should be the principle of our duties towards ourselves. This means that our actions must be in keeping with the worth of man. [5]

Kant's line of reasoning here is echoed and clarified in the *Groundwork of the Metaphysic of Morals*, where he argues that the content of our duty is determined by the categorical imperative. In its second formulation this states that we should always act so as to treat humanity, whether in our own person or in that of another, as an end, and never as a means only [6]. It is because human beings should be treated in a certain way, that we have obligations to ourselves *qua* human beings. His emphasis is thus on the preservation of human worth, and he depends on a notion of certain acts as intrinsically degrading. If we indulge in them we lose our worth.

This view, as we shall see, is open to the objection that there is widespread disagreement as to what counts as degrading.

However, there are alternative concepts of morality which can allow for duties to oneself. For example, any view which sees morality as concerned with the flourishing of human life in general (with the possibility of expanding to show concern for other species) should be able to account for moral obligations towards ourselves. For a view which says that the object or point of morality is to promote the flourishing of human beings (however this is interpreted) can surely include the promotion of one's own flourishing [7].

2. The Mind–Body Problem

A further difficulty about speaking of duties to oneself is that any such idea of duties to the self must be able to account for the 'self'. What is this supposed to mean?

We cannot escape this problem simply by asserting that in the present context we are concerned with duties towards one's own body, for to speak of duties towards the body raises problems of its own, e.g. the mind–body problem. If I say I have duties towards my body it might naturally be thought that I see myself, as moral agent, as distinct from my body, thus taking a dualist view.

Kant seems to want to operate in the *Lectures on Ethics* with an idea of the completeness of the whole person, a concept of the person as necessarily embodied. In the Lecture on 'Duties towards the body in regard to life' he says:

> Our life is entirely conditioned by our body, so that we cannot conceive of a life not mediated by the body and we cannot make use of our freedom except through the body. [8]

He frequently says that the person is a unity. My finger is thus an integral part of me. But that does not imply that it does not make sense to ask whether I have an obligation not to cut it off. Such a question does not commit me to a dualist view.

This seems right, but even if we accept that it makes sense to speak in terms of obligations to my own body I need to have some idea of the extent of my obligations, where 'extent' is understood in a physical sense. What are the boundaries of my own body? This is not always clear, and it is a problem not discussed by Kant.

An obvious example is the case of Siamese twins. The boundary between one twin and another is not precisely fixed. Possibilities of bodily transfer, discussed in the context of problems of personal identity, also raise difficulties for the suggestion that we have clear and precise ideas of the boundaries of our own bodies.

In less bizarre cases we have to face the possibility of losing whole limbs. Does this produce a change in the boundaries of one's body? If so, does that mean that if there are duties towards our own bodies, there are no longer any obligations towards the amputated part?

The answer to this question will depend on the reasons for holding that we do have obligations to our own bodies. If the reason is that this body is the embodiment of this person, then the question will turn on the extent to which bodily continuity is necessary for personal identity. On the most plausible version of the bodily continuity view, it is the continuity of the brain (or at least, a sufficient part of it) that is held to be crucial [9]. Then we can accept the loss of a limb without thinking that we are sacrificing anything essential to our personal identity. Kant is willing to countenance amputation in some circumstances, as we shall see. But if we thought we had duties towards our bodies *as such*, then the question of the proper treatment of an amputated part could be a proper cause for concern [10].

So to sum up, there do not seem to be insuperable obstacles in the way of speaking of duties towards one's own body, if we agree with Kant that morality is concerned with how human beings, including oneself, are to be treated, and that human beings are necessarily embodied.

Let us now look at what Kant actually says about duties towards the body and their implications for medical ethics.

B. Selling the Body

The main argument of Kant which we need to consider concerns the impermissibility of selling the body or any part of it, which has relevance for the current trend towards traffic in bodily parts.

Kant in *Lectures on Ethics* says:

> a human being is not entitled to sell his limbs for money, even if he were offered ten thousand thalers for a single finger. [11]

What are his arguments for this view? The first is as follows:

(a) If he were so entitled, he could sell all his limbs [12].

This seems to be an instance of a slippery slope argument. If I can sell one part of myself, I can sell the whole (which could result in slavery, if I sold myself all at once, or in death, if I sold myself in a succession of mutilations).

Let us follow Jonathan Glover's distinction between logical and empirical versions of this type of argument, and see how they work out [13].

In *The Guardian*, 23 November 1984, there was an article entitled 'Debtors sell their kidneys to pay loans'. This article described how people in Japan were selling kidneys to avoid being subjected to violence from loan sharks who were anxious to recover what was owed to them.

Now it seems clear that if I have sold one kidney, thinking it justifiable so to do, that does not commit me, logically, to thinking it justifiable to sell the other. There is a very relevant difference between selling one kidney and selling two, viz., that I can survive with only one but not with none.

Whether any empirical research has been carried out on people who have surrendered one kidney I do not know, but from the psychological point of view, if I know that I have only one kidney left, it seems likely that that fact will make me more, rather than less, anxious over the fate of the other one.

So if I can sell one part of myself it does not at all follow that I can legitimately sell all of myself, or that I am likely to.

However, Kant has further considerations to adduce.

(b) We can dispose of things which have no freedom but not of a being which has free will [12].

The reason why it is wrong, according to Kant, to sell oneself, even a part of oneself, is that we are beings which have free will, and beings of this sort are not to be sold.

What exactly is the objection here? There are various possibilities.

(i) The objection might be that in selling myself I make it impossible to exercise my freedom in future. Thus one objection to the exercise of a free choice to sell oneself into slavery is that such a choice would close the door on future freedom of choice. But does selling a finger have the objectionable consequences that it leads to a loss of freedom? It is difficult to see how it could have such catastrophic consequences.

(ii) Kant elaborates upon his argument:

A man who sells himself makes of himself a thing and, as he has jettisoned his person, it is open to anyone to deal with him as he pleases. [14]

In selling myself I make of myself a thing. Once I have placed myself in a position where I can be bought and sold then people can treat me as an object.

But does it follow from the selling of a finger that I can be treated in any way anyone happens to feel like treating me? Kant may be relying implicitly here on an argument, not merely that if I can sell a part I *can* sell the whole (shown to be implausible in (a) above), but that if I sell a part I *do* sell the whole. If so, this argument is equally implausible: the conclusion simply does not follow.

(iii) Kant seems ultimately, however, to invoke a notion of what is intrinsically degrading to human beings. What he seems to be saying is that human beings, having free will, are simply not the sorts of things that should be bought and sold, and if you offer any part of yourself for sale then you have made yourself into an object for other people's pleasure.

Kant unfortunately has not explained here why we should accept that to sell one's finger is intrinsically degrading. For example, is it any more degrading than selling one's labour in menial employment?

(c) Kant has a further argument for the impermissibility of selling one's body. He says, in 'Duties towards the body in respect of sexual impulse'

Man cannot dispose over himself because he is not a thing; he is not his own property; to say that he is would be self-contradictory; for in so far as he is a person he is a Subject in whom the ownership of things can be vested, and if he were his own property, he would be a thing over which he could have ownership. But a person cannot be a property and so cannot be a thing which can be owned, for it is impossible to be a person and a thing, the proprietor and the property. Accordingly a man is not at his own disposal. He is not entitled to sell a limb, not even one of his own teeth. [15]

The argument is that the would-be seller is involved in a contradiction. But Kant himself is not consistent in the use he makes of this type of argument. For in *The Doctrine of Virtue* at 417 he says that there is the following possible objection to duties to oneself:

If the obligating I is taken in the same sense as the obligated I, the concept of duty to oneself contains a contradiction. For the concept of duty contains the notion of being passively necessitated (I am obligated). But if the duty is a duty to myself, I conceive myself as obligating and so as actively necessitating ... hence a contradiction. [16]

He goes on to assert that *nevertheless* man has duties to himself. It seems open to the would-be seller of a kidney to retort as follows: if a man can both owe and be owed a duty to himself, why cannot he be both owner and property?

The difference between the two cases must rest, not on the existence or non-existence of a contradiction, but elsewhere. Kant needs to find other reasons for saying that one is not 'entitled' to sell a limb.

He claims that 'a man is not at his own disposal'. But this itself contradicts what he says elsewhere. He is prepared to admit that in some circumstances we do have rights of disposal over our own bodies. In the Lecture 'Suicide', Kant says,

We may treat our body as we please, provided our motives are those of self-preservation. If, for instance, his foot is a hindrance to life, a man might have it amputated. To preserve his person he has the right of disposal over his body. [17]

But if I can have my foot amputated to save my life, why not sell my kidney to pacify the loan sharks from whom I am in fear for my life? After all, it may be from motives of self-preservation that I feel the need to sell a part of myself.

For Kant, it seems, if the disposal amounts to a selling, it is ruled out, because of the arguments outlined above. But the arguments, as we have seen, do not provide the support he needs for his claims.

C. Rom Harré: the argument revised

In an article in *Cogito*, Rom Harré has attacked Kant's arguments and argued for an alternative way of looking at obligations towards the body. Harré proceeds to look at the similarities and differences between things and bodies. He starts from the premiss that in general the owner of a thing owns its parts and has rights of transfer of ownership. However, even in the case of things, such as works of art or classic cars, these rights are limited. In the case of such objects Harré argues that they are limited by the value of artistic integrity. However, when one tears out illuminations from a manuscript, Harré argues, one does not only an aesthetic but a moral wrong, partly because such an act deprives other persons of the possibility of seeing them [18].

In the case of one's body, there is an organic, rather than an aesthetic value. If rights of disposal were not restricted then the organic value of the maintenance of life would be under threat. This is a moral point because the maintenance of life is necessary for the survival of persons.

So Harré suggests a tightened up version of Kant's argument.

If to be this person is to be embodied in this body then the maintenance of the body's organic integrity boils down to a defence of the person. [19]

However, if we are talking about the maintenance of life, then Kant's view, that one cannot dispose of even a finger, is too extreme, because such a disposal does not put the life of the person at risk. I take Harré here to mean that even if the disposal includes selling the finger, it need not be ruled out.

Harré adds the proviso that any disposal of a bodily part should lead to its being put to a 'proper' use; i.e. "a fate commensurate to the dignity and moral standing of the person from which it came" [20]. So Harré, like Kant, seems ultimately to need some concept of what is intrinsically fitting to human beings.

One of the consequences of both Kant's and Harré's views appears to be that we do not have obligations to the body as such. For it turns out that we have obligations to the body only in order to serve the interests of the person whose body it is.

Harré would like to go further, for this account, he says, fails to meet the need for an account of the kind of talk that goes on in Fitness Clubs and magazines, where the body is spoken of as if it had moral claims in itself. Harré thinks that "the force of this talk seems to depend on the trick of personifying the body, on treating it as other than oneself, with its own moral qualities" [21]. Harré wants to look at whether there is anything in this.

His suggestion is that there is one category of organic being to which we have accepted an obligation despite their non-personhood, and that is pets. He suggests that the human body is to be seen as a pet with a permanent live-in master or mistress.

Rather than solving anything, this account seems to introduce more difficulties. For one thing, it is not at all clear why I should regard my own body in the same way that I regard a distinct entity, a pet. The way in which we own our pets seems quite unlike our relationship to our own bodies. Harré's only argument in support of this account is that here we have a category of organic non-persons to whom we have obligations. But there must surely be different considerations pertaining to whether it is justifiable to sell a pet from those which arise in considering whether I can sell my own body. Harré's view fails to take into account the fact that a pet dog, for example, is a sentient being with a consciousness of its own. Further, as Harré himself admits, looking at the issue in this way does seem to involve a reintroduction of Cartesian dualism, the problem we mentioned in section A.2.

Harré also, however, does not want to be committed to saying that our obligations to our bodies reduce to our obligations to ourselves *qua* persons; he thinks this conclusion 'dull'. But in fact if we are forced to adopt that conclusion it is far from dull, because there are still very difficult and interesting questions about how our obligations to ourselves as persons affect what we may do to our bodies.

Both Kant and Harré think that there are restrictions here: they both have two principles which are similar but different. Let us express Kant's first principle as follows:

> It is a necessary, but not a sufficient, condition of a right of disposal of a bodily part that it is done from the motive of self-preservation.

We may compare Harré's position, interpreting it in the following way:

> It is a necessary, but not a sufficient, condition, of a right of disposal over a bodily part that it does not actually undercut the maintenance of the body's organic integrity.

These are not sufficient conditions because both Kant and Harré think that we have to add a proviso to the effect that there are certain modes of treatment of the body which are incompatible with the dignity of human beings. Though they share this second principle they come to different conclusions in practice, Harré thinking the selling of a tooth may be acceptable, Kant wanting to go further and rule even this out.

The first principle, the necessary condition that any disposal must be compatible with the preservation of life, will be too strong for anyone who wants to admit the possibility that suicide is justifiable in some circumstances, e.g. when there is no likelihood of future flourishing for a human being [22].

The second principle is unhelpful because it leads Kant and Harré to different conclusions. There is little agreement on what is intrinsically degrading, and the principle assumes what is at issue, viz. that there are certain ways of treating the body which must be ruled out. Clearly more needs to be said.

D. Disposing of Bodily Parts

While Kant wants to rule out the selling of a bodily part, could he approve of the *donation* of a bodily part, e.g. the donation of a kidney to a sibling? His principle that any disposal must be carried out from the motive of self-preservation seems to exclude this possibility. But if we compare this with the first principles of Kant's moral philosophy, this is not what we would expect. If one may have a kidney removed in order to preserve one's own life, but not to preserve the life of another, this seems to introduce a partiality which is inimical to Kant's view of ethics.

There are two possible sources of difficulty here. First, it may be the case that Kant does not deal with this aspect of the issue because he is thinking only of how one may treat one's own body, and one's duties to it, and it alone. But second, he simply did not have the possibility of organ transplants to think about.

But having clarified that limitation, we still need to know whether there are good reasons, as he thought, for ruling out the selling of bodily parts.

Individual and Collective Ownership

A large part of the problem turns on the question of the sense in which one can be said to 'own' one's body. Kant's view seems to be that this body is not 'mine', it is me. But there is a sense in which it is clearly mine as opposed to anyone else's (ignoring, for present purposes, problems about personal identity), and even Kant recognises some rights of disposal, which as Harré points out usually go with the concept of ownership.

In the individualistic market-oriented society in which we live, ownership of the body may perhaps naturally be thought of in terms of rights to buy and sell. It is therefore not surprising that the idea of trafficking in bodily parts is becoming more common.

Some writers have suggested that we should, instead, think more in terms of collective ownership of bodies, at least after death [23]. For example, the proposal that there should be an 'opting out' scheme for kidney donations, rather than an 'opting in' scheme, rests on the assumption that we should presume that people's kidneys may be used to help others unless the 'owner' registers an objection, rather than the other way round. This proposal has as yet not really caught on [24].

Some people may fear the extension of this idea and the development of a society where schemes such as John Harris's 'survival lottery' might become a reality [25].

At one extreme we have an individualistic account that holds that we have complete rights of disposal over our own bodies, which includes the freedom to sell them. At the other we have a collectivist account which takes away our freedom to deny the use of our bodies by others when they are needed for the pursuit of social goals.

Although these two accounts seem to be at different extremes, they actually have a lot in common. That is, they both view the human body as a set of resources, to be exploited either by the individual 'owner' or by the collective.

This may be because our concept of ownership, as Harré points out, is very much interpreted in terms of rights of transfer. We are so used to thinking in terms of the institution of private property that we think of ownership of our bodies in the same way. But this is a mistake, because there are clear differences between our bodies and possessions such as tables and chairs. If we abolished the institution of private property we should still, in some sense, own our bodies. If we recall Strawson's arguments in *Individuals*, in order to have a concept of myself as an individual person I have to be able to distinguish between my body and those of others [26].

This body belongs to me *if* to anyone (for present purposes I shall ignore problems of personal identity and bodily transfer). So I may think that if anyone has the right to sell its parts, then I do. But that issue is not settled by saying it is mine, because that depends on seeing ownership of the body in terms of the institution of property, which it is not clear we should do.

So what is the way forward? Our bodies are, as Kant pointed out, the embodiment of persons. A significant thing about persons is that they have desires, feelings and interests. In general people do not like to be treated as objects. There is plenty of evidence for this, e.g. in women's attitudes to being regarded as sex objects. It is difficult if not impossible for people to flourish when they feel they are treated as just bodies or objects [27].

For Kant, the realisation that one thinks that one should oneself be treated as an end, and not as a means, led via the application of universalisation to the conclusion that all rational beings should be treated as ends.

Now one undesirable consequence of the selling of our own bodies is that it contributes towards a society in which the bodies of persons are regarded as resources. The action of selling one's own body contributes to the prevailing ethos of everything being for sale, everything having a price. It reinforces the ethic of the market. The seller of bodily parts encourages the purchaser to think that everything is available, for a price. Kant's remark that the seller makes himself into a thing in the purchaser's eyes is expressing this insight. The potential effects on the purchaser may be as undesirable as the effects on the seller.

The above considerations provide reasons for the view that it is morally undesirable for people to sell their organs. But the following objections may be raised.

(1) What if someone actually wants to sell their organs? If the purchaser is acting in accordance with the seller's desire, how is the seller treated as an object? For the autonomous wish of the seller is surely then being respected. What of the person who is in that position where he or she feels there is no alternative, such as the accused in Italy or the debtor in Japan?

The answer to this is that what are really objectionable are the social conditions in which these sorts of situation arise. For it is not comfortably off people who sell their organs, engaging in an undertaking which involves non-negligible risk to health and life. It is people who find themselves in situations where they cannot flourish, and where the sale of an organ appears to be a way out. For the seller at the time it may be the lesser of two evils, but any such selling reinforces the social conditions in which people are forced by economic necessity into this type of transaction. This provides a reason for opposing it.

(2) It might be objected that any commercial transaction reinforces the market ethic and is therefore, on this argument, to be avoided. But not every transaction for buying and selling has as its object a person or part of a person, nor does it involve the threat to life and health mentioned above. (It might be said that some forms of selling one's body are difficult to distinguish from selling one's labour, and that needs to be worked out, but here I want to confine my attention to actually selling parts of one's body.)

(3) It might be suggested that there is a distinction to be made between the disposal of a renewable part of one's body, such as blood, and a non-renewable one, such as a kidney. Would selling renewable ones avoid the above difficulties?

This is too simple. Richard Titmuss, in his book *The Gift Relationship*, argued for voluntary blood donation rather than a system of paid donors, partly on health grounds, but also on the grounds that once the market ethic pervades that relationship it will have dire consequences for society's values as a whole. At the time he wrote he thought there was a correlation between the values of the voluntary blood donor system in Britain and those of the National Health Service. With the undermining of the latter in the late 1980s, and the consequent dangers of creeping commercialism, it is even more important to uphold donation as opposed to selling [28].

E. Conclusions

It might be thought that the account I have given here gets away from the idea of duties to oneself, because I have spoken in terms of consequences for human society as a whole.

This is not, however, incompatible with the view that it makes sense to speak in terms of a duty to oneself. Whereas Kant has spoken of what is intrinsically degrading (as has Harré), I have spoken in terms of the conditions in which people can flourish. If I have a duty to promote the flourishing of human beings in general, then I have a duty to promote my own, as a member of the class of human beings.

Of course, the point that I am a *member* is significant. I am one person among others. My duty to promote my own flourishing will not always take priority, but on my view it at least makes sense to speak of a duty, other things being equal, not to sell my organs, if to sell would contribute to the diminishing likelihood of my own flourishing. What is it to flourish? It seems clear, at least, that you do not flourish if you feel undervalued and used by others. If to refuse to sell one's organs would help to avoid such an outcome, one has a duty, other things being equal, to do so.

That, however, is not the whole story. It is not simply a question of the duty of the individual, when deciding to sell or not to sell. We have to consider the social context in which such decisions are made. If we have a situation in which poor Third World people sell organs to the West, or where individuals in capitalist societies sell organs to extricate themselves from debt, we need to ask to what extent individuals are free to make a choice, and to what extent the values of the market are overriding other values, to the detriment of all.

Thus if contracts for the sale of organs are undesirable from a moral point of view, it may not be enough to suggest, for example, that they be unenforceable or illegal: the underlying economic forces and the values on which they rest need to be exposed and questioned, to see to what extent they provide the conditions in which people can flourish and act to promote their own flourishing.

Ruth F. Chadwick, School of English Studies, Journalism and Philosophy, University of Wales, College of Cardiff, P.O. Box 94, Cardiff CF1 3XE, United Kingdom.

NOTES

I am grateful to Robin Attfield for comments on an earlier draft, and to members of the Cardiff Philosophy Society, particularly Andrew Belsey, for points made in discussion.

[1] See, e.g., J. L. MACKIE (1977) *Ethics: inventing right and wrong* (Harmondsworth, Penguin), Ch. 5.

[2] See PETER SINGER (1981) *The Expanding Circle* (Oxford, Oxford University Press), esp. Ch. 1.

[3] I. KANT (1963) *Lectures on Ethics* (translated by LOUIS INFIELD) (New York, Harper & Row), p. 121.

[4] Ibid., p. 117.

[5] Ibid., p. 124.

[6] I. KANT (1948) *Groundwork of the Metaphysic of Morals* (translated by H. J. PATON as *The Moral Law*) (London, Hutchinson), p. 91.

[7] For this view of morality see, e.g., MACKIE op. cit., p.193, where he takes "general human well-being or the flourishing of human life as the foundation of morality".

[8] KANT, *Lectures on Ethics*, pp. 147–148.

[9] DEREK PARFIT (1984) *Reasons and Persons* (Oxford, Oxford University Press), pp. 202–204.

[10] It might be suggested that we should speak in terms of duties regarding our own bodies, rather than in terms of duties to them. If we were satisfied that we do only have duties to treat our bodies in certain ways in so far as they are the embodiment of persons, this might be a less misleading way of speaking in that it would avoid the implications of mind-body dualism. But I shall continue to speak in terms of duties towards the body, as there is a view of duties towards the body as such which has to be considered.

[11] KANT, *Lectures on Ethics*, p. 124.

[12] Ibid.

[13] JONATHAN GLOVER (1977) *Causing Death and Saving Lives* (Harmondsworth, Penguin). Glover calls the argument he discusses the wedge argument.

[14] KANT, *Lectures on Ethics*, p. 124.

[15] Ibid., p. 165.

[16] I. KANT (1964) *The Doctrine of Virtue* (Part II of The Metaphysic of Morals) (translated by MARY J. GREGOR)(Philadelphia, PA, University of Pennsylvania Press), p. 79.

[17] KANT, *Lectures on Ethics*, p. 149.

[18] ROM HARRÉ (1987) Body obligations, *Cogito*, 1, pp. 15–19.

[19] Ibid., p. 16.

[20] Ibid.

[21] Ibid., p. 18.

[22] To discuss suicide in detail would take us too far from our present concerns. Kant does of course have objections to suicide, e.g. that the suicide is involved in a self-contradiction, but I would argue that this argument is no more successful than the attempt to show that the position of the seller of bodily parts is self-contradictory.

[23] Harré actually discusses the possibility of collective ownership of the bodies also of living people, in the context of surrogate motherhood.

[24] R. A. SELLS (1979) Let's not opt out: kidney donation and transplantation, *Journal of Medical Ethics*, 5.

[25] JOHN HARRIS (1975) The survival lottery, *Philosophy*, 50, pp. 81–87.

[26] P. F. STRAWSON (1959) *Individuals* (London, Methuen), Ch. 3.

[27] This argument is of course open to what might be called the 'contented slave' objection, that some people do not feel unhappy about what others might regard as exploitation, e.g. slavery, treating people as sex objects. But I shall not discuss that, or the standard 'false consciousness' reply, here.

[28] RICHARD G. TITMUSS (1970) *The Gift Relationship: from human blood to social policy* (London, Allen & Unwin).

27

A Fortnight of My Life is Missing: a discussion of the status of the human 'pre-embryo'

ALAN HOLLAND

ABSTRACT *Summed up in the coinage of the term 'pre-embryo' is the denial that human beings, as such, begin to exist from the moment of conception. This denial, which may be thought to have significant moral implications, rests on two kinds of reason. The first is that the pre-embryo lacks the characteristics of a human being. The second is that the pre-embryo lacks what it takes to be an individual human being. The first reason, I argue, embodies an untenable view of what it is to be human. The second reason exploits certain logical difficulties which arise over the possibility of twinning. I question the relevance of the appeal to such difficulties and conclude that there is no good reason for denying that a human being begins to exist from the moment of conception.*

The 'missing fortnight' of my title is the first fortnight of human life [1]. Members of the medical profession, embryologists and philosophers, have begun to employ a new concept—the concept 'pre-embryo'—when speaking of this stage of human life [2]. The term is intended to carry the implication that a human being, as such, does not begin to exist at the moment of conception, but only at some later stage of human life. It may therefore appear to licence this important conclusion among others, that experimentation on embryos at a sufficiently early stage is of little or no moral consequence. My contention is that the capture of such moral ground by this conceptual manoeuvre is indefensible.

I

In one of his contributions to a meeting on the subject of human embryo research held at the Ciba Foundation in November 1985, Bernard Williams observed that: "An embryo which, if all goes well, will develop into a human being is certainly a human embryo, but that does not imply that it is itself a human being" [3].

Undoubtedly, the fact that something *will develop* into a human being does not imply that it *is* a human being. (What it implies, if anything, is that it is *not* (yet) a human being.) And if a human embryo is no more than an embryo which, if all goes well, will develop into a human being, then the fact that something is a human embryo does not imply that it is a human being. Yet, the claim that a human embryo is no more than an embryo which, if all goes well, will develop into a human being is surely open to question. For, the fact that something is a human embryo certainly seems to imply that it is an embryonic human being; and the fact that something is an embryonic human being certainly seems to imply that it is a human being. Therefore, the fact that something is a human embryo certainly does seem to imply that it is a human being. Here, then, is a counter-argument to Williams's view.

True, both premises of the counter-argument might be challenged. Take, first, the premise that if something is a human embryo then it is an embryonic human being. This cannot be supported by an appeal to the more general claim that for any X, a human X is an X-ish human being, because the more general claim is false. A human sample, for instance, is not a sample human. However, there is, I suggest, a *prima facie* case for claiming that the term 'embryo' belongs to a restricted range of 'developmental' concepts for which this conversion does, in general, apply. 'Embryo', 'infant', 'adolescent', 'adult': all admit both an adjectival and sortal noun form. A human adult is an adult human being, a human adolescent an adolescent human being, a human infant an infant human being. The logic of the concept 'embryo' seems to parallel exactly the logic of the concept 'adult' and the rest. Surely, therefore, some argument is needed to support the contention that 'human embryo' does not convert, simply, into 'embryonic human being'.

Next, take the premise that if something is an embryonic human being then it is a human being. This, too, cannot be supported by an appeal to the general claim that for any X, an X-ish human being is a human being. Neither a future, nor a would-be human being *is* a human being. And as regards the use of 'embryonic' in other contexts, it would seem to be debatable whether, for example, an embryonic idea or theory *is* an idea or theory. But if it were allowed, once more, that 'embryonic' belongs with the restricted range of developmental concepts cited above, then the premise would stand. For an adult human being *is* a human being, as is the adolescent and infant. So therefore, on this model, is the embryonic human being.

It might be objected here that the concept 'embryo' is in fact unlike the other developmental concepts in that, whereas infant, adolescent and adult are all stages of the fully-formed human being, the embryo is not yet a fully-formed human being. But such an objection is open to the reply that the infant is not fully-formed either, since it is not yet capable of reproduction. To the further objection that the embryo is not merely not fully-formed but is not yet 'organised' in any way, the further reply is that this is false and, even if it were true, would constitute precisely the kind of difference for which the term 'embryo' was devised. What is true is that, naturally enough, it is not organised along the same lines as the adult human [4]. But, even as a single cell, it certainly does have functioning parts, such as membrane, nucleus and chromosomes.

I somehow doubt, however, whether purely conceptual exchanges of this kind can, or will, be allowed to be decisive. Anne McLaren, for example, whose views I shall later be discussing, could accept my conceptual claims entirely, while at the same time agreeing with Williams on the point of substance. For she denies that, during the first fortnight or so of its existence, the fertilised egg *is* an embryo. It is better described, she thinks, as a 'pre-embryo' [5]. Her move indicates a belief that 'embryo' *does* carry the implication I have suggested, but at the same time it completely defeats the object of my argument. For even accepting that the human embryo is a human being, it will not follow that a human being exists from the moment of conception. Setting aside verbal manoeuvres, the question of substance is: whether human life, from the moment of conception, constitutes a human being. It is becoming clear that to reach anything like an informed position on this question we need to look much more closely at the actual details of early human development. But we also need to decide, as further discussion of Williams's position will bring out, how exactly the term 'human being' is to be understood.

II

There are two related presumptions about what it is to be human which militate against the claims of the embryo to be counted as a human being [6]. They appear to be widely accepted and come to the surface, briefly, in Bernard Williams's remarks. Yet there is good authority for rejecting them both.

The first presumption surfaces when Williams endorses a point attributed to Jonathan Glover. Arguing against someone who, presumably, believed that human life constitutes a human being from the moment of conception, Glover had mischievously suggested that his opponent would be considerably put out if, having been invited to a dinner of chicken he were served with an omelette made of fertilised eggs. This rather brutal joke, comments Williams, outraged the opponent, but "made an entirely valid point" [7]. He adds that we do not naturally regard viable acorns as oak trees, or caterpillars as butterflies, because we do not ascribe to items which merely have the potentiality of developing into a mature form of a given species the term appropriate to that mature form. The presumption is that the 'proper' form of a human being, or indeed of the member of any species, is the one which is found in the mature adult member of the species. Becoming a human being is, on this view, a matter of coming to acquire a certain form: an embryo is a cell, and then a collection of cells, which gradually takes on human form.

However, as long ago as 1945, the eminent biologist J. H. Woodger had delivered this stern admonition: "Another type of linguistic shortcoming [in biology] is illustrated by the persistence of our tendency to identify *organisms* with *adults*". Glover and Williams, I suggest, succumb to this tendency. "It is not just adults we classify", he continues, "when we classify organisms ... We can speak of the egg as the primordium of the future adult, but not [as the primordium] of the future organism because it already is the organism" [8]. Applied to human beings, the implication is clear. We can speak of the embryo as the future adult, but not as the future human being because it already is the human being.

In truth, if Williams were correct to imply that 'human being' is the term appropriate to the mature form of the species, then the alleged fact that an embryo is not referred to as a human being would be quite irrelevant. For the issue is not whether an embryo is a mature member of its species (it obviously isn't), but at what stage we can say that an organism of a particular kind has come into existence. Terminology is hardly consistent across species for the very good reason that different species exhibit different patterns of development. This makes the use of analogies with other species unsafe. Lepidopterans are a case in point because they, like other orders of insects, pass through a larval stage in which they manifest very different characteristics from those of the adult form. It is natural therefore that the larval and adult stages should have acquired distinct labels. But terminology is also not particularly rigorous and in other cases—perhaps including that of humans—species terms seem to perform a role analogous to that of both 'butterfly' and 'lepidopteran'. Elvers are not eels, nor cygnets swans. Yet elvers *are* (baby) eels and cygnets *are* (baby) swans. (A 'count' of swans on a stretch of river would include cygnets.) Appeal to the fact that we talk of 'fertilised eggs' rather than 'chicken' is particularly unsafe because of the suspicion that this is 'table talk'. Biologists at any rate, referring to the organism at this stage, tend to favour 'chick embryo'—a term which gives absolutely no handle to the kind of point which Glover was originally attempting to make.

At the back of the presumption that the 'true' human form is that exemplified in the mature adult lies a second presumption, which is: that being human is a matter of satisfying a (possibly) disjunctive check-list of characteristics. Individual human beings and, indeed, the members of any species are seen, on this view, as the instances, specimens, or exemplars of a type, specifiable by general description [9]. Natural kinds of living things are likened to artefacts, fashioned according to some blueprint. Abnormal instances of the kind are even treated as 'mistakes' or at least as products of 'mistakes' [10].

Such a view is both pre-Darwinian in all essentials and untenable. It would appear innocent of the admirable work being done by theoretical biologists such as Ernst Mayr and Michael Ghiselin towards realising the full implications of Darwin's radical conception of species [11]. According to these interpreters, species are, in effect, historical particulars rather than types. This explains, among other things, why dodos (natural kinds) are said to have become extinct whereas bronze axes (artefacts) are not. Thus, to do justice to the Darwinian conception of species, the move away from essentialism with respect to natural kinds has to be far more radical than many philosophers seem prepared for. According to this new conception, species concepts refer primarily to particular historical groups or populations which form a reproductive community. The term 'human' is presumably no exception. Human characteristics are, simply, whatever characteristics are exhibited by one such population—those which happen to belong, contingently, to a particular group ultimately identifiable perhaps only as 'this crowd'. To be sure, in almost all species there is considerable uniformity among their members. Why this is so constitutes a fascinating and challenging problem for the theory of evolution, and perhaps there would not be such things as species if it were not so. But it remains a contingent fact that an individual member of a species has the characteristics which it has. Individuals are human not by virtue of their intrinsic properties but by virtue of their extrinsic relations with each other. The criterion of origin rules. An alien from another galaxy who is indistinguishable from some particular human being is nevertheless not a human being, because what counts is lineage, and the lineage is wrong [12].

Against this background, I submit that one is bound to be unimpressed by the complaint that human embryos lack the characteristics required of a human being; first, because there are no defining characteristics of the sort required; second, because in any case the embryo ought not to be required to have the characteristics of the adult; third, because it satisfies the only criterion which counts. In short, the view which disqualifies the embryo from being counted as a human being for as long as it bears little or no resemblance to a miniature adult is ill-founded and ought to be abandoned.

A rather different argument for the conclusion which I wish to reject is advanced by Michael Lockwood [13]. Lockwood argues, first, that in the event of brain death you or I would cease to exist, even though a living human organism might for a while continue to exist [14]. His second point is that the identity of the individual must be supposed to follow the fortunes of the brain, or at least "some crucial part" [15] of the brain, rather than of the rest of the body, in an imaginary case where these are supposed to become separated [16]. Identifying the individual that you or I are essentially—what we can neither become nor cease to be, without ceasing to exist—as a *human being*, he believes that these considerations force a distinction to be drawn between a *human organism* and a *human being*, and infers specifically that the individual human being cannot be said to come into existence until the brain is formed [17]. Once again, then, we arrive at the conclusion that the early human embryo is not yet a human being.

Both of Lockwood's key claims—that you or I would cease to be, in the event of brain death, and that we would be associated exclusively with the brain in the event of its separation from the body—can, it seems to me, be challenged. But I do not need to challenge them here. The only point I need to make is that the identification of you and me as essentially human beings (although I happen to agree with it!) stands unsupported. Without that identification (supposing instead, for example, that you and I are essentially *persons* rather than *human beings*), then, although he is entitled to conclude that *you or I* do not begin to exist until the formation of the brain, he is not entitled to conclude that a *human being* does not begin to exist until the formation of the brain. I should want to argue that, *given his other beliefs*, he is not entitled to the view that you and I are essentially human beings.

III

For Anne McLaren and others, the view that the early embryo is not yet a human being has quite a different basis: it is derived from a detailed examination of the early stages of human development. In outline, the argument is that the newly conceived embryo is not yet a human being, *not* because it as yet lacks the 'proper' form of a human being, but because it has not yet become an *individual* human being. To appreciate the point, one needs some understanding of the details of early mammalian, and in particular human, development, which I shall briefly review, basing my account partly upon the Warnock Committee's Report [18] and partly upon McLaren's article "Prelude to Embryogenesis" [19].

At fertilisation the egg and sperm, each already genetically unique after a division prior to fertilisation known as *meiosis* which halves their respective chromosome numbers, unite to become a single relatively large cell with a full and unique complement of 46 chromosomes. This single cell is totipotential. From it, in other words, all the different types of tissue and organs that make up the adult human body are derived, as well as the tissues that become the placenta and fetal membranes during intra-uterine development. After a day or so it begins to divide into first two, then four, then eight smaller cells and so on, by a process called cleavage. During the earlier stages of cleavage each cell retains its totipotential capacity. Thus, if separation of the cells occurs at the two-cell stage, each cell may develop to form a separate embryo. Such separation leads to identical twins. The collection of cells now developing is known as a *morula*. At around the sixth day a fluid-filled space forms in an eccentric position within the morula and the collection of cells has reached the stage when it is known as a *blastocyst*. A small group of cells within the blastocyst develops to become the inner cell mass (ICM), a subsection of which forms into a plate-like structure—the embryonic disc. At one end of the structure there appears finally, on the fourteenth or fifteenth day after fertilisation, as a heaping up of cells, what is known as the primitive streak. This is the first identifiable feature of what the Warnock Report terms the 'embryo proper'. For here, in a strictly localised process, is formed a groove, folds, and the beginnings of the organic differentiation which is to mark the adult form. The remaining cells of the embryo—by far the larger part—go to provide the nutritive and protective life-support systems for the 'embryo proper'. Two primitive streaks occasionally form in a single embryonic disc. This is the latest stage at which identical twins can occur.

In the light of this detailed picture of early human development Anne McLaren, focusing on the question of origins, remarks: "To me the point at which I began as a total whole individual human being was at the primitive streak stage" [20]. She gives as a reason that: "If one tries to trace back further than that there is no longer a coherent entity. Instead there is a larger collection of cells, some of which are going to take part in the subsequent development of the embryo and some of which aren't" [21]. In the interests of clarity she urges the adoption of a new terminology, stated to have been first suggested by Dr Penelope Leach (a member of the Voluntary Licensing Authority for embryo experiments) reserving the term 'embryo' for what the Warnock Committee calls the 'embryo proper', and introducing the term 'pre-embryo' for the collection of cells which constitutes human life up until the formation of the primitive streak. Her justification seems to incorporate two separate points: (a) that the 'pre-embryo' does not have the wherewithal to be counted as an individual (not a "coherent entity"); and more especially (b) that it does not stand in the required relationship to the subsequently developing human individual for it to be counted as the same individual.

Let us consider, first, the suggestion that the 'pre-embryo' lacks what it takes to be counted as an individual. It is variously described as a 'population', 'cluster', 'collection' or 'clump' of cells. Now, without more ado, one might insist on taking the relaxed line that populations, clusters, collections and clumps are as a matter of fact, perfectly respectable individuals. But this invites the response: how can a collection of cells—even if it is a kind of individual—be the same individual as an adult human being, who seems to be a different kind of individual? One might point out that human beings are collections of cells anyway, but I guess that this comment is not quite to the point. What is being asked is: how can something which is a *mere* collection of cells be the same individual as something which is not a *mere* collection of cells?

In response, it can be pointed out that provided there is *some* covering concept, our notion of what counts as the same individual over time does allow for considerable transformations. The collection of pieces which lie on the watch-repairer's bench is surely the same individual watch as the one that I sent off for repairs. A given caterpillar and a given butterfly may surely be identified as one and the same lepidopteran. There will only be a problem in the case of the 'pre-embryo' and the human adult if we are deprived of the covering concept 'human being'; and the case for that remains to be made. Suppose we forget for a moment what is supposed to hang on the question of the status of the early embryo. There is something just a little perverse about treating the fascinating insights we have gained into the early stages of human life as if they amounted to the 'discovery' that what is there is not really a human being at all. (What difference would it make if the 'pre-embryo' was of microscopic adult form?) It needs to be added, moreover, that the 'pre-embryo' appears not to be a *mere* collection of cells in any case—such as a barrel of apples, for example, united only by spatial proximity. Warnock likens the morula to a blackberry [22]. And surely that's good enough. A blackberry, after all *is* a reasonably *bona fide* individual. A great deal remains to be learnt about the very early stages of mammalian development. But certainly in the case of the mouse embryo, from the stage known as compaction onwards (which in humans begins at the eight-cell stage), J. M. W. Slack reports that the individual cells cease to be readily identifiable and, moreover, that junctions form between the cells allowing diffusion of low-molecular-weight dyes *throughout the embryo* [23]. I cite this as evidence that the 'pre-embryo' is apparently an integrated structure.

But I fancy that the point which is uppermost in McLaren's mind and chiefly leads her towards distinguishing the embryo from the 'pre-embryo' is a different one. It is quite simply that the vast bulk of the cells that go to make up the 'pre-embryo' are such that neither they nor their progeny are fated to form the later fetus, which emerges from but a small part of the whole. "Once implantation is completed," she writes, "the only cells not committed to an extra-embryonic fate [i.e. to a purely supporting role] are a group of a few thousand in the epiblast layer of the embryonic plate. It is in the embryonic plate that the primitive streak is formed ... Since we now have a spatially defined entity that can develop directly into a fetus and thence into a baby, we are for the first time justified in using the term 'embryo' " [24]. A similar point is made by Slack when he remarks: "Up to the present, however, mammalian embryology is really 'pre-embryology', since it deals with the formation not of the embryo body plan but of various extracellular membranes which are necessary to the support and nutrition of the embryo proper" [25].

A natural response to this point is what one may call the 'I'm-in-there-somewhere' response. For, of course, the 'pre-embryo' will at all times *contain* cells which are ancestors of those cells which are eventually differentiated to form the later fetus. Indeed, the further back one traces this ancestry the higher the proportion they form of the total 'pre-embryo' population, until one reaches 100%, possibly at the 16-cell stage and certainly at the initial single-cell stage. The fact of spatio-temporal continuity between 'pre-embryo' and fetus on which this response depends is, of course, crucial to an attempt to establish identity. If the 'pre-embryo' were but a cradle, as it were, in which the embryo appears as if from nowhere, or as if from somewhere else, there would be no question of identity. But the facts are quite otherwise. Prior to implantation, indeed, embryonic development proceeds quite without the benefit of any foreign material whatsoever, not even in the form of nutrition. The pre-implantation embryo, bouncing down the fallopian tube, is a veritable free spirit. Never again are we to be quite so self-contained as in our first six days of existence. Cell lineage is still a matter of considerable uncertainty, but if we take the 16-cell stage for purposes of illustration, two extremes can be envisaged for the derivation of the cells that constitute the later embryo (when it begins to show organic differentiation). One is that they derive from all 16 cells; the other is that they derive from only one. There are any number of possibilities in between. My impression from reading the embryologists is that the actual pattern or patterns of derivation are not yet known, nor yet is it known how much variation there may be from case to case. A similar picture holds for the cells, however many there are, that form the inner cell mass in its early stages. By this time, none of the cells making up the rest of the 'pre-embryo'—these form what is called the *trophectoderm*—will in fact belong to the ancestry of the later embryo. They are committed, as McLaren has it, to an 'extra-embryonic fate'.

There are two important points to be borne in mind in assessing this 'I'm-in-there-somewhere' response. The first, if I may be permitted such an obvious remark, is that we live forwards not backwards. The very question, 'When did I begin?', encourages one to overlook this simple fact. Care is needed to avoid conflating the legitimate project of tracing an individual's identity back in time (where it is in the tracing only that one moves 'backwards') with the illegitimate picture of life's actually being lived in reverse. Shorn of this latter insinuation the 'I' who am in there somewhere can be a very shadowy existent indeed. One way to see this is to try identifying the 'I' in question should it die after just nine days. The other point is that no cell in the early stages of development is earmarked for a particular future role. Cell-commitment is a gradual process. The 'potency' of a cell, i.e. the total of all the things into which it can develop if put in the appropriate environment, becomes more and more restricted as development proceeds in response to external stimuli ('inductive signals') [26]. Slack comments upon the paucity of terminology to describe the intermediate stages between totipotency and complete determination. We are driven, he says, to "referring either to positions ('anterior mesoderm', 'posterior mesoderm') or to the future organ ('limb field', 'eye field') ... " [27]. In other words, these labels do *not* mean that a cell is already earmarked 'limb' or 'eye', only that its progeny will form part of the limb or eye if left undisturbed [28]. Taken together, these facts considerably reduce the intuitive attraction of the 'I'm-in-there-somewhere' response. Indeed, McLaren's implicit allusion to the lack of a 'spatially defined entity' so far as the 'pre-embryo' is concerned, may well be predicated upon, and be a response to, the 'in-there-somewhere' position. The 'in-there-somewhere' entity, given the indeterminacy of the 'pre-embryo's' cell states, certainly does lack clear spatial definition. It seems, then, that the attempt to identify the 'you' or 'I' of the first fortnight of existence with some *portion* of the 'pre-embryo' has to be abandoned.

Yet, there still remains an entity which *is* spatially defined—namely the whole 'pre-embryo'; and we have yet, to my mind, to be given convincing reasons against identifying the *whole* 'pre-embryo' as the same individual (human being) as the later fetus.

The notion that the bulk of the 'pre-embryo' is committed to an extra-embryonic fate, if we look here for the decisive reason, appears susceptible to two rather different interpretations. If we emphasise the extra-*embryonic* character of the fate of these cells or their progeny, then we seem to face once more what I have deemed a mere prejudice—namely, the view that only something beginning to approximate to a miniaturised adult human is entitled to count as a human being, or even as an embryo. But an alternative interpretation is to see the remark as directing our attention to the fact that only a very small proportion of the pre-embryonic cells carry their progeny through to the future individual, irrespective of whether this has the form of a miniaturised adult or not [29].

In its own right the point is rather difficult to assess. We surely do allow identity to continue through very considerable variations in bulk. Many cells and many of their progeny are destined to be shed. But this does not lead us to discount, say, the layers of outer skin which are destined to be shed as not part of the adult human. But the point is, it might be argued, that the progeny are not simply destined to be shed but are destined to be part of a structure which is not part of the future individual. This does seem to beg the question, however, with respect to the fetal human: we have not yet agreed to count only the miniaturised adult form, shorn of placenta, umbilical cord, etc., as the future individual [30]. We should not imagine that we can draw clear lines around the human individual even at the adult stage. Where exactly do *we* end, and our environments begin? Do *we* include our skin, hair, finger and toe-nails—all dead tissue? Do we scrape off the sweat, do we scoop out the saliva, mucus and about 3 lb or so of bacteria which make a living in our gut, before we get down to the real, neat, naked us? We had better not, for if we literally did that, then in a short time that real, neat, naked 'we' would be dead. Moreover, and this is the main point, what the progeny of a given set of cells *will be*—say, the set that makes up the trophecto-derm—hardly seems decisive as to the status of those cells *now*. In baby photos of the future, with cameras able to operate inside the human body, why should we not find ourselves saying: 'Look, here I am 5 days after conception, when I was part trophectoderm, part ICM?'

IV

But now the facts seem to throw up another equally or more formidable obstacle, which is this [31]. So far as the internal constitution of the 'pre-embryo' is concerned, it is not finally decided whether there will be one fetus or two until the primitive streak stage. In that case, if the 'pre-embryo' is not determinately either one or two human beings, *how can it be any number of human beings at all?*

An initial response might be to say: 'although it does not appear determinately either one or two human beings, it *will be* either one or two. Let us say then that if it will be one, it is now one; and if it will be two, then it is now two'. But here again it has to be remembered that we live only forwards. For suppose it will not be either one or two because it will die before the time of commitment arrives. In that case it would not now be determinately either one or two. So there would be a worrying asymmetry among otherwise indistinguishable 'pre-embryos' between those which will die and therefore fail ever to be human beings, and those which will survive and therefore manage to be either one, or two, human beings from the moment of conception. Furthermore, it would become possible, by killing something, to make it never have been a human being. An even greater objection faces the suggestion that if a 'pre-embryo' will be twins, it is now twins. For this seems to be a straight violation of the principle that no two individuals of the same kind can occupy the same place at the same time. Suppose we evade this last impossibility by treating twins as a special case, and deferring the starting point of a twin's life until the formation of the primitive streak. We should be left with the asymmetry—some 'pre-embryos' are human beings while others are not—and should have acquired in addition the anomaly that twins begin *their* lives a fortnight later than anybody else does.

The pressures to succumb to McLaren's position appear considerable, if not overwhelming. Yet a nagging doubt remains. Can it be for *this* reason alone (I assume, for the purpose of argument, that I have shown all the other reasons to be inadequate)—namely that the single 'pre-embryo' may on occasion yield two primitive streaks—that we are to withhold the epithet 'human being' from the 'pre-embryo'? Is the worm to forfeit its wormly identity just in case the ploughshare might make it two?

Suppose for the moment, taking our cue from the worm, that we resolve the asymmetries and anomalies the other way and make the 'pre-embryo' in all cases a single human being. (It is important to understand, for the line of reasoning which follows, that, so far as is known, twinning is the result of some concatenation of circumstances which is in an important sense as 'accidental' as those which result in a worm's being divided.) Applied to the case of identical twins this would involve supposing that each of a pair of identical twins exists at a time when neither is separately identifiable because, for the first fortnight, they share a common life. He or she might say: 'I did exist then and I was identifiable then; but I was not separately identifiable'. Each would point to the 'pre-embryo' and say, 'that's me'. For the first fortnight of their lives identical twins would be the same human being.

Such a proposal does not involve violating the principle that no two individuals of the same kind can occupy the same place at the same time, since what is proposed is that the 'pre-embryo' is not two individuals, but one. However, the proposal does appear to fall foul of another logical principle—the transitivity of identity. If we insist that the 'pre-embryo' is one human being, that the ensuing twins are two human beings, and that the 'pre-embryo' is the same human being as each ensuing twin, then we challenge the principle that if $a=b$ and $a=c$, then $b=c$.

It would appear that this difficulty, if it should prove real, must be decisive. I do not deny that it is a real difficulty. But I do deny that it is decisive, for the simple reason that analogous conceptual problems of bifurcation occur in cases where a 'solution' clearly cannot be sought by withdrawing from the item prior to its bifurcation the covering concept which generates the problem, as it is proposed to withdraw the covering concept 'human being' in the case of the 'pre-embryo'. One such case is much discussed in recent literature on personal identity—the hypothetical case of brain-bifurcation. If one person's brain were to be divided, as is said to be logically and in principle even technically possible, in such a way that each portion of brain tissue was capable of functioning passably as part of a person (in different bodies, let us say), the relation of the subsequent 'persons' to the original person would be highly problematic. The problem is a vexed one to which I do not pretend to know the 'answer'. But two points at least seem reasonably clear. One is that there are very strong pressures, in this particular hypothetical case, in favour of a solution which postulates the retention of *some* form of identity between the subsequent 'persons' and the original person, despite the violating of the transitivity of strict identity that is entailed. The other is that the option of denying personhood prior to the bifurcation is simply not available.

In case 'person' should seem to be a concept of a special kind, from which it would be unwise to extrapolate, it is worth observing that, arguably, exactly the same points can be made concerning the brain itself whose bifurcation underlies the bifurcation of the person. The brain too, becomes two brains, each enjoying some measure of identity with the original. No doubt there is a temptation here to say that the brain is *halved*—which would certainly dissolve the problem in this case since there is nothing puzzling about an object's being rendered into two, or more pieces. But it ought to be noticed that whether or not that option is available depends crucially on whether or not the brain is construed as a substance. For individual subtances are *indivisible*. (This is a property of all substances, not a mysterious property of immaterial ones.) This does not mean that you cannot take pieces out of substances, for of course you can. What it means, rather, is that, if the brain is construed as an individual substance, then the notion of 'half a brain' is a nonsense, just as much as it would be a nonsense to speak of 'half a squirrel', 'half an oak tree', or 'half a human being'. What should be said, rather, is that the material constituting the brain is halved; the brain itself becomes two brains.

If one should demur over the hypothetical nature of the cases so far cited, or be in doubt about whether the brain is a substance, then both of these sources of scepticism might be removed by reverting to the case of the bisected earthworm. Despite the fact that we commonly refer to a worm's being cut in two, this is certainly an incorrect way of speaking, since a worm certainly is an individual substance and *cannot* therefore be halved. It is the worm's body that is divided in two, one half of which is a worm without a head, the other half of which is a worm without a tail—situations soon rectified by the remarkable process of *regeneration*. The worm, in short, becomes two worms; one substance of a given kind becomes two substances of that kind.

In the above case, it may be that the pressures favouring a solution which postulates the retention of some form of identity through the bifurcation are beginning to disappear. They have disappeared entirely when we come to the cases of fission undergone by many forms of protozoa, such as the amoeba, the stentor and the like [32]. In such cases, the 'solution' to the problem of bifurcation is, of course, to give up identity entirely and to start talking instead of 'reproduction'. It should not be imagined, however, that these labels really solve anything very much. Asexual reproduction is so different from full-blown mammalian sexual reproduction that the label itself is hardly helpful.

The apparent gap between regeneration and asexual reproduction is something of an illusion and it is almost certain that there is an evolutionary connection between them. Regenerative phenomena "are closely related to the devices for asexual reproduction that have evolved in the various groups" [33]. Further, as Elizabeth Hay remarks: "there is no reason to believe that the actual mechanisms of growth are any different in the two cases" [34]. Thus, the relation between 'offspring' and 'parent' among the protozoa is by no means so straightforward as facile talk of reproduction would lead one to believe. What bears remark yet again is that although (perhaps I should say, because) in this case the supposition of individual identity being preserved through the bifurcation is yielded up, there is no question but that the individual prior to bifurcation is a substance of the same kind as the individuals subsequent to bifurcation.

In briefly reviewing these various cases of bifurcation, I have not meant to suggest for one moment that they are all of a kind, or that any of them exactly parallels the case of the 'pre-embryo'. None of them, for example, quite shares the ontogenetic character of the latter. What I do mean to suggest is, first, the general point that it is likely to be within the context of a general theory of developmental biology that this family of cases, *including* the case of the bifurcating 'pre-embryo', will eventually achieve conceptual clarification. Nor should it be the occasion of surprise if, under a broadly evolutionary perspective, human development, in its very early stages, should exhibit features similar to those found in the development of simple life-forms But what I mean to suggest, more particularly, is that although it would 'solve' the problem of the 'pre-embryo' becoming twins if we should withdraw the epithet 'human being' from the 'pre-embryo' prior to this event's taking place, this solution would be totally *inappropriate*. (Furthermore, if it were conceded that the 'pre-embryo' was any *kind* of individual at all, rather than a mere piece of tissue, then there would *still* remain the substantial problem of saying what exactly the relationship is between this individual and the resulting human twins.) If this charge is justified, then it follows that the difficulty about twinning is not a *reason* for withdrawing the epithet 'human being' from the 'pre-embryo'. If this is not a reason and if, as I have tried to show, there is no other good reason, then it follows that there is no good reason for denying that a human being begins to exist from the moment of conception.

V

'Pre-embryos' die naturally, unnoticed and unmourned, in their thousands. Why then, if these are human deaths, is there not an outcry at such tragedy, as there is when any large number of human beings is stricken prematurely? I do not see this, however, as an argument for denying that these are human deaths, but merely as a reminder, should we need one, that nature holds human life as cheap as she holds any other form of life. We do not have to follow nature in this regard, although, in the light of these naturally occurring deaths, excessive regard for the life of the 'pre-embryo' might well seem misplaced. For this and other reasons, the moral ground of those who think that experimentation on early embryos should be permitted may well prove to be defensible. But I have sought to show that it should not be defended by relying upon the metaphysically dubious notion of the 'pre-embryo'. We should shun at all costs the capture of moral ground by verbal manoeuvres. You and I are human beings. There is only one concept of 'human being'—the biological one. A human being is simply a living organism of the species *Homo sapiens*. In contemplating embryo research we must describe accurately, honestly and without sentimentality what it is that we propose to do. We must not hide from ourselves (what I believe to be) the fact that when we experiment on human embryos we experiment on human beings.

Alan Holland, Department of Philosophy, Bowland College, University of Lancaster, Lancaster LA1 4YT, United Kingdom.

NOTES

[1] In calling it 'my life' I take the liberty of assuming, without defending it here, that what you and I are essentially are human beings.

[2] A recent (1987) publication by the British Medical Research Council, for example, has the title: *Why Pre-Embryo Research? What You Need to Know.*

[3] BERNARD WILLIAMS (1986) Types of moral argument against embryo research, in: G. BOCK & M. O'CONNOR (Eds) *Human Embryo Research: yes or no?* (London, Tavistock), p. 192.

[4] A point which is carefully registered in the *Encyclopaedia Britannica* (1980) 15th edn, 5, p. 626 sbv. Animal Development: "After fertilization, the zygote undergoes a series of transformations that bring it closer to the essential organization of the parents".

[5] ANNE MCLAREN (1986) Prelude to embryogenesis, in: *Human Embryo Research*, pp. 5–23, esp. p. 12.

[6] For the moment I retain this term to refer to human life from conception.

[7] WILLIAMS, op. cit., p. 192.

[8] J. H. WOODGER (1945) On biological transformation, quoted in DAVID WIGGINS's monograph *Identity and Spatio-Temporal Continuity* (1967) (Oxford, Basil Blackwell), p. 69.

[9] It thus becomes possible to subscribe to the principle that all human beings are morally considerable in advance of knowing which individuals count as human beings, and, in particular, whether embryos do. But, on the view taken here, the question whether all human beings qualify for moral consideration should wait upon an answer to the question whether embryos are human beings rather than be used to determine the answer.

[10] JONATHAN GLOVER (1984) *What Sort of People Should There Be?* (Harmondsworth, Penguin), p. 31.

[11] MICHAEL T. GHISELIN (1987) Species concepts, individuality, and objectivity, *Biology and Philosophy*, 2, pp. 127–143; ERNST MAYR (1987) The ontological status of species: scientific progress and philosophical terminology, *Biology and Philosophy*, 2, pp. 145–166.

[12] Conversely, to hazard a dramatic, if fictional example, the hero of Kafka's tragic story *Metamorphosis*, provided he underwent a genuine metamorphosis and not some magical switch, must be held to have remained a human *after* the alteration in his circumstances; for Mrs Samsa remained his 'mum'.

[13] MICHAEL LOCKWOOD (1985) When does a life begin? in: M. LOCKWOOD (Ed.) *Moral Dilemmas in Modern Medicine* (Oxford, Oxford University Press), pp. 9–31.

[14] Ibid., p. 11.

[15] Ibid., p. 19.

[16] Ibid., p. 17.

[17] Ibid., p. 19.

[18] MARY WARNOCK (1984) *A Question of Life* (Oxford, Basil Blackwell), pp. 58–60.

[19] MCLAREN, op. cit., pp. 5–23.

[20] Ibid., p. 22.

[21] Ibid., p. 22.

[22] WARNOCK, op. cit., p. 59.

[23] J. M. W. SLACK (1983) *From Egg to Embryo* (Cambridge, Cambridge University Press), p. 139.

[24] MCLAREN, op. cit., pp. 11–12.

[25] SLACK, op. cit., p. 136.

[26] Ibid., pp. 19, 25.

[27] Ibid., p. 7.

[28] Cells from the prospective neural plate (brain, spinal cord) of an amphibian embryo, if grafted early enough to a different region, will form epidermis (skin).

[29] On the other hand, the original cell (*all* of it), and possibly all of the first 4, 8, or 16 cells, will have descendants destined for an *intra*-embryonic fate.

[30] Until the mouth and lungs come into operation after birth, for example, the nutrition and support system effectively functions as mouth and lungs.

[31] The problems are canvassed with great force by G. E. M. ANSCOMBE (1985) Were you a zygote? in: A. PHILLIPS GRIFFITHS (Ed.) *Philosophy and Practice* (Cambridge, Cambridge University Press), pp. 111–116.

[32] These phenomena may be judged closer than those previously cited to the case of the 'pre-embryo' in that they happen naturally rather than being a violation of some natural process or condition. At the same time it ought to be observed that twinning is judged to be an *abnormality* in humans: *Encyclopaedia Britannica* (1980) 15th edn, 6, p. 748 sbv. Human embryology.

[33] ELIZABETH HAY (1966) *Regeneration* (New York, Holt, Rinehart & Winston), p. 1.

[34] Ibid., p. 10.

28

Defining Death

ALISTER BROWNE

ABSTRACT   *Modern technology has made it uncertain as to when exactly death occurs, and this has put us in a quandary over when we can initiate behaviour traditionally deemed apt if and only if a patient is dead. In the light of this, there is general agreement that death should be redefined, but wide disagreement remains about how. I argue, against this, that it is a mistake to redefine death in any way: (1) redefining death will not help to settle the question of when traditional death-behaviour becomes appropriate, (2) any attempt to redefine death is attended with significant disutilities and no compensating utilities, and (3) the practical problems generated by the indeterminacy can be better handled in other ways.*

Death is customarily regarded as a time of great behavioural significance. For example, it is thought that we cannot rightly do such things as mine an organ donor's body for transplantable organs, begin an autopsy, use the body for certain experimental or teaching purposes, or routinely withdraw all life-support systems from patients before death occurs, but can quite properly do them as soon as it does. Now certainly we can, in an utterly unproblematical way, identify some people as dead and others as alive. But, owing largely to innovations in medical technology, there are also some cases in which we cannot make such a determination, and thus are left with the problem of how to treat them. This had led some to regard the question of defining death as a practically important one that urgently stands in need of an answer; hence the spate of recent efforts to provide such a definition.

This literature is characterized by general agreement on the need to redefine death, but wide disagreement on how it should be redefined. Some advocate a whole-brain definition, others a higher-brain definition, and still others a heart-lung definition. I want to argue, against all this, that it is a mistake to redefine death in any way. I will contend that redefining death will not help to settle any questions of when behaviour becomes appropriate; that any attempt to redefine death is attended with significant disutilities and no countervailing utilities; and that the practical problems generated by the indeterminacy can be better handled in other ways.

I want to begin, however, by claiming agreement with the redefinists on one point: the ordinary concept of death is indeterminate. It will be useful to describe how. This is needed not only to show that there is a genuine issue over whether to redefine death, but also because the full scope of the indeterminacy has not always been recognized, and this had led to some oversimplified accounts of how it can be remedied.

Uncontroversially, death is the loss of some function or set of functions. But when we try to be more precise, we meet two kinds of indeterminacy. First, we cannot provide a topic-neutral definition that adequately captures it, and second, even if we could, we would not be able to supply content to that definition in an unproblematical way. We will take these claims in order.

It is plausible to think that there is some property or set of properties, P, which is related to the state of being dead in such a way that that state can be analysed in terms of P. Thus the question arises: What is the relation between death and P? One way of answering this is to say that a being, A, is dead if and only if A at one time possessed P, A now lacks P, and A cannot be brought to repossess P. For example, suppose that P=spontaneous heartbeat and respiration. On this view, we would not call a being dead unless it had at one time exhibited these vital signs: it is logically impossible for an entity that has never lived to be dead. But the loss of those properties is not a sufficient condition of death; in addition, it must be the case that those properties cannot be restored. The question now arises as to how we are to understand the "cannot" in the last clause of this formula.

One way of reading it is to take it to express logical impossibility [1]. But this view has two odd consequences. First, it yields the result that we can never know that a person is dead; for, according to it, we can only know that a person is dead if we know that it is logically impossible for him to repossess P, and that is something we cannot know. It is not logically impossible that a person for whom all mental and bodily functions had ceased for 2000 years be brought to repossess the same. So, on the view we are now considering, we cannot know that the person is dead. Secondly, if it is a conceptual truth that death is in that sense permanent, stories of the miraculous raising of the dead should be self-contradictory. But they are not. Miracle stories may strike us as fantastic or unlikely, but they are not conceptually incoherent. There is no contradiction in saying that at T_1 Lazarus was dead, really dead, and that at T_2 Lazarus was alive, really alive, again. To claim to discover a covert contradiction in this is to read something into the concept of death that is not there; certainly no one can insist that any competent speaker of the English language must conclude from the fact that Lazarus was alive at T_2 that he could not have been dead at T_1.

But we need not read the 'cannot' in the formula under consideration as expressing logical impossibility; there are two other ways of understanding it. One is to take it to express empirical impossibility. On this construal, a person lacking P is dead if and only if it is contrary to the laws of nature that he be brought to or come to repossess P. Alternatively, we can take it to express technical impossibility. On this account, a person lacking P is dead if and only if it is beyond the current technological capacity of medical science to bring it about that he repossess P.

Neither of these accounts, however, is entirely satisfactory. The technical impossibility reading has the consequence that two persons may be in identical states at different times, yet because of differing technology, one may be described as dead and the other as not dead. And this sounds odd: if, as is *ex hypothesi* the case, they really are in identical states, it seems that they should either both be dead or both be alive. But, on the other hand, odd consequences follow from linking death to the empirical impossibility of bringing a person to repossess P. For if we make death contingent on the claim that it is contrary to the laws of nature that a person regain P, to the extent to which we cannot substantiate that claim we cannot be sure that a person is dead. And in so far as all the laws of nature are not disclosed to us, it is difficult to say firmly in any case that it is incompatible with the laws of nature for a person in a particular state to regain P. So, on the empirical impossibility account, our judgements of death can only be tentative; we can never say with certainty that a person is dead. Future discoveries may force us to revise our judgement that Socrates died.

One way of avoiding both of these odd consequences is simply to drop the clause containing the modal term, and to say that a person, A, is dead if and only if A at one time possessed P and A now lacks P. This has the virtue that we can say with certainty that a person is dead, and do so in a way that does not make that judgement relative to the technology of the age, thus enabling us to avoid certain problem cases. But the view is not entirely free from difficulty. If we restrict the range of possible values of P to things like spontaneous heartbeat, monitorable brain activity, etc., and exclude things like *ability* to be revived, *ability* to regain spontaneous heartbeat, etc., then this account has the consequence that a person can die many times. Many people find this consequence repugnant, yet many others willingly embrace it: occasionally we find, often in the *Reader's Digest*, stories written by people who describe themselves as having died (sometimes multiple times) on the operating table. And not only in the *Reader's Digest*; as L. C. Becker puts it in a quite different sort of periodical, "People die, but sometimes can be revived" [2]. It would be a high-handed piece of verbal legislation to insist that those who speak in this way are speaking either loosely and improperly or metaphorically. Such descriptions may sound a little odd, but there is nothing downright wrong about them. It would, however, be downright wrong to say that when one says that a person is dead he could not sensibly mean anything more than that person lacks a certain property such as spontaneous heartbeat, respiration, etc.; sometimes we do mean more.

I have just discussed what I think are the only plausible topic-neutral definitions of death that can be offered, and have argued that none of them adequately captures our ordinary concept of death. This is one way in which that concept is indeterminate. There is also another one. Even if we could specify the sense in which death is the loss of P, the question would arise as to what the value of P is. What exactly is the property or set of properties that a person must lose if that person is to count as dead? Three possible answers come to mind: higher-brain (or, as it is sometimes alternatively put, neocortical or cerebral) function, whole-brain function, and heart-lung function.

The first of these can be dismissed fairly quickly. Whatever virtues the higher-brain account [3] may have as a redefinition of death, there can be no doubt that it fails grotesquely as an explication of our ordinary concept of death. On this account, Karen Ann Quinlan should have been declared dead as soon as it was determined that her higher-brain centres which sponsor consciousness had been permanently destroyed. But the fact that she exhibited spontaneous heartbeat and respiration due to the activity of the lower-brain makes such a judgement odd: as far as our ordinary concept of death goes, spontaneous breathing and cardiac activity are incompatible with calling a patient dead. Since this is so, and since such activity is compatible with the permanent loss of higher-brain function, the permanent loss of the latter function could not be a sufficient condition for pronouncing death.

The whole-brain account [4] does something to meet this problem, for according to it a patient is dead if and only if the lower-brain as well as the higher-brain has shut down, and thus there is no question of calling anyone with spontaneous heartbeat or respiration dead. But while we may well agree that we can call people dead *only if* they do not have spontaneous heartbeat or respiration, it is not clear that we can do so *if* they lack those functions. Suppose we have an individual on a respirator such that his respiratory and cardiac systems are functioning, but not functioning spontaneously. How should we describe the case? Do we have before us a case of simulated life or artificially supported life? It is unsatisfactory flatly to say (as does David Lamb [5]) that since the great organ systems have shut down, and will never again function naturally, what we have before us is a corpse being ventilated. It is not a fact of science or of ordinary language that one who has suffered whole-brain death is dead. One could perhaps correctly say that if such a patient is not on a respirator—if blood is not circulating, food metabolizing, wastes being eliminated, etc.—then he is dead. But if he is on a respirator, and these processes are occurring—albeit artificially supported—one cannot claim it to be an obvious or indisputable fact that he is dead. Science, and ordinary language, are silent on the question of whether vital functions must occur naturally if an organism is to be counted as alive. So the heart-lung account [6] according to which there must be absence of all spontaneous and nonspontaneous respiration and heartbeat before a patient is counted as dead, cannot be summarily dismissed. And if we adopt such an account, then we would regard a whole-brain-dead individual on a respirator as an instance, not of simulated life, but of artificially supported life. But I know of no way of resolving any disagreement that may arise over the correct way to describe the case. The fact that the great organ systems are functioning may well incline us to say that the person is alive, but the fact that they are not functioning on their own may tempt us to say that he is dead. And there is nothing to which we can appeal to decide the matter.

We thus find that ordinary language speaks with an uncertain voice on the exact boundaries of the concept of death. This should not take us by surprise. The concept of death developed during a time when absence of heartbeat, absence of respiration, and irreversible coma all occurred at roughly the same time, and the technology of the day rendered it senseless to distinguish between spontaneous and artifically supported heartbeat and respiration, as well as reversible and irreversible absences of those functions: the absence of those functions in any way soon led to irreversible coma. It is thus only to be expected that when technological innovations prise these traditional criteria apart and force finer distinctions on us that the ordinary concept of death be unresponsive. We are put in exactly the same situation as when the presence of the anatomical features that normally go with a woman are found together with the chromosomal count that normally goes with a man and are asked whether we have a man or woman before us.

But even granting that the present concept of death is indeterminate, that important legal, moral, and medical consequences flow from the determination of death, and that it is undesirable to be left in limbo on these matters, it still does not follow that we ought to make precise the definition of death. There remains the alternative of leaving the definition of death in its present indeterminate state, and going on to specify what can be appropriately done to whom when. Thus, for example, we could have rules such as: "No transplant proceedings can be initiated until all spontaneous and nonspontaneous respiration and heartbeat have irreversibly ceased"; "Life-support systems may be routinely terminated as soon as an individual is irreversibly comatose, even if spontaneous respiration and heartbeat still occur"; "Any person who intentionally causes another to lose his capacity to function as an integrated conscious being shall be punished by the most severe sanction available in this jurisdiction"; and so on. I do not want to insist that these particular rules ought to be adopted; my point is only that we can remove any uncertainty in practical affairs without fiddling with the definition of death [7].

Is there, then, any advantage in redefining death? The temptation to make precise the definition of death surely rests on one of two beliefs. First, one may think that since certain behaviour is deemed appropriate if and only if a person is dead, if we could determine when a person is dead, we would thereby determine when that behaviour becomes appropriate. This is perhaps the main motivation in the rush to redefine death, and it exemplifies an approach to the problems of medical ethics which has become popular. Since science is successful in solving problems in a way in which ethics is not, it is enormously tempting to convert questions concerning matters of ethics into those concerning matters of fact in the hope of being able to set them to rest in a clear and objective way. We thus find the question of when treatment can be properly withheld or withdrawn made contingent on whether the treatment is ordinary or extraordinary, the question of how we can appropriately bring about the death of patients on whether what we do is an instance of killing or letting die, and the question of whether abortion is morally permissible on whether the fetus is a human being. We are accordingly encouraged to think that if we can only get clear about the ordinary/ extraordinary, killing/letting die, and human/non-human being distinctions, the moral problems of when certain behaviour becomes appropriate will likewise be resolved. Similarly, the thought is that by redrafting the life/death distinction we will thereby resolve some knotty questions about the appropriateness of behaviour. Secondly, one may not believe this, but nonetheless think that there is utility in having a clear and crisp line dividing the living from the dead. On this view, the advantage in redefining death derives just from having a useful shorthand way of referring to a time of great behavioural significance. If one did not hold either of these views, it would be hard to see why one would want to redefine death. I will, however, argue that both these beliefs are false, and hence that death should not be redefined.

Whether we can resolve any questions about the appropriateness of behaviour by making the definition of death precise depends on *how* we can make it precise. The first thing we must recognize is that we cannot remove the indeterminacy by any amount of empirical research. Neurophysiologists can provide ways of diagnosing the occurrence of higher-brain death, whole-brain death, and heart-lung death, but they cannot tell us which of these states should be identified as the death of the organism. That is a question which will still persist even after all the neurophysiological facts are in, and settling it is a conceptual, not a scientific, matter. What conceptual moves can be made to remove the indeterminacy in question? So far as I can see, there are four.

First, one can try to equate death with the loss of valuable life, and then go on to suggest that if we can specify those features which make human life significant, we will be able to identify death as the loss of those things [8]. But this formula will not uncontroversially yield any determinate definition of death, for what makes life valuable is a disputed question, and, depending on what one thinks that is, one will be led to define death in terms of anything from the earliest time at which one could accurately diagnose permanent loss of consciousness, to such a loss of personal identity, to such a loss of all interests. There is, however, a more fundamental objection to be made. The equation of death with the irreversible loss of that which gives life value is faulty in as much as it makes perfectly good sense to describe a person as alive but not living a life worth living or preserving. On the face of it, loss of valuable life is one thing, loss of life quite another, and unless some advantage can be presented sufficient to set aside this commonsense distinction, this way of making precise the definition of death must be rejected.

Secondly, one could try to argue, as Michael Green and Daniel Wikler [9] recently have, that death can be equated with the permanent loss of personal identity. Suppose we can separate the brain from the body and keep it functioning so that it shows consciousness and psychological connectedness and continuity with the erstwhile person. If we now ask, "Which entity is the person?", the natural reply is that the brain is, and the body is not. Thus if the brain were to be destroyed, the person would be no more, and hence we can confidently say is dead. But if so, this should be our judgement when the brain remains in place and merely permanently ceases functioning, either in whole or in those parts which sponsor the psychological states which constitute personal identity. So far, so good; the problem comes when one tries to infer from the fact that the *person*—the entity having self-awareness—is dead that the *patient*—the organism occupying the hospital bed—is dead. Consider the following sequence: Jones first falls prey to the early stages of Alzheimer's disease; then he slips into a deep dementia; then suffers higher-brain death, followed by whole-brain death, and finally heart-lung death. Clearly Jones the person went partly out of existence at the first stage, and wholly so at the second. But it would be wrong to say the same of Jones the patient. The organism occupying the hospital bed clearly continues to exist for some time after personal death has occurred, and continues to be properly referred to as 'Jones': it is *Jones* who has suffered permanent memory loss, higher-brain death, heart-lung death, and whom we eventually bury. Not only does Jones continue to exist after personal death, he continues to be alive past that point. No one want to say that patients in end-state Alzheimer's are dead, and few that those in the state which made Karen Ann Quinlan famous are so. Just when the patient Jones died in the above sequence of events is still to be determined, but we clearly cannot settle the matter by identifying the point at which personal identity is permanently extinguished.

The third way of removing the indeterminacy consists in treating the concept of death as an evaluative concept, and making its definition consequential on our judgements of when it would be appropriate to engage in certain behaviour. On this way of proceeding, we would first determine when it would be appropriate to perform death-behaviour—i.e., behaviour which is traditionally (but not therefore necessarily correctly) deemed appropriate if and only if a patient is dead—and say that death occurs at that time. Thus, for example, if we were to say that it is appropriate to engage in death-behaviour if and only if an individual has irreversibly lost whole-brain function, then we would say that a patient is dead when that state of affairs exists.

The fourth possible way of fixing the definition of death is by arbitrary stipulation. One may want to treat the concept of death as a strictly biological/factual concept. If so, how can one go about making its definition precise? To what can one appeal to settle the question of whether or in what sense death is permanent, or whether or in what sense vital organs must have ceased to function spontaneously? Consulting ordinary usage will not help. There are no conceivable biological discoveries which will resolve the issue. Appeal to the concept of personal identity is of no avail. Utility of consequences cannot be taken into account without importing considerations of value. It thus seems that the only way left of fixing the definition and yet keeping it value-free is by arbitrary stipulation: we must simply decide where the life/death boundary is to be drawn.

These last, it seems to me, are the only two viable ways of making the definition of death precise. But if so, we can see that making that definition precise will not help us to settle any questions about when certain behaviour becomes appropriate. If we make the definition precise by arbitrary stipulation, those questions will remain *after* the definition of death has been settled, for we cannot rightly resolve such questions by arbitrary fiat. And if we fix the definition by treating the concept of death as an evaluative concept in the way described, the questions have to be resolved *before* the definition of death can be decided [10]. It is thus apparent that any hope of resolving questions about the appropriateness of behaviour by redefining death is forlorn, and hence the first reason one may have for wanting to redefine death turns out to be a bad one.

If the above is right, the exact moment of death is not a time which can be *discovered*; it must be, in one way or another, *decided*. In this respect, the question, "When does death occur?" is more like the question, "What is the age of maturity?" than like the question, "What is the half-life of uranium?" And, like that question, it is worth deciding only if there is some advantage in doing so. Is there?

Given the foregoing, the only advantage one could possibly seek from redefining death is to secure a useful shorthand way of referring to a time of great behavioural significance, and hence we are led to the second reason one can have for redefining death. If we could find some point at which all or most traditional death-behaviour can properly be initiated, by redefining death to coincide with that time we could, simply by calling someone dead, economically communicate that certain behaviour is now apt which was not before. But, of course, this advantage can be secured only if it turns out that there is some single point at which all or most traditional death-behaviour becomes appropriate, and that is not clearly the case. When the behaviour we now commonly refer to as death-behaviour came to be wedded to the time of death, death was, as noted before, characterised by absence of respiration, absence of heartbeat, and irreversible coma all occurring at the same time, and no attention was paid to the spontaneous/artificially supported or reversible/irreversible distinctions. It would be remarkable and fortuitious if all or most of that behaviour which became appropriate if and only if all three of those features occurred also became appropriate if and only if some precisely stated subset of them did.

And it does not seem to. When we ask when the various items of death-behaviour become appropriate, the answers we receive splay them over the full spectrum of possible definitions of death. Some say that we can terminate all health-care services at the time of higher-brain death. Others contend that while we can remove or withhold all medical procedures at that point, we must continue to provide nutrition and hydration until whole-brain death has occurred. But few of those who hold the former view will say that we can at that time also initiate other traditional death-behaviour such as harvesting transplantable organs or using the body for certain teaching purposes. It is common to hold out for at least whole-brain death for organ-harvesting, and many claim that even this is too early, maintaining that we must switch off the respirator and allow heart-lung death to occur before excising the organs. And heart-lung death is most commonly held to be a necessary condition for using a body for teaching or experimental purposes.

If all the individual's interests were foreclosed at a single point, and there were no other factors to be taken into account, it would be easy to condemn any opinion which pegged different items of death-behaviour at different times. But neither of these is the case. While there is a significant reduction in a patient's interests at the point of irreversible coma, he typically will have interests concerning respectful and dignified treatment of his body which extend beyond that time, and even beyond the time at which he can be uncontroversially pronounced dead. We also have to take into account the sensibilities of others, as well as the utility from the point of view of transplant procedures, teaching advantages, costs, etc. of initiating certain behaviour at one time rather than another. When all these factors are taken into account, it is not clear what the appropriate dating of death-behaviour is—that remains an unresolved problem— but it is far from obvious that there is some single instant at which all or most of it becomes apt.

But even if all or most death-behaviour did coalesce at some one time, there would still be a problem. If we fix the definition in this way, judgements of death encapsulate value-judgements. However, since to say that a person is dead certainly does not sound like a value-judgement, but a hard, cold, scientific fact, we will be involved in misrepresentation: we will pass off value-laden judgements as value-free ones.

But this is not sufficient warrant to dismiss the proposal, for as Green and Wikler have contended [11], truthfulness to the facts, while it may be a cardinal virtue in theoretical work, need not be so in questions of framing social policy. There truth must give way to utility, and dishonesty in this case has advantages. First, if we say that we can initiate traditional death-behaviour at a particular time and make it clear that the basis of this is (as it must be) an evaluation based on the kinds of factors adumbrated above, there will be a hue and cry about who has the right to make such judgments about human life. But if we call the patient dead at that point we will avoid this, and hence the misrepresentation will help to entrench certain practices concerning the timing of behaviour (which we may here for the sake of argument agree are desirable) as public policy. Secondly, as Green and Wikler have argued [12], the misrepresentation does something to arrest a possible slide down a slippery slope. If we make it clear that our policy to terminate treatment of persons at a certain time is based on a value-judgement, the public will perhaps start to think about extending the policy. If today we can aptly do it in cases of those who have suffered whole-brain death, why not tomorrow on those who have suffered higher-brain death? And then why not, in following days, on the senile, the moderately retarded, the unproductive, and so on? However, if we disguise this value-judgement and say that we are terminating treatment because an individual is dead, this train of thought with all its dangers does not get started.

I do not find these advantages sufficient [13]. If, as the first has it, we pass off a value-laden judgement as a value-free one on the ground that the public otherwise would not accept the initiation of certain behaviour at that time at all, or would not accept it as easily, we not only show deep disrespect for public opinion, but foster very bad habits in legislators. We do not want to encourage legislators to misrepresent public policy when they think good will come of it. That kind of patronising manipulation is incompatible with a self-governing community, and since the misrepresentation in question will promote that, there is a hefty counterweight to any advantages we may so secure.

The second alleged advantage also has this drawback, and other problems as well. Let us begin by confronting our fears: what exactly are we afraid might happen to the vulnerable people in question? That they will not get maximally aggressive lifesaving treatment? That, in non-life-threatening situations, they will not get optimal care? That positive steps will be taken to exterminate them? Whatever we may think of the latter two possibilities, we cannot reasonably recoil from the first, unless we are prepared to say that we must bend every effort to maintain the life of an anencephalic infant, or to resuscitate a senile septuagenarian with a formidable array of serious health-problems who one day stops breathing, or to treat aggressively any life-threatening infection a patient who has suffered higher-brain death develops. But these are not reasonable proposals, and in so far as we reject them we have already compromised the principle that there is no such thing as a life not worth living or preserving, and thus already opened the door to the dangers in question. If we are unprepared to close that door, the proposal that we should redefine death to prevent an unwanted slippery slope loses its point. A statute allowing termination of all health-care services on the whole-brain dead (as opposed to a statute defining death as whole-brain death) does not raise any new dangers, or, so far as I can see, exacerbate existing ones. Not only does this proposal lack the utility claimed for it, it threatens a substantial disutility. Insofar as it does anything to serve its alleged purpose it must dampen discussion of euthanasia. But less public discussion of that is the last thing we need, given the current state of confusion and disagreement. Debate rages over the exact conditions under which treatment can be foregone, whether we can withhold food and fluids as well as medical treatment, and the appropriateness of active euthanasia. I do not know of any way of resolving these important issues except by full, open, and vigorous public debate. Taboos have never served us well, and there is no reason to think this case will be an exception.

I thus think that the legislative option sketched earlier is preferable to that of providing a statutory definition of death in point of clarity, honesty, and utility. At the same time, given the already-widespread adoption of the whole-brain definition, hopes for that proposal are dim. But what still can be non-quixotically insisted on is that by so redefining death we do not thereby settle any of the pressing moral questions which prompted the exercise. In so far as we treat that redefinition as the outcome of the settling of those questions, we must judge it to be premature, and thus unfit to serve that question-settling function; and in so far as we treat that redefinition as a non-moral matter, it cannot have any implications for morality.

Alister Browne, Department of Philosophy, Vancouver Community College, 100 West 49th Avenue, Vancouver, B.C. V5Y 2Z6, Canada.

NOTES

[1] This view is held by L. W. SUMNER (1976) A matter of life and death, *Noûs*, 10, pp. 145–171, see esp. p. 154.

[2] Human being: the boundaries of the concept, *Philosophy and Public Affairs*, 4, p. 357.

[3] This account is advocated by ROBERT VEATCH (1975) The whole-brain-orientated concept of death: an outmoded philosophical formulation, *Journal of Thanatology*, 3, pp. 13–30.

[4] The most famous supporting document of this is that of the Ad Hoc Committee of the Harvard Medical School to Examine the Definition of Brain Death, 'A definition of irreversible coma,' *Journal of the American Medical Association*, 205, pp. 337–340.

[5] Diagnosing death, *Philosophy and Public Affairs*, 7, pp. 144–153, esp. p. 147.

[6] A proponent of this account is HANS JONAS Against the stream: comments on the definition and redefinition of death, in his (1974) *Philosophical Essays: from ancient creed to technological man*, pp. 132–140 (Englewood Cliffs, N.J., Prentice-Hall).

[7] This alternative to redefining death is advocated by ROGER DWORKIN (1973) Death in context, *Indiana Law Journal*, 48, pp. 623–646.

[8] VEATCH op. cit., tries to make the definition of death precise in this way.

[9] Brain death and personal identity, *Philosophy and Public Affairs*, 9, pp. 105–133.

[10] Two comments: (1) The ways of making precise the life/death distinction which foist these alternatives on us are also, I submit, the only ways of making precise the ordinary/extraordinary, killing/letting die, and human being/non-human being distinctions. Thus the argument which shows that one hope in redefining death is forlorn can be adapted to show that the corresponding hopes in these cases are so too. (2) Strictly, I do not need to claim that arbitrary stipulation is the only viable alternative to treating the concept of death as an evaluative concept in order to arrive at the conclusion of this paragraph. Given the Humean doctrine that we cannot extract a moral conclusion from any matter of fact alone, no non-moral way of making the definition precise will serve to settle the question of the appropriateness of certain behaviour. So we can get the same conclusion out of the wholly uncontentious claim that we must proceed to make the concept of death precise by treating it either as an evaluative or as a non-evaluative concept.

[11] Op. cit., p. 129.
[12] Op. cit., Sec. IV.
[13] The objections which follow are anticipated, but not responded to, by GREEN & WIKLER, op. cit., p. 130, n. 43.

Society for Applied Philosophy

The Society for Applied Philosophy provides a focus for philosophical research with a direct bearing on areas of practical concern which are capable of being illuminated by the critical, analytical approach characteristic of philosophy, and by direct consideration of questions of value. Areas of concern include environmental and medical ethics, the social implications of scientific and technological change, philosophical and ethical issues in education, law and economics.

The Society's aim is to foster and promote philosophical work which is intended to make a constructive contribution to problems in these areas.

Enquiries should be addressed to the Hon. Secretary, Susan Mendus, University of York, York, YO1 5DD, UK.

Journal of Applied Philosophy

The *Journal of Applied Philosophy* is the journal of the Society for Applied Philosophy and reflects its interests and aims.

Editorial Correspondence to:
The Editors, Stephen Clark and Brenda Almond, *Journal of Applied Philosophy*, University of Liverpool, PO Box 147, Liverpool, L69 3BX, UK.

Index

Printed and bound by CPI Group (UK) Ltd, Croydon, CR0 4YY

24/10/2024

01778279-0013